Gynaecological Care

Gynaecological Care

Helen Farrer RN RM

Churchill Livingstone

MELBOURNE EDINBURGH LONDON AND NEW YORK 1987

CHURCHILL LIVINSTONE
Medical Division of Longman Group UK Limited

Distributed in Australia by Longman Cheshire Pty Limited, Longman House, Kings Gardens, 95 Coventry Street, South Melbourne 3205, and by associated companies, branches and representatives throughout the world.

First edition 1979 (Pitman Publishing Pty Ltd)
Second edition 1985
Reprinted 1987 (Churchill Livingstone)

ISBN 0-443-03910-0

Produced by Longman Singapore Publishers Pte Ltd
Printed in Singapore

Foreword

I am delighted again to be invited to proffer an introduction for the second edition of Helen Farrer's acclaimed nursing textbook, *Gynaecological Care.*

The need for a second edition underlines not only the popularity of the original text, but also the substantial strides made in gynaecology during the last decade. I believe it is almost fair to say that gynaecology has the fastest growth rate of any of the modern day specialities of medicine. The claims it makes on the nurse are demanding, for what other speciality in medicine can at the same time boast of the simultaneous explosive advances in reproductive biology, genetic engineering, intracellular endocrinology, infinitesimal perinatology, therapeutic oncology, in-vitro fertilisation and cryo-embryology, to name a few?

Despite this excitement, we still must be involved in old fashioned but still present conditions like genital prolapse, fibroids and endometriosis not to mention menstrual abnormalities, premenstrual tension, the climacteric and of course genital tract cancer.

Discourses on all of these are aggregated handsomely in the following pages and one feels a debt to Helen Farrer for bringing the subject up to date. I am sure the second edition will rapidly outsell the first edition of this now established book which is specifically presented for nurses involved in caring for those special problems which occur only in women.

Ian A McDonald
MGO (Melbourne), FRCS (England), FRCOG, FRACS, FRACOG
Consultant gynaecologist, Royal Melbourne Hospital
Past Australian President, RCOG

Contents

Foreword v

Preface ix

Part I Introducing gynaecology

1 'To begin with . . .' 1
2 The language of gynaecology 4
3 The main symptoms and their significance 8
4 The anatomy of the female reproductive system 20
5 The physiology of the female reproductive system 32
6 Changes in the life of a woman 40

Part II The gynaecological examination

7 'What we are here for' 53
8 The gynaecological examination 61
9 Common gynaecological treatments and investigations 76

Part III Diseases and disorders of the reproductive system

10 Intersex conditions 86
11 Developmental disorders 92
12 Disorders associated with menstruation 97
13 Pelvic infections, sexually transmitted diseases 111
14 Pruritus vulvae 136
15 Dyspareunia 142
16 New growths 146
17 Endometriosis 170
18 Displacements of the pelvic organs 174
19 Urinary problems in gynaecology 182

Part IV Gynaecological surgery

20 Common operations, their indications and implications 190
21 Gynaecological surgical care 200

Part V Conditions related to pregnancy and conception

22 Family planning 211
23 Abortion, ectopic pregnancy and hydatidiform mole 226
24 The infertile couple 240

Further reading 251

Index 252

Publisher's note

A decison had to be made on the gender of pronouns in this book. Of course there are both male and female doctors and nurses. Simply to avoid confusion, or the clumsy or repetitious use of he/she, doctors are referred to as 'he', nurses as 'she'.

Preface

This new edition of *Gynaecological Care* has been updated to include the many developments that have taken place in gynaecology over the past few years. Ultrasound has replaced a number of the older methods of investigation, and new forms of treatment have been developed for several gynaecological conditions. Some gynaecological infections, eg herpes genitalis, have become more widespread and therefore needed to be covered in more detail.

The revision of *Gynaecological Care* has given me the opportunity to adapt and adjust the text in response to the many letters I received from users of the first edition, particularly nurse educators, throughout Australia. I am grateful to all these people for their helpful comments. Mrs Barbara Moxon of the Royal Women's Hospital, Melbourne, deserves special mention as she examined the first edition with great care and suggested several changes.

Thanks are due to those who have assisted in gathering and assessing the new information. Mr Ian McDonald, Mr Graeme McLeish, Dr Cliff Flower, Dr Raphael Kuhn, and Dr Coral Tudball gave their time and critical help, as did Miss Sue Giffney, Ms Jane Hall and Mrs Pauline Walker.

I would also like to thank Dr Howard Welch and Miss Marie Lunt for their help and encouragement from the very start.

I am grateful to St Vincent's Hospital, Melbourne, the Royal Women's Hospital, Melbourne, and Mr Colin Woodward for providing the photographs that appear in this edition.

Despite the advances in medicine and the changes in society, the needs of our gynaecological patients remain: to be nursed with understanding, skill and care.

Helen Farrer
January 1985

Part I Introducing gynaecology

I 'To begin with . . .'

Gynaecology is a special branch of medicine. It takes a special kind of doctor and a special kind of nurse to really understand and care for a gynaecological patient. The word 'gynaecology' simply means the 'study of woman' but this word is commonly used specifically in relation to the functioning and malfunctioning of the female reproductive organs.

It would be easy (and possibly even boring) for nurses to learn just the facts about the reproductive system, the common conditions and their treatments, and the pre- and post-operative care required for the patient who has an operation on her pelvic organs. It is less easy to apply this learning to the person who is *not* in our care specifically as a gynaecological patient but whose behaviour and condition can be understood only by a knowledge of how the emotions, the sex hormones, childbearing and aging may affect a woman. The behaviour of any woman who is admitted to hospital for almost any disease or operation, from a tonsillectomy to the stripping of varicose veins, can be affected by some factor associated with her reproductive system and by her attitude to it.

The following situation may demonstrate this:

> Mrs Green is admitted to a general surgical ward for a gall bladder operation. She has suffered from moderate stress incontinence for a number of years, but has told no one. When the nurses encourage her to do deep breathing and coughing exercises post-operatively, how *can* she co-operate? She knows that she could wet the bed, but she is worried what they might think of her if she tells them. She has overheard them when they were changing the bed of the little lady in the corner. The nurses are really very nice but wet beds *do* seem to upset them. A nurse who has a good knowledge of gynaecology and a sensitive approach to

women has an insight into the problem. She can ask herself, 'Why won't Mrs Green try to cough? I've shown her how to hold her suture line. Coughing shouldn't hurt her too much. She is quite alert and usually very eager to please. What can it be about coughing that worries her?' The nurse can then go to Mrs Green and ask her this last question. She may also add something more specific: 'Is it because a little bit of urine sometimes dribbles away?'. The nurse has understood. She has put it into words, but not made it sound so terrible. Mrs Green feels immensely relieved. She can then explain everything to this nurse who is not going to disapprove of her. 'I usually wear a pad inside a pair of pants, but when I came in here they told me that I had to wear just my nightgown in bed. I didn't like to tell them about the wetness. *It's not all the time you know!'*

A nurse, not in a gynaecological ward, looking after a patient whose main diagnosis was quite unrelated to gynaecology, has nevertheless used her knowledge and understanding of this subject to assist someone who needed help.

Gynaecological nursing is not usually full of drama and excitement. There are not many opportunities for demonstrating one's efficiency with manual skills or for operating complicated medical machinery. The range of operations performed is not large; the types of patient may not seem to vary from one week to the next. Many gynaecological complaints can be dealt with at an outpatient level—the doctor sees her, then she goes home. What can the nurse contribute in that situation?

This book aims to show what a nurse *can* do, how she can help and why she needs to know gynaecology. It aims to provide a full picture of the problems that a woman may have in relation to her reproductive system—in health, in sickness and in her particular culture. It covers the normal functioning of, and then the diseases and disorders affecting, the female reproductive system. Because the majority of nurses working in this field are female, it aims to make these nurses aware of the importance of their approach to their patients and the significance of their own femaleness—that they are in fact potential or possible gynaecological patients themselves. The women with the problems, hopes and fears could be ourselves, our mothers or our grandmothers. In this light it is not always easy to be objective about the subject or symptoms of gynaecology.

It is easier to avoid getting too close. It is easier to avoid the difficult and embarrassing conversations that might arise. So we may give our gynaecological patients excellent physical care and endeavour to keep them cheerful at all costs, but miss out somewhere simply *because* most of us are women and because we may have the same fears and misconceptions as women the world over.

This book is written for student nurses and therefore aims to give information at a level suitable for students. However, student nurses are going to be qualified nurses and so need to be equipped for that role. Most nursing teachers have had students inform them that only the qualified staff do some of the things that have just been told to them. But what are nurses training for? Very soon, as qualified nurses, it will be their task to plan the nursing management of their patients. Soon it will be their opportunity to enlighten and dispel the fears of a woman who is worried about the effects of an operation upon her femininity and her marriage. To do this the nurse must be aware of the multitude of misconceptions and fears that abound *as well as* having a clear knowledge of the facts. In addition to studying her textbooks and attending lectures she needs to read and interpret the many magazines and papers that purport to inform the world at large about the mysteries of the reproductive system. She must listen to her mother, her friends and acquaintances, and to her patients, and encourage them to talk about problems in these matters. She may be able to set them on a course of action—to consult a doctor rather than remain worried and continue with self-medication.

Most nurses have, at one time or another, been approached by people who say something like 'You're a nurse—you'll know!'. We *are* expected to know. But, more than that, we are expected to understand. It is hoped that the material in this book will be an aid to our understanding of this most important subject—the study of women.

2 The language of gynaecology

A student nurse was once heard to say just before her first lecture in gynaecology 'I don't think that I want to learn any of this. There are too many long and horrible words involved!'

Some of the more specific language of gynaecology is given here so that when the text is read this list may be consulted quickly, before the reader is overwhelmed by it all. In places, the non-medical substitute for a word or term is included, as well as the more formal or medical definition.

abortion: the termination of a pregnancy before the foetus is viable. The term miscarriage is often substituted, especially when referring to spontaneous abortion

adenomyosis: glandular tissue (endometrium) present in the muscle wall (of the uterus)

adnexae: appendages; the uterine adnexae are the fallopian tubes and the ovaries

amenorrhoea: the absence of menstruation

androgen: a masculinising hormone

aplasia: failure of tissue to grow or develop

apareunia: inability to practise sexual intercourse

atrophy: decrease in size or wasting of normally developed tissue or organs

azoospermia: the absence of spermatozoa in the semen

carneous: fleshy(carneous mole)

caruncle: a small fleshy growth or eminence

chancre: the primary lesion of syphilis

chancroid: a non-syphilitic sore, but one which is also usually sexually transmitted

chromosomes: small rod-shaped bodies present in the nucleus of each cell. They contain the genes or hereditary factors

climacteric: the specific symptoms which accompany the cessation of ovarian function; the 'change of life'

coitus: to go together—sexual intercourse

colpo: a fold or hollow—pertaining to the vagina

conception: the union of male and female germ cells to begin a new organism

cone excision: a circular tapering excision of the tissues of the external os of the cervix
congenital: existing at the time of birth
cystocele: herniation and descent of the bladder (through the anterior wall of the vagina)
cytology: the study of cells, especially for malignant changes
decidua: that which is shed. Decidua is the name given to the lining of the uterus during pregnancy
dermoid: resembling the skin and its related tissues
douche: the administration of a stream of fluid into a cavity, eg the vagina
dysmenorrhoea: pain associated with menstruation
dyspareunia: pain or difficulty with intercourse
ectopic: out of place. An ectopic pregnancy is one in which implantation of the fertilised ovum occurs outside the body of the uterus
embryo: the name given to the unborn baby, from the third to the eighth week of development
endocervix: the mucous membrane lining of the cervical canal
endometriosis: the presence of functioning endometrium in a site other than the lining of the uterus
enterocele: herniation of intestines (through the upper posterior vaginal wall)
episiotomy: an incision into the perineum to enlarge the vaginal orifice during the delivery of an infant, in order to prevent tearing
erosion: eating away; cervical erosion—ulceration of the superficial cervical tissues at the squamo-columnar junction
fertilisation: the union of the spermatozoon with the ovum; also called conception
fibromyomata: fibroids; benign growths of fibrous and muscular tissue
fimbriae: fringe-like (ends of the fallopian tubes)
foetus: the unborn child from the eighth week of pregnancy until birth
follicle: a little bag or sac; ovarian follicle—sac within the ovary containing the ovum and fluid
fundus: that part of the uterus above the points of insertion of the fallopian tubes
gamete: a reproductive cell capable of fertilising or being fertilised to produce a new individual, ie an ovum or a spermatozoon
genitalia: the reproductive organs
gestation: the development of an individual from conception to birth
gonad: a sex gland—the ovary or the testis
gonadotrophin: a substance which stimulates the gonads to function

gravid: pregnant; **gravida**—a pregnant woman
hirsutism: abnormal growth of hair
hydatidiform: resembling drops or small sacs
hypoplasia: incomplete growth or development of tissues or organs
hystero: pertaining to the uterus or womb
inclusion cyst: a (usually) small vulval cyst caused by some epithelial tissue being caught up in an episiotomy
infertile: unable to conceive or maintain a pregnancy
insufflate: to blow into (tubal insufflation)
intercourse: communication between individuals; sexual intercourse—coitus
introitus: entrance (to the vagina)
karyotype: the chromosome make-up of a cell
lactation: secretion of milk by the breasts
leucorrhoea: non-blood-stained vaginal discharge
leukoplakia: the presence of thickened white patches on a mucous membrane surface, eg the vulva
menarche: the first episode of menstrual bleeding
menopause: the last episode of menstrual bleeding
menorrhagia: heavy or profuse menstrual bleeding
menstruation: the periodic shedding of blood and the functional layer of the endometrium from the non-pregnant uterus
metrorrhagia: irregular or unusual bleeding from the vagina, occurring at times other than menstruation
motility: ability to move spontaneously (motile sperm)
oophor: pertaining to an ovary
os: a mouth (cervical os)
ovulation: the process in which an ovum is released from the ovary. Ovulation should occur fourteen days before the next menstrual flow is expected
ovum: the female germ cell
oxytocic: an agent which acts to contract the uterus
parity: the childbearing status of a woman
parturition: the act of childbirth
perineorraphy: repair(by suturing) of the perineum
pessary: 1 an article placed into the vagina to support prolapsing structures; 2 a medicated vaginal suppository
placenta: the 'afterbirth'. An organ which develops from the outer cells of the fertilised ovum and which acts to provide nourishment, oxygen and protection for the growing embryo or foetus
postcoital: after intercourse
primipara: a woman in the process of having, or who has just had, her first viable infant
prolapse: a falling forward (or down)
pruritus: itching

pseudocyesis: false pregnancy
puberty: the stage in life at which a person's reproductive organs mature and at which he or she is potentially able to reproduce
rectocele: herniation of the rectum (through the posterior vaginal wall)
retroflexed: bent backwards—the body of the uterus may bend backwards from the cervix
retroverted: turned or tilted backwards—the body *and* the cervix of the uterus are tilted backwards
semen: seminal or 'seed' fluid—that fluid which is discharged from the male during intercourse and which carries the spermatozoa
speculum: an instrument which, by displacing adjacent tissues, allows visualisation of an internal organ or structure
spermatozoon: the male germ cell
sterility: inability to produce germ cells
stroma: tissue which forms the ground work or basis of an organ
tampon: a pad or plug of absorbent material used in the vagina
thrush: a fungal condition caused by *Candida albicans*
tubo: pertaining to the fallopian tubes
urethrocele: herniation of the urethra (through the anterior vaginal wall), with displacement of the bladder neck
vaginismus: strong and usually painful contractions or spasms of the vaginal muscles during intercourse
venereal: sexually transmitted
vesicle: a small fluid-filled sac or blister
viable: capable of independent existence after birth; capable of surviving. In Australia a birth must be registered if the foetus weighs at least 400 g or is known to be of 20 weeks gestation (the exception to this is the ACT which follows the World Health Organisation's criteria of 500 g or 22 weeks).
vulvovaginal: a condition or treatment which involves both the vulva and the vagina
womb: the uterus
zygote: an organism produced by two gametes. The fertilised ovum before cleavage

3 The main symptoms and their significance

Symptoms are changes in the physical or mental state of a person—changes that he or she is able to recognise and bring to the attention of some other person.

The symptoms associated with a woman's reproductive system are often difficult for her to describe objectively. The way in which these symptoms are described to the doctor or nurse depends on her feelings about the symptoms, her attitude to sexual matters and her previous experience in talking about her symptoms with other people. *Any* symptom is of some importance to a woman, no matter how she talks about it. It may be thrown in at the end of a medical consultation as a 'by the way ...' Often these 'by the way' symptoms are the real reason for the woman's visit to the doctor, but are left until the end to give the impression that they are not really worrying her. It is our serious responsibility as nurses to listen to every word that our patients say to us, and to remember that little worries can grow large if nothing is done at the time of their appearance.

Difficulty in communication may arise when the symptom has been experienced before and has been minimised or brushed aside by the doctor or nurse. She may then have to exaggerate her problem in order to gain their attention and help. She may not return for a further appointment if she is made to feel that she has wasted their time. If the symptom is new or unfamiliar to her, she will probably worry about how people will respond to hearing her story.

Sometimes she feels out of control at the interview. She may not be given time to tell the story at her own pace or in her own way. Sometimes words other than the ones that she would have chosen are suggested to her by the doctor or nurse. These professional people are very confident in their knowledge of all the right terms and phrases. She may find herself agreeing to something that is not quite correct to her, or that she really does not understand, but she is unable to express it any more clearly herself.

Often the problems are complicated by her reluctance to speak about embarrassing subjects. She may think that once she has revealed her concerns about her reproductive system or her sexual activity to a doctor or nurse, their respect for her as a person will be lost. How can you tell other people that your vagina and vulva itch constantly and that you have been scratching 'down there'? How can a widow of sixty calmly describe a vaginal discharge that stains her pants and smells foul? How can a woman of fifty explain how it hurts to have intercourse—when the doctor or nurse appear to be about the same age as her own sons or daughters, when all the advertisements show sex as important only for the young, and when she has never used the word intercourse before and doesn't really know what to call it?

The woman who is in hospital usually sees the nurse as the one who will listen to her symptoms. It is the nurse who is there during the night when the woman is unable to sleep. It is the nurse who performs, or should perform, without embarrassment, the sponging and toilet procedures. It is the nurse who can, or should be able to, understand the words that the woman uses and who can translate them into medical terms. And, probably most important of all, the woman sees the nurse as the one who will have the *time* to listen to her.

The woman who is not in hospital—who comes as an outpatient or goes to the doctor's room—may have even more need of someone who can understand her symptoms and her reason for making the appointment. The nurse is there while the woman is waiting (and worrying); the nurse is usually there after the doctor has finished and gone. It may be the encouragement and gentle handling given by the nurse that make the whole experience of the gynaecological examination easier for the woman.

All nurses differ and all patients differ. The marital status and sexual knowledge of both patients and nurses must influence their response to the discussion of gynaecological symptoms. If we are to help people by understanding some of the associated problems, then we must be ready to look beyond the first stated complaints and think about how the daily life of the woman, her partner and her family, may be influenced by those symptoms.

The major symptoms of gynaecology, how a woman may respond to them, and some of the effects that they may have, are discussed in this chapter. A fuller coverage of the causes, investigations and management of each of these symptoms will be given when discussing the diseases and disorders of the various organs of the reproductive system.

Dysmenorrhoea—'Ghastly periods'

Menstrual periods can be painful. A girl or woman with dysmenorrhoea feels awful, but is often unable to state *how* awful. It may be because of her own reluctance to speak of her periods or because she senses that others will be embarrassed if she does. If she uses other words: 'I'm feeling really rotten', and people respond with 'I hope it's nothing serious?', she is then almost obliged to either tell them in one way or another that it is 'just a period'. 'Just a period' has another common response—'Oh, is *that* all it is?'. Most of us probably try to minimise the effects of pain and irritability often associated with menstruation. It is not going to last forever. But while it is there, while it is making her double up and feel unable to cope with any effort at all, it is more than 'just a period'.

Most books and magazines urge women to have an enlightened and healthy approach to menstruation. 'Sensible women take it in their stride.' If there is *discomfort* and one *is* able to stride, that is excellent. Unfortunately, excessive discomfort becomes pain and pain may reduce the stride to a very slow shuffle. The right attitude and healthy approach to having periods has to be handed down from mothers or handed across by friends. Some girls almost inherit dysmenorrhoea; the mother suffered, so does the daughter. She *expects* it to be bad. The discomfort of a period is not lessened when that particular period is unwelcome, as it is when a woman wants to be pregnant. The period hurts, she resents it, it hurts more.

At institutions where the majority of the population is female, complaints of dysmenorrhoea may not be received kindly. 'We are all women here and we all have to put up with it.' Boarding schools for girls and even hospitals and schools of nursing may be examples of this. If the girl or woman simply cannot carry on with her work or study, if she can find no sympathy and is not allowed any modification of her work load, or if she is unable to even talk to her seniors about it, she will very likely perform poorly, both physically and mentally.

Despite the fact that dysmenorrhoea is a common problem, the person who suffers from this symptom should not be ignored. She should be listened to with care and sympathy, and appropriate symptomatic relief given. At the same time she should be urged to seek medical advice *before* the next period is due, to be shown how this pain can be understood and relieved. If dysmenorrhoea is not managed well, the woman who really suffers from it is certainly not able to initiate and maintain a sensible and healthy outlook.

Menorrhagia—'It absolutely pours'

Excessive menstrual loss is one symptom that prompts most women to consult a doctor early. There is no shame and not really much embarrassment in talking about excessive blood loss. Most doctors will agree with the woman that her coming to see the doctor was the proper thing to do.

How does a woman judge her menstrual loss to be normal or heavier than normal? What is the normal amount? Most textbooks state that only about 50–100 mL are lost over a period of three to five days in the average case. Nurses, who are experienced in measuring fluids in both small and large amounts, are often surprised at this because the appearance of the loss on the pad is deceptive—it appears to be much more than it actually is.

Many women have no idea of the amount that is regarded as average. What they do understand is the often untimely messiness and stickiness involved with menstruation. Most women can manage to cope with the normal flow fairly well. But some women who are particularly fastidious may regard the normal as excessive because they cannot bear to feel messy at all. If the period is a real annoyance to her, in her work or social life, it may seem to require too much attention and go on for too many days. As in the case of dysmenorrhoea, if the period is unwelcome because of a desire for pregnancy, she may not regard it as normal. It will seem to be 'so much blood'.

There are a number of reasons why the menstrual flow may be heavy. These are discussed in Chapter 12 under the heading 'Menorrhagia'. Whatever the cause, the fact remains that the woman has to cope with a heavy loss and she may worry that she has not enough protection; that it will show through her clothes or stain the sheets and bedclothes. When she is out shopping she cannot try on clothes. When she is attending lectures, sporting activities or social functions and has to leave her bag in a locker or cloakroom some distance away, it is a nuisance and an embarrassment to have to get her bag, find a toilet, change the tampon or pad or whatever and dispose of it. She feels obvious doing all this. When the flow is not heavy, the tampon or pad will be satisfactory for normal occasions and she will be spared all this fuss.

Chronic excessive menstrual loss will eventually lead to iron deficiency anaemia. This gradually brings on an extra set of symptoms to cause added anxiety. The woman may be tired all the time and find that even small everyday tasks are almost beyond her. She will wonder why she is not coping.

Although pallor can be hidden by cosmetics, she often feels that somehow she does not look her best. This is especially distressing for the woman to whom appearance is of some importance. But the fatigue that also accompanies anaemia may lead her to care less about this; it can become a drag to do any more than run a comb through her hair or to think about wearing anything apart from a few old clothes and sloppy shoes. Eventually the combination of a lowered image of herself and the feeling of exhaustion at the end of an ordinary day's work may result in the loss of energy or inclination even to think about any sort of sexual activity. Over a period of time this can have a profound effect on her partner and their relationship.

When she does organise herself enough to make and keep an appointment to see a doctor about her menorrhagia, she will need understanding and encouragement to go through whatever course of treatment is recommended. If she is admitted to hospital for investigation or removal of the cause, she will expect relief from her symptoms. She will also know that inside herself she is not the person she appears to be but may, in her attempts to be a good patient, be unable to relax. It is not our role, nor is it our right, to label her as 'another gynae neurotic' because we cannot really understand how she has been affected in her life or work by this problem of excessive and, in some cases, chronic blood loss.

Metrorrhagia—'I suppose it's nothing to worry about'

Irregular or unusual bleeding (or bleeding at times other than those when a period is expected) nearly always makes a woman suspect an abnormality but not always does it make her seek advice. The bleeding may be slight, and unaccompanied by other symptoms. She may ignore it and decide to consult a doctor only if it gets worse. If the bleeding has occurred during or after intercourse she may try to avoid having intercourse rather than have to tell the doctor. She may suspect something very serious, such as cancer, and be reluctant to have her suspicions confirmed.

If the couple abstain from intercourse when the woman is bleeding, eg during the menstrual flow, because of either aesthetic or religious reasons, they may find their sexual relationship severely restricted. This is an additional problem when the only method of child-spacing or family planning available to, or suitable for, them is centred around knowing days and dates and predicting the time of ovulation. In such cases, unless the couple are able to obtain expert advice easily, the only thing to do would be to practise prolonged sexual abstinence, or to worry. Neither alternative is good if a healthy relationship is to be maintained.

On the other hand, there are a number of women who are very vague about the dates of, and intervals between, their menstrual flows. In such a case, the woman may not be sure of what is normal and what is not normal about her vaginal bleeding. At the beginning, and particularly towards the end, of the reproductive years there is often a disruption to the normal regular pattern of menstrual cycles. Many women know that there will be this change as they approach the menopause and don't worry. The problem comes when they continue to be unconcerned about, or even ignore, bleeding or spotting that occurs after the menopause has happened.

When we hear 'It's such a little thing and I don't want to bother the doctor; he's so busy', we can only reply, 'He will be made a great deal busier if things get worse. See about it *now*, while it's little!'.

Amenorrhoea—'My periods haven't come'

When menstruation is expected and does not occur there are three possible reactions.

The first is: 'Am I pregnant?'. There are not many adult women in our society who do not know that missing a period is one of the first signs of pregnancy. Pregnancy may be greatly desired and if so the sign is a welcome one. But pregnancy might be greatly feared and this fear of pregnancy may, through the complex hypothalamic-pituitary-ovarian relationship, itself be a cause for amenorrhoea.

The second response is: 'Something is wrong'. To the woman who is fairly confident that there is no possibility of pregnancy having occurred, the cessation of periods is an abnormality. The fact that the doctor is almost obliged to do a pregnancy test and await the results before embarking on any course of treatment may be disconcerting to a woman. She may feel that he does not believe her and with this in mind is likely to lose some of the trust and confidence which is so important in the relationship. If it is a case of primary amenorrhoea (where menstruation has never occurred) the girl will most likely be anxious because she is behind her friends in an important milestone. Possibly she feels different, and cannot share in their discussions. She probably also senses her mother's anxiety about this problem.

At the other end of the reproductive span is the menopause. If amenorrhoea occurs before a woman feels that she is ready to give up her potential to be pregnant, before she feels old enough to enter a new phase in her life, she may prefer to think that there is something wrong with her reproductive system.

The third reaction is a hangover from the olden days. Menstruation was thought to have an excretory function, a regular emptying out of poisons and maybe even 'stale seed' from the body. Although there is now widespread education, in at least the basic facts of reproductive physiology, the way that the subject of menstruation is shunned as an acceptable topic of conversation—spoken about in whispers or euphemisms or not at all—does give the impression that there is something rather nasty about it. As well, the point of exit of the menstrual flow is right between two other outlets, both excretory. So a woman not passing this sticky, bloody mess may well be frightened that it is building up inside her and that this will be affecting her body in other more serious ways. Such a woman may find it very difficult to wait, without worrying, for weeks between appointments.

Leucorrhoea—'An awful discharge'

Vaginal discharges other than blood are collectively termed 'leucorrhoea'. It is known and accepted that there is some moisture in and around the vagina. To have a dry vagina would be like having a dry mouth—it would be uncomfortable. There is a physiological increase in the amount of moisture at certain times and this too is generally understood. Most women are not worried by this increase but a few will be bothered by it. In some cultures a great emphasis is placed on feminine attractiveness and so even the normal, natural secretions will be attacked by a host of douches, sprays and towellettes. These may then cause further problems because they could upset the natural defence mechanisms, or cause localised inflammations.

When the natural secretions are increased beyond the normal limits, how does a woman react? Often by trying to cope on her own, using self-medications in an attempt to clear the discharge before going to a doctor. She may worry about the source of the discharge—how did she get it? A vaginal discharge is associated in the minds of many people with the fear of veneral disease. There may even be a fear that her partner has passed on an infection. The shame associated with almost any sexually related disease may make a woman reluctant to seek advice. 'You must think I'm awful!'

If the discharge is, or seems to be, foul smelling the woman may stay away from other people if she thinks that they will notice it. Going to the doctor about it involves taking off the clothes and pads that are at least keeping the smell under cover. It is inevitable that a woman with this problem will be looking for our reactions and will be sensitive to the slightest gesture or expression which could be interpreted as distaste or disgust on our part.

If the discharge is associated with itching or burning, even the thought of sexual intercourse will not be pleasant, and so she will probably avoid it. If the woman relies on a form of family planning centred around observation of the cervical mucus, the mucus may be obscured by the discharge. These factors may cause problems in their relationship, especially if she and her partner find sex a difficult matter to discuss.

A large number of factors, quite unrelated to a woman's current sexual activity, may be the cause of vaginal discharge. It is our duty to know why these discharges arise and persist so that we can tell a woman that she is not 'awful' and so that we can describe simply the various factors that may have caused this symptom.

Pruritus vulvae—'This dreadful irritation'

Pruritus vulvae is an irritative condition of the vulva—an itch—which brings about an intense desire to scratch. The first effect is discomfort; the woman wants to scratch to relieve the discomfort because she knows that scratching will take away the itch. In civilised societies, however, uninhibited scratching is not acceptable and neither (to many people) is touching 'down there'. Those who suffer from this symptom, and it is estimated that at least one woman in ten who visits a gynaecologist does suffer from pruritus to some degree, usually do not know how to manage the itchiness. Very few spontaneously tell of the itching or the scratching.

If the doctor's questions do not lead to a discussion about itching a woman may have to resort to a 'by the way' method of introducing the subject as she is on her way out. That is, if she has the courage. This brief mention of the symptom might produce but a brief response and perhaps a quickly written prescription. In contrast, a thorough discussion of the factors that might be adding to the intensity of the itch and a full investigation of the initial causes of the irritation can have dramatic results in terms of relief from this very unpleasant symptom. Self-medication is often resorted to, with varying success.

Although the skin of the vulva and lower vagina is meant to be sensitive, it is not meant to be the site of itching and burning. If the vulval tissues are scratched and damaged, they are slow to heal. This may be because of their location, which does not have light, air or freedom from moisture. It may also be because the area is warm and this warmth heightens the sensitivity so that there is more awareness, more itching and so more scratching.

The itching is often at its peak at night. A combination of warmth, weariness and lack of distractions can result in the woman being far more aware of the discomfort. This may prevent sleep and so affect her proper functioning during the day. Itching is another cause of difficulty with intercourse; if the symptom and her reaction to it by scratching make her feel ashamed she may begin to avoid her previous spontaneous and relaxed approach to sexual activity. As well, if the vulval skin is irritated and damaged, intercourse is likely to hurt. Her partner will not want to hurt her, she will not want to be hurt; this results in a tendency for both of them to make excuses. This simple problem may thus become a complex problem, demanding both medical and nursing skills and understanding of a very special kind.

A lot of the management of pruritus vulvae is sheer common sense. When the ways of minimising the itch and controlling the urge to scratch are pointed out, the usual response is 'Of course! Why didn't I think of it myself?'. Why she didn't think of it herself is because when the vulva is itching the mind is not thinking. At least, it is not thinking rationally about the symptom.

Dyspareunia—'It hurts when I go with my husband'

Dyspareunia is the term used to describe pain or difficulty with intercourse. Most women find it hard to talk about this problem. Once again the reluctance to mention, let alone discuss, one's sexual activity is there. If she has to talk to somebody who appears to be just as embarrassed as she is, she may feel that she shouldn't talk about it at all. Yet she may have been sent specifically to talk about it.

Dyspareunia can have real consequences on the lives of the couple involved. It affects both of the partners in the relationship and, if it goes on for any length of time, it can seriously harm that relationship. There can be feelings of guilt in one or both of the partners. If either has had previous sexual experience with another partner, comparisons, conscious or unconscious, will be made, and if blame is laid the current relationship must suffer. A sad but not uncommon effect of dyspareunia arises when the problem has started after the birth of a baby. The baby becomes the source of blame for the changed relationship and, until the condition is cured, may be resented because of this.

There are many causes of dyspareunia and most of them can be treated effectively. Almost every couple experiences occasional difficulty or pain with intercourse, but usually it is transient and the next attempt is without problems. The real difficulty emerges when the symptom persists and the couple are unable to find anyone who will listen to them and who will be capable of finding the right way or the right people to help them.

Incontinence of urine—'The water runs away'

Being out of control of any part of any one of our functions which is normally under our control is difficult for most people to cope with. Urinary incontinence is no exception. Even if it is the mildest degree of stress incontinence, the fact that it does happen can have a profound effect on a woman's comfort and life style. If every time she coughs, sneezes, laughs, jumps or runs, a dribble of urine is likely to run away, she is unlikely to be able to relax and enjoy life. One woman who had suffered from stress incontinence for a few years told of the problems that she had encountered.

> It wasn't much of a bother at first, though each night when I was undressing there was a wetness on my pants and unless I soaked them overnight they would be stained and look nasty after an ordinary wash. After a while I realised that I was actually losing some urine at certain times. Then I went to a friend's home one evening. It was a social gathering for the church ladies' guild and there were some items and a very funny sketch sending up every single one of us. We laughed until we nearly burst, then all of a sudden I felt something wet. I sat in the chair and felt terrible. It was a beautiful green brocade upholstered chair which matched their lounge suite. I stayed there until most of the people had gone, trying to think of a way to get up and see if it had gone through to the chair. How would I tell my friend what had happened? My husband came to collect me and I had to get up. There was a mark there—a big ugly wet patch. I couldn't tell my friend then. The next morning I started to dial her telephone number but couldn't do it. After all, the chair might have dried without staining so it would be silly and embarrassing to talk about it if she hadn't even noticed. All the same I couldn't face her or the other ladies after that. I didn't go to church or to the ladies meetings for the next few weeks, then I just got out of the way of it and found other things to do at home. The priest came to see me and tried to find out if he could help me to come back. Had I told him the truth then I am sure that he would have sorted things out, but it was too late. I told him we were a lot busier now and would come back when things settled down. Two of the ladies came to call one afternoon but I didn't even ask them in; I just spoke to them through the fly-wire door. I miss them all. I especially miss going to church. I watch the service on television but it's not the same. And I'm scared to get involved in another parish—what if the same thing happened there?

This woman also left her bowling club after discovering a wet stain on the back of her white bowls dress. She started to wear sanitary pads most of the time but hated buying them. She could feel the chemist's assistant looking at her. Then her vulval area started to feel sore and chafed. She tried several creams and lotions but it was hard to clear up because the wetness came back such a lot. The whole business was miserable. She took to staying at home most of the time, dreading invitations to functions and gatherings, feeling bored and lacking energy. Luckily this course of events was arrested by the intervention of a visitor, her granddaughter, who had just completed her nursing course. The granddaughter discovered a tear-off strip from a self-adhesive pad in the bin in the bathroom, and asked her grandmother why she needed to wear the pads. On hearing the reason, the nurse was then able to help her grandmother make an appointment with a doctor. This then led her to undergo special treatment which tightened up some muscles, and she is now completely free of the problem.

There are other forms of urinary incontinence which have the same potential effects, the embarrassment and the feeling that others know about it by seeing or smelling. There is a tendency to stay in familiar places where the woman knows the whereabouts of the toilets. She may attempt to keep her bladder as empty as possible by going to the toilet every hour or even more often, a practice which could lead eventually to a contracted bladder with a lowered capacity.

Not every woman who suffers from urinary incontinence is going to have the same set of problems. But if we know something about some of the effects of this symptom, and can show her that we do understand, she is more likely to listen as we encourage her to seek treatment or to continue with it.

Infertility—'Why can't I get pregnant?'

Infertility is the final symptom to be discussed in this chapter. It is not really a symptom, rather it should be termed a state or a condition. Whatever it is called, infertility has a profound effect on the lives of the two people involved. But it is the woman who does not become pregnant and it is she who has to make the first move in the attempt to solve the problem.

The pressure on a normal young couple to have children can be enormous. A couple who do have children and delight in them will naturally want to urge their childless friends to have a family. They will not want their friends to miss out on the joys and pleasures that they are experiencing. Others might not have the same pure motives. There may be jealousy of their freedom, and of the quietness and orderliness that is not always a feature of the houses where children live. Potential grandparents generally want to 'live to see their children's children'.

A couple who have deliberately decided not to have children can usually cope with this sort of pressure if they are secure in their decision and in their relationship. But imagine the feelings of those who want to have a family yet are unable to become pregnant. How much it must hurt when their well-meaning friends and parents urge them to 'get going before you're too old to enjoy them', or when they feel that others think that their childless state is deliberate and selfish—so that they can advance in their careers and financial status.

To begin with nobody knows where the 'fault' of the infertility lies, unless either partner has produced a pregnancy by someone else in the past. Even if this situation exists, the previous partner may have been highly fertile, while the present relationship might consist of a couple who both have a low fertility rating.

When a pregnancy does not occur after the couple have been trying for some time they will want to know why. The woman may feel unfulfilled. She wants to be a mother. She loves her partner and thinks that there ought to be more people like him. Who would be more like him than his own children? The man likewise is not free from the effects of infertility. He would like to be a father. Both partners (probably unconsciously) want to leave something of themselves behind in the world when they leave it. A long-standing family profession or business may die out or go to others if there are no children. Wills may be written on condition that the couple have children. In some cultures, a man must be buried by his son to fully achieve the afterlife.

Once infertility investigations are underway, the couple may be able to relax a little, knowing that they are at least starting to solve the problem. But the tests themselves are not simple. They may involve months of watching temperature charts and deliberately timing intercourse. They can include complicated X-rays preceded by pelvic examinations by doctors who are strangers to them. A sperm count and analysis is often required and the obtaining of this specimen may cause consternation to the couple. The couple may suddenly stop being investigated because they do not want to know whose fault it is.

If a definite cause for the infertility is found the couple may react to the findings with a change in behaviour. Some sad and extreme reactions have been seen in such practices as baby-snatching. A somewhat less frightening reaction, and one which is probably an attempt to dismiss their infertility altogether, is for the couple to undergo a change of attitude about the whole business of having children. They attempt to convince themselves that children really are a nuisance. They may seek only the company of people who do not have children or who do not query why they have none.

We have to show extreme care in this area of our work. It is our role to listen, to explain and to support, but it is not our right to probe into an area that can be extremely private and often painful.

4 The anatomy of the female reproductive system

The whole reproductive system is designed with one ultimate aim—reproduction. Each organ and structure has a specific contribution to make to the achievement of this aim, from the structures which aid in sexual arousal and vaginal lubrication, through to the muscular powers which expel the foetus at term. Some structures have a protective role—to prevent infection from ascending and thus possibly causing blockage of the fallopian tubes. Other structures are designed to support the uterus in the best position for spermatozoa to enter, and to continue supporting it as it increases enormously in size and weight during pregnancy.

Any disease or disorder of the reproductive organs will, to some extent, have an effect on a woman's reproductive ability. In order that we may fully understand this system and be able to adequately explain its workings, a careful review of the anatomy and physiology involved is essential.

Each structure is described as it appears during the period of reproductive maturity; that is during those years between puberty and the climacteric.

External genitalia

Vulva

The vulva is the name given to the external genital structures (Figure 4.1). The word means a cover or wrapper. The vulva extends from the mons pubis anteriorly to the perineum posteriorly, and it is bounded each side by the labia majora. Within these boundaries are included the labia minora, the clitoris, the vestibule and the fourchette. Opening into the vestibule are the urethral orifice and the vaginal orifice, and also the ducts of the paraurethral (Skene's) glands and Bartholin's glands.

Mons pubis

The mons pubis is the pad of fatty tissue lying above the symphysis pubis. It is covered by skin and pubic hair. The mons has a cushioning effect during sexual intercourse. The skin contains specialised sweat glands, the secretions of which have a characteristic odour. These secretions, held in some degree by the pubic hair, are believed to be of some sexual significance to the male.

Labia majora

The labia majora ('large lips') are two folds of skin with underlying fat which continue down as extensions of the mons pubis and merge into the perineum. The labia majora have hair and glands on their lateral aspects, but the inner surfaces are smooth.

Their function is protective—they close the entrance to the vagina and their fatty padding acts as a cushion.

Labia minora

The labia minora ('small lips') are two much thinner folds of skin lying inside the labia majora. They are joined at the front, forming the prepuce over the clitoris. Posteriorly they rejoin to form the fourchette. The labia minora have no subcutaneous fat. Their inner surfaces are normally in contact with each other and thus they add to the guarding of the entrance to the vagina.

Clitoris

The clitoris is a small projection of erectile tissue which is the homologue of the penis. It is situated within the anterior junction of

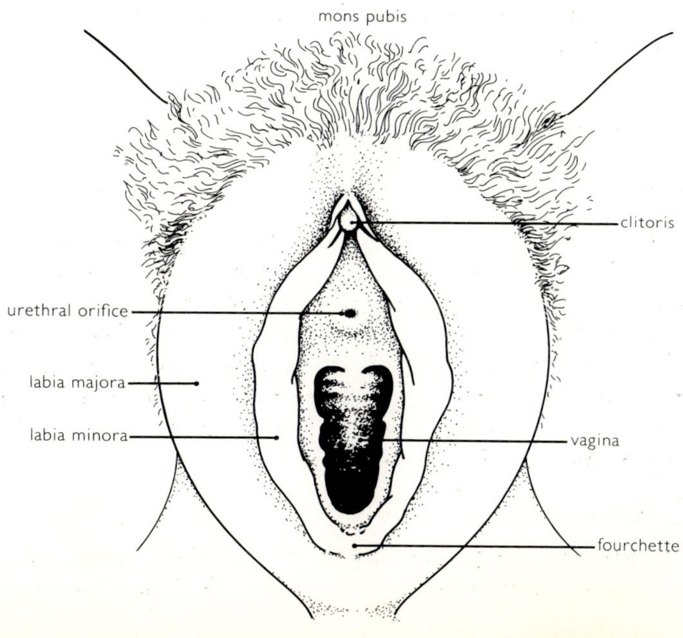

Figure 4.1
The vulva

the labia minora. The clitoris is richly supplied with blood and nerves, and it is one of the major erotic zones of the female.

Vestibule

The vestibule is the name given to the space enclosed by the labia minora. The urethral orifice opens into the vestibule just below the clitoris. The ducts of the two paraurethral or Skene's glands open into the vestibule, one on each side of the urethral orifice.

The vaginal orifice also opens into the vestibule. It is surrounded by a fold of thin membrane, the *hymen*, which does not completely close off the entrance to the vagina. After either the first act of intercourse, digital interference or the insertion of tampons, the hymen is usually torn or stretched open. Following the vaginal delivery of a child the hymen disappears except for a few tags of skin known as *carunculae myrtiformes*. The function of the hymen is a protective one—to guard the entrance to the vagina during the prepubertal years.

The ducts of the Bartholin's glands open outside the hymen, one on each side, just posterior to the vaginal orifice. The two Bartholin's glands secrete a mucoid lubricating substance especially during sexual excitement.

Perineum

The perineum is made up of the perineal body—the central junction of the muscles of the pelvic floor, covered by the perineal skin. It extends from the fourchette (the posterior junction of the labia minora) to the anus.

Internal genitalia

The pelvic organs are shown in Figure 4.2.

Vagina

The vagina is an elastic fibromuscular canal which extends upwards and backwards from the vulva to the uterus. The cervix or neck of the uterus is inserted into the upper end of the vagina. This area is known as the vaginal vault. The anterior vaginal wall measures approximately 7·5 cm and the posterior vaginal wall measures 9 cm. These walls are normally in close contact but can be separated easily. The lining of the vagina is arranged in folds (rugae). This allows the vagina to expand enormously, as it needs to, to accommodate the foetal head.

Structure

The vaginal wall has four layers:

- a lining of stratified squamous epithelium. There are no glands but some fluid seeps through the epithelium to provide moisture

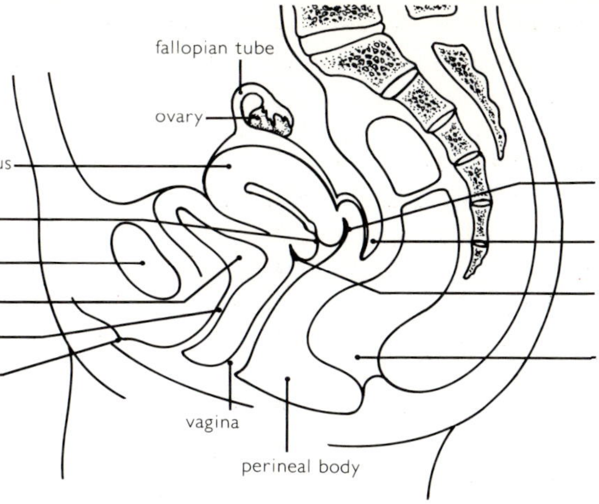

Figure 4.2
The pelvis—sagittal section

- areolar connective tissue, well supplied with blood vessels
- smooth muscle tissue of longitudinal and circular fibres
- an outer layer of white fibrous connective tissue which blends with the surrounding pelvic fascia.

Fornices

Fornix comes from the latin word for gutter. Where the cervix dips into the vaginal vault, a gutter is created surrounding the cervix. As the vaginal canal slopes backward and the uterus normally turns forward, there is a larger space at the posterior part of the gutter. The gutter is divided into four sections: a posterior, anterior and two lateral fornices.

Relations

Anterior vaginal wall: the bladder base is related to the upper anterior vaginal wall, and the urethra to the lower anterior vaginal wall.

Posterior vaginal wall: the pouch of Douglas (or uterorectal cul-de-sac), the lowest point of the peritoneal cavity, lies directly behind the posterior vaginal fornix—the rectum lies behind the upper two-thirds of the vagina. The perineal body lies behind the lower third of the posterior vaginal wall.

Secretions

The vaginal epithelium does not contain glands but there is a transudate or seepage of fluid through the vaginal wall to provide moisture. This is increased by the constant breakdown of superficial epithelial cells and the consequent release of glycogen. The glycogen is acted upon by Doderlein's bacillus, a normal inhabitant of the vagina, to produce lactic acid. In the normal healthy adult woman the vaginal pH varies from 5·4 to 4·3 at different times of the menstrual cycle.

Functions

The vagina has four main functions:

- a passage for spermatozoa; they are deposited during sexual intercourse into the space provided by the posterior fornix
- an outlet for the foetus and the other products of conception during labour
- an outlet for the menstrual flow
- by its acid secretions, it provides a barrier to ascending infection.

Uterus

The uterus is a thick-walled, hollow muscular organ, lying between the bladder in front and the rectum behind (see Figure 4.3). It consists of two parts, the corpus or body, and the cervix or neck. The cervix constitutes the lower third of the uterus, half of the cervix projecting into the vagina.

Figure 4.3 The internal reproductive organs—cross-section, viewed from behind

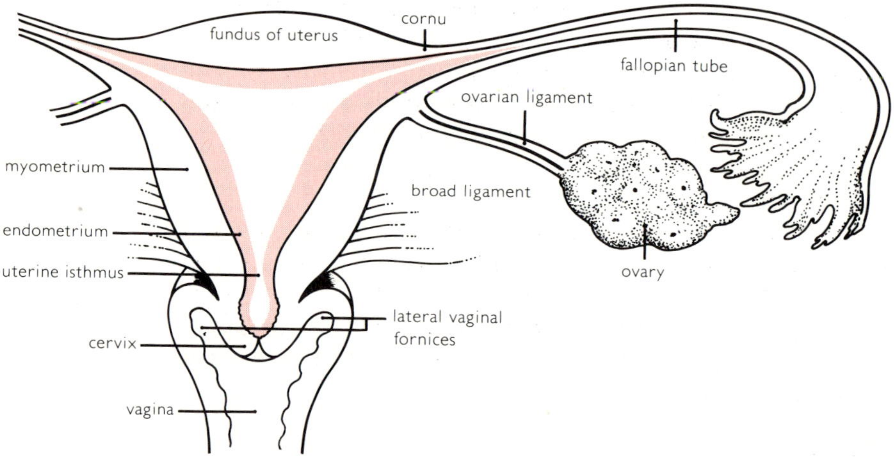

The uterus measures approximately 7·5 cm in length, 5·5 cm in width and 2·5 cm in depth. The walls are very thick, about 1·2 cm, thus the hollow cavity is extremely small.

Projecting laterally from the upper uterus are the fallopian tubes or oviducts. The points of insertion of these tubes are termed the cornua (or horns) of the uterus. That part of the uterus which is above the cornua is known as the fundus, while the junction of the cervix and the body of the uterus is called the isthmus uteri.

The hollow part of the cervix is called the cervical canal. The opening of the cervical canal into the vagina is called the external os and the opening of the canal at the level of the uterine isthmus is called the internal os.

Structure

Lining

The body of the uterus is lined by *endometrium*, which is epithelial tissue containing glands and stroma. The endometrium has a surface layer which is built up and then shed during each menstrual cycle, and a basal layer which remains constant.

The cervical canal is lined with columnar epithelium, and contains large glands secreting a clear mucus which forms a protective 'plug' at certain times, especially during pregnancy.

The vaginal projection of the cervix is lined with stratified squamous epithelium, continuous with the lining of the vagina. The junction of the columnar and squamous epithelium approximates to the external os. This is an important zone, for the majority of cancers arise here.

Muscle layer

The middle layer of the uterine wall is muscular and is termed the *myometrium*. There is an outer longitudinal, middle oblique and inner circular arrangement of muscle fibres, interspersed with a small amount of fibrous tissue. The lower cervix contains a much greater amount of fibrous tissue in proportion to muscle tissue.

Outer coat

The outer layer of peritoneum, or the *perimetrium*, covers the anterior and posterior surfaces of the body of the uterus. The posterior fold forms a cul-de-sac (the pouch of Douglas) which lies close to the posterior vaginal fornix where its contents may easily be palpated. The peritoneum then extends in a fold to the lateral pelvic walls as the broad ligament.

Functions

The functions of the uterus are to:

- prepare a suitable place for a fertilised ovum to embed
- provide protection and nourishment for the embryo/foetus until it is mature
- expel the foetus and placenta in labour
- control bleeding from the placental site by the contraction of the interlaced muscles—the 'living ligatures'.

Fallopian tubes

The fallopian tubes are also known as the oviducts and sometimes as the uterine tubes. They extend, one on each side, from the cornua of the uterus towards the lateral pelvic wall. They are covered by the peritoneum forming the broad ligament. They are about 10 cm long, but do not stretch straight out—they bend and turn posteriorly. Their distal ends open out into the peritoneal cavity and can move freely. The ends are fimbriated, and these fimbriae embrace the ovary at ovulation thereby helping to attract the ovum into the tube. The lumen of the fallopian tube is very narrow, especially where the tube enters the uterus. At this point, the interstitial part of the tube, the lumen is less than 1 mm.

Structure

The tube is lined by ciliated and secretory cells arranged in many folds. Some of the cells secrete a serous fluid which may nourish the ovum.

Outside the epithelial lining, separated by a fine layer of connective tissue, are two muscle coats, an outer longitudinal layer and an inner circular layer.

The peritoneum forming the broad ligament, covers the tubes.

Functions

The fallopian tubes provide a passage for sperm to meet the ovum, where fertilisation can take place. They also propel the ovum through to the uterus by their muscular action, aided by cilia and fluid.

Ovaries

The ovaries are the female gonads or sex glands. There are two ovaries, one on each side lying within the abdominal cavity, behind the broad ligament near the fimbriated end of the fallopian tube. They lie within the peritoneal cavity. They are grey-white structures, with an irregular surface, measuring about 3 cm by 1·5 cm.

Both ovaries are attached to the uterus by the ovarian ligaments which run from the posterior surfaces of the uterus close to the cornua. There is extra support from the infundibulo-pelvic ligaments which extend to the side walls of the pelvis.

One surface of the ovary is in contact with the posterior surface of the broad ligament suspended by the mesovarium. At the centre of the mesovarium is the hilum, and it is through this gateway that the ovarian blood vessels, lymphatics and nerves pass.

Structure

The ovary consists of a medulla and a cortex. The medulla is the inner portion, containing blood and lymphatic vessels supported by connective tissue. The cortex is the outer portion containing the ovarian follicles or egg cells, embedded in stroma.

The ovary is not covered by true peritoneum. It has instead a modified form of peritoneum—the germinal epithelium (Figure 4.4).

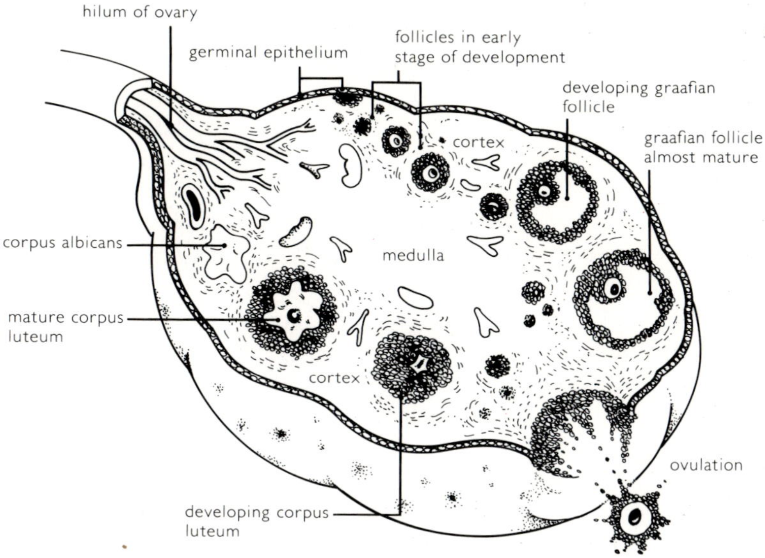

Figure 4.4
The ovary

Functions

The functions of the ovaries are:

- the production, storage and ripening of ovarian follicles and the release of ova
- the production of the ovarian hormones, specifically oestrogen and progesterone.

Pelvic supports

Although the cervix of the uterus is fixed, the body is free to rise and fall with the filling of the bladder, and free to grow to accommodate a pregnancy.

Uterine ligaments

The pelvic connective tissue supporting the uterus consists of the broad ligament, the round ligaments, the uterosacral ligament and the pubocervical ligament.

Broad ligament

The broad ligament is a raised fold of peritoneum and fibromuscular tissue stretching from the uterus to the side wall of the pelvis.

The broad ligaments give very little support to the uterus, but at the base of these ligaments the fascia becomes dense, to form the cardinal ligaments, from the cervix to the lateral pelvic walls (Figure 4.5).

Figure 4.5
The cardinal ligament

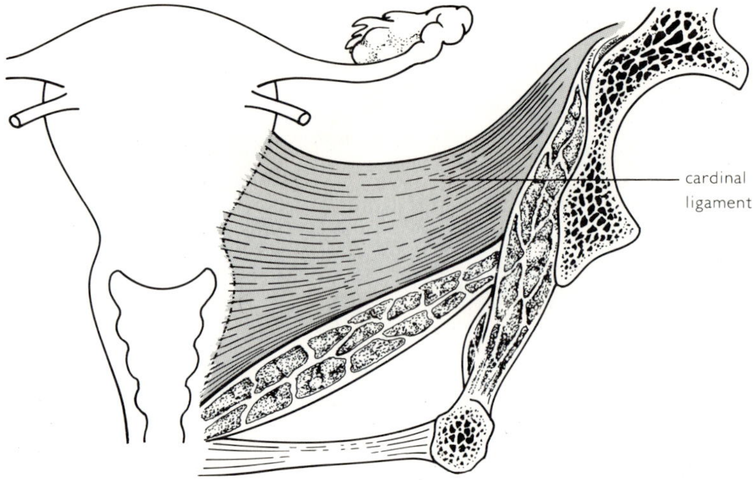

Round ligaments

The round ligaments pass from the anterior cornua of the uterus forward and down through the inguinal canal to be attached to the subcutaneous fat in the labia majora. They aid in holding the uterus anteverted or turned forward.

Uterosacral ligament

The uterosacral ligament (Figure 4.6) extends backwards from the cervix and the cardinal ligaments to the sacrum. It divides to pass

Figure 4.6
The uterosacral ligament

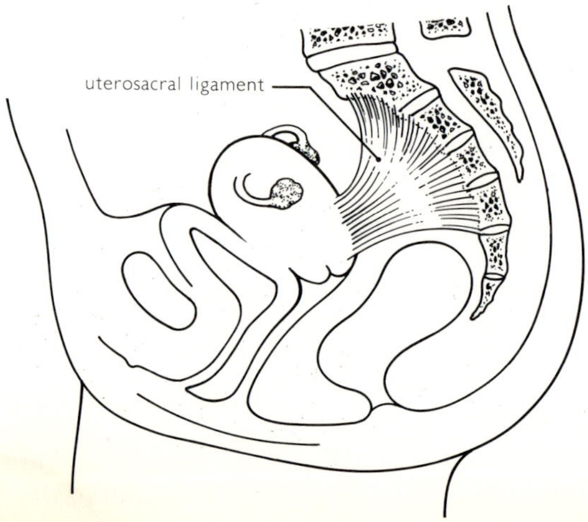

around the rectum, then reunites. By pulling the cervix back and up, it also helps to maintain anteversion of the uterus.

Pubocervical ligament

The pubocervical ligament runs from the front of the cervix forwards to the back of the pubic bone. It also divides to pass around the urethra.

Pelvic floor

The term 'pelvic floor' includes all of the tissues which fill the pelvic outlet and support the organs above (Figure 4.7).

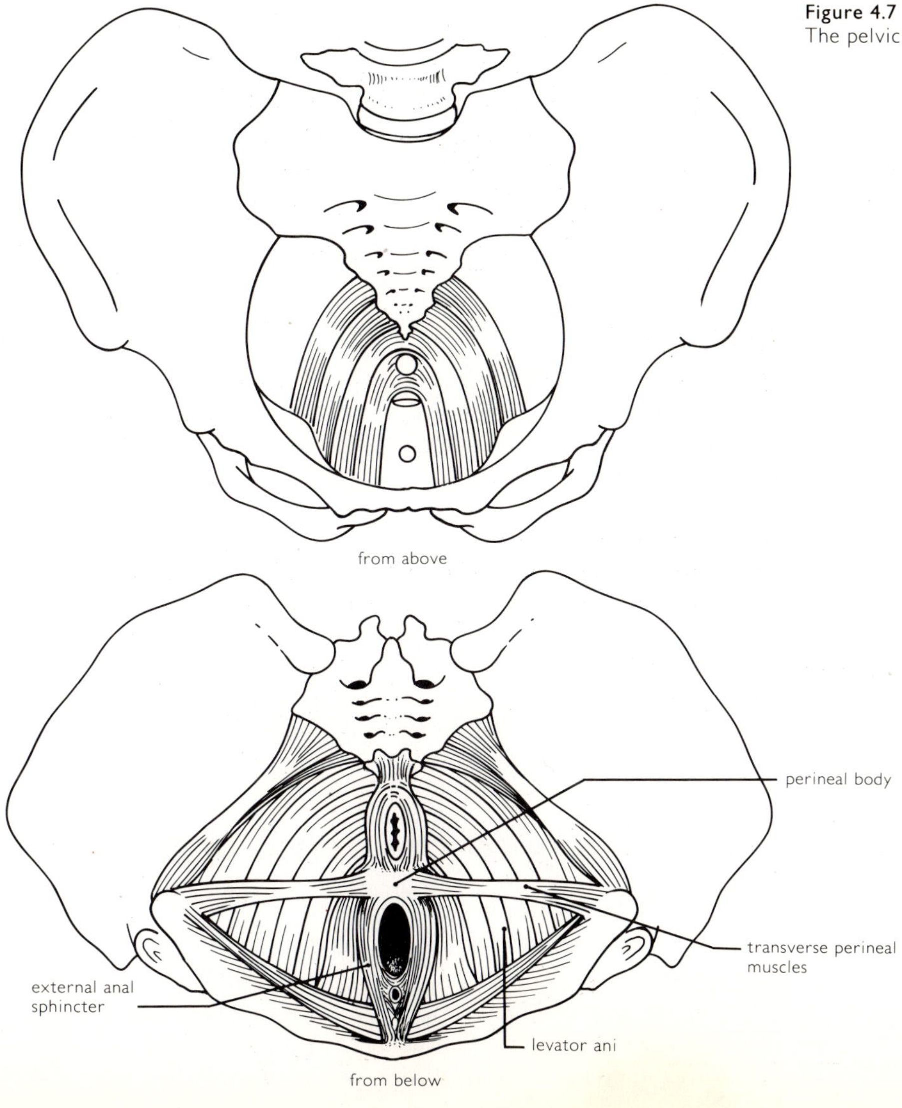

Figure 4.7
The pelvic floor muscles

Levator ani muscles

The levator ani are the strongest supports of the pelvic floor. These muscles form a broad sheet from the back of the pubis to the sacrum and coccyx, extending to the lateral pelvic walls. From the side walls, they sweep down and inwards to meet in the centre. The urethra, vagina and rectum pass through this muscular sheet. This weakens it to some extent, but it is normally an adequate support for the pelvic contents when a woman is standing erect.

Superficial perineal muscles

These lie below the levator ani sheet. They come in from the pubis, the sacrum and the lateral pelvic walls to unite between the vagina and the rectum, thereby forming the superficial half of the perineal body (Figure 4.8).

Figure 4.8
The muscles of the pelvic floor—sagittal section

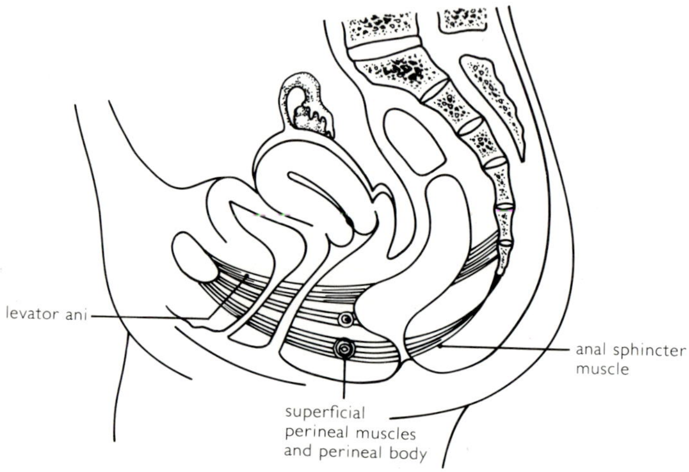

Perineal body

The perineal body lies between the lower vagina and the lower rectum. It is a wedge-shaped body of muscle made up of the inferior surface of the junction of the levator ani muscles and the junction of the superficial perineal muscles.

Blood supply to the pelvic organs

Arteries

The arteries supply blood to the internal and external genitalia in the following ways.

The uterus gets its blood supply from two large arteries on each side. It is essential that the uterus receives a large blood supply to cope with the great demands during pregnancy.

The *uterine artery* branches from the internal iliac artery. It runs through the base of the broad ligament to the internal os. It then divides and one branch goes upwards to the fundus with coiled branches, to allow for uterine expansion, going off to enter the uterus all along its length. A separate branch goes down to supply the cervix and vagina.

The *ovarian artery* is a branch of the abdominal aorta. A large branch enters the ovary and then the ovarian artery continues across to anastomose with the uterine artery.

The vulva is supplied by the *internal pudendal artery*, which is another branch of the internal iliac artery.

Veins

The veins of the pelvic organs normally travel beside the arteries of these organs, an exception being the left ovarian vein which usually drains into the left renal vein.

Lymphatics

The pelvic lymph drainage follows the blood vessels. The lymph channels drain into groups of nodes near the major arteries of the pelvis. There is a cross-drainage from one side of the vulva to the other, which is why both inguinal lymph nodes are removed when there is a malignant lesion on only one side.

Pelvic nerves

The vulva, perineum and lower vagina are innervated from the pudendal nerve (somatic nervous system). The skin of the vulva is very sensitive; perineal injuries are usually quite painful. The lower vagina is sensitive but the upper vagina is insensitive to ordinary stimuli.

The uterus, cervix and upper vagina are innervated by the sympathetic nervous system via the presacral plexus. Diseases such as vaginitis, ulcers and carcinoma of the upper vagina do not, in themselves, cause pain.

The cervix is able to be cut, pierced or diathermied without discomfort. It is, however, extremely sensitive to stretch—it is the dilating of the cervix which contributes to much of the pain of labour.

The ovary is insensitive except to squeezing (as in bi-manual examination). This explains why ovarian cysts may grow and not be noticed until they are very large.

The fallopian tubes are, unlike the ovaries and uterus, sensitive to cutting, touching, crushing and stretching.

5 The physiology of the female reproductive system

The functioning of the female reproductive system is dependent upon the maturation of ovarian follicles and the production of the ovarian hormones oestrogen and progesterone. These ovarian activities in turn depend on stimulation from hormones secreted by the anterior lobe of the pituitary gland. The production of the pituitary secretions is governed by a combination of the hormone releasing factors sent down by the hypothalamus and a 'feed-back' arrangement from the level of ovarian hormones in the blood. The levels of circulating ovarian hormones also send 'feed-back' to, and so affect, the hypothalamus.

As well as this purely chemical system of hormonal control, there is a direct influence upon the hypothalamus from the cerebral cortex, and so emotional factors can also affect the course of the normal workings of any of the structures involved.

It is obvious then that an understanding of the 'menstrual cycle' and menstrual disorders involves far more than just knowing about the changes that occur in the uterine lining. It has to be thought of as the hypothalamic-pituitary-ovarian-endometrial relationship. It is presented here as simply as possible in order not to confuse; but it is a complex topic and its finer points are still not fully understood.

The physiology of the reproductive system is discussed under the following headings:

- ovulation
- the menstrual cycle
- actions of the ovarian hormones
- changes caused by aging and childbearing.

Ovulation

At birth, the ovaries of a baby girl contain something like 200 000 primary ovarian follicles. These lie in the cortex of the ovary, just below the germinal epithelium. During the very early years, there is little activity associated with these follicles. After the girl is seven or eight years old a gradual awakening of activity occurs in response to a pituitary hormone, follicle stimulating hormone (FSH). It is not known exactly what triggers off the initial release of FSH but it is believed to have some connection with the output of the pituitary growth hormone. By an awakening from the time of the first releasing of FSH onwards, oestrogen is produced by the primary follicles, in very small amounts at first but gradually increasing. Between the ages of eleven and sixteen, when enough of the follicles have been stimulated to mature, the effects of oestrogen on its 'target' organs become evident, and the first ovarian follicle ripens to become a *graafian follicle* which will rupture to release its ovum, ie ovulation.

Several hundreds of follicles probably start to ripen each month (once the cycle is established), each producing a certain amount of oestrogen. At some stage during this ripening process, one follicle is more advanced than the others and it produces a much greater output of oestrogen. This causes all those other ripening follicles to stop production and to atrophy; they simply disappear into the substance of the ovary. The one follicle which has continued to grow and produce hormones is called, at this stage, a graafian follicle (see Figure 4.4).

The mature graafian follicle consists of a layer of granulosa cells surrounding a space filled with follicular fluid. At one side of this space is the ovum. When the follicle is fully mature and is bulging out from the ovarian capsule, the outer cells of the follicle rupture and the ovum is discharged, along with most of the fluid, directly into the peritoneal cavity. From here it should be picked up by the fimbriae of the fallopian tubes which almost embrace the ovary at the time of ovulation.

Following the release of the ovum, the cells of the ruptured follicle join together to form a ring. They immediately start to grow and swell under the influence of another pituitary hormone, the luteinising hormone (LH), which has been released in response to the high levels of oestrogen, to form the *corpus luteum* (yellow body). The corpus luteum produces large quantities of progesterone and also continues oestrogen production. It has, however, a limited life span of about ten to twelve days. It can be maintained by the hormone chorionic gonadotrophin which is normally produced only by the outer cell mass of a fertilised ovum. If there is no embedded fertilised ovum, the corpus luteum will degenerate and the levels of its hormone secretions will fall. The degenerated corpus luteum atrophies to remain as scar tissue on the surface of the ovary and is then known as a *corpus albicans* (white body).

Menstrual cycle

Approximately every twenty-eight days, the adult female body is prepared for pregnancy. It should be noted here that twenty-eight days is the *average* length of established menstrual cycles. There can be variations from between twenty-one days and thirty-five days which are considered normal for those who experience these intervals regularly. The cycle days are always counted from the first day of bleeding until the first day of bleeding of the next cycle.

The menstrual loss is usually about 50–100 mL in amount, spread over a period of three to five days. It is usually moderate on the first day and heavier on the second day, after which it gradually tapers off. The blood loss should not contain clots. It is believed that an enzyme, released from the endometrium, prevents this blood from clotting. If the flow is heavy and fast, the enzyme may be insufficient in amount or too slow in action to prevent clots from forming as the blood reaches the vagina.

Hormonal control

This is shown diagramatically in Figure 5.1. Follicle stimulating hormone is released when there is a low level of oestrogen in the bloodstream; it is inhibited by a high level of oestrogen.

Luteinising hormone is released in response to a high or rising level of oestrogen in the bloodstream. Its output falls when the progesterone level rises.

FSH stimulates the follicles to ripen and as they ripen they produce oestrogen. This oestrogen reaches a certain level to which the body responds by releasing LH and inhibiting FSH. After ovulation, if the corpus luteum is not maintained by pregnancy, the levels of both oestrogen and progesterone will fall. FSH is once again released in response to the lowered level of oestrogen and the cycle is continued.

Changes in the lining of the uterus

The endometrium consists of a basal layer and a functional layer. It is the latter which changes in response to the production and withdrawal of oestrogen and progesterone.

Following menstruation, the functional layer starts to grow up from the basal layer as the oestrogen level starts to rise. This continues until ovulation occurs, and is known as the *proliferative phase*. The endometrium is repaired and rebuilt, and the tiny blood vessels swell and fill with blood. Once ovulation has occurred and the level of progesterone rises, the glands of the endometrium come into action and begin to secrete mucus, glycogen and other substances specifically to aid in the embedding and nourishment of the fertilised ovum. This is known as the *secretory phase*.

Here it is important to understand that there is probably a 'threshold' for bleeding, dependent on the level of oestrogen in the bloodstream. If the amount of oestrogen is insufficient to cause the building up of the endometrium, no bleeding will occur. If the amount of oestrogen is kept above a certain level, it will maintain

Figure 5.1
Hormonal control of the menstrual cycle

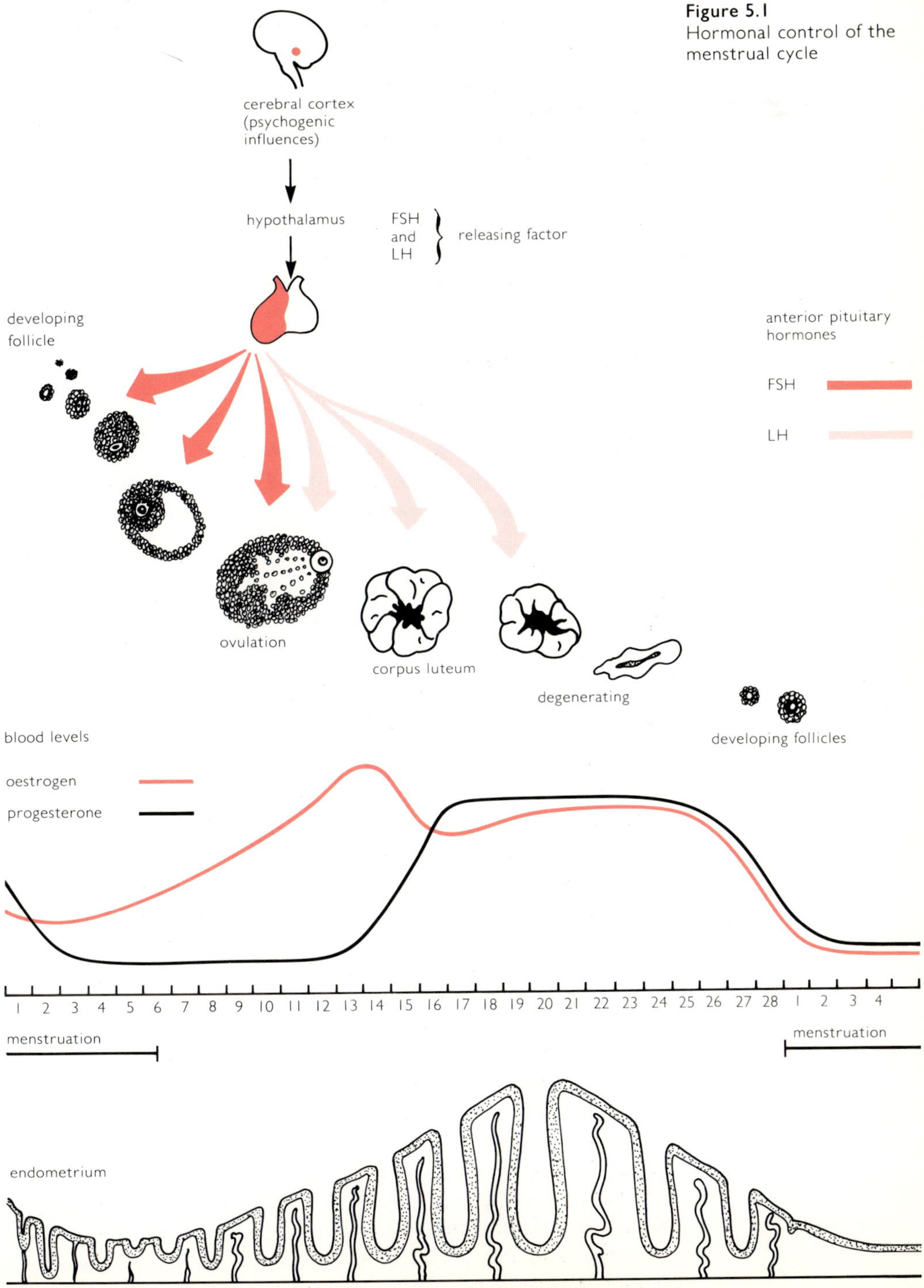

the endometrium and so no bleeding will occur. It is when the endometrium has been primed with sufficient oestrogen and then the level of oestrogen falls that bleeding occurs. When the oestrogen level is high enough to stimulate endometrial growth but not high enough to maintain it, breakthrough bleeding occurs.

In a normal cycle, after ovulation, the corpus luteum produces sufficient oestrogen to inhibit the endometrium from breaking down. If the corpus luteum does not degenerate at the usual time, that is if it is maintained by a pregnancy, oestrogen continues to be produced; the oestrogen level is kept above the bleeding threshold and *amenorrhoea* is one of the first signs of that pregnancy.

In the absence of a pregnancy the corpus luteum, with its limited life span, will degenerate and stop producing its hormones, and the level of oestrogen will fall below the threshold. When deprived of the hormonal support the endometrial growth and secretion cease. The arterioles go into spasm resulting in ischaemia of the surface layer. As the cells die from lack of blood, small haemorrhages occur into the endometrium. It begins to break down, more bleeding results and the whole functional layer is shed. This, together with blood, is the menstrual flow, or menstruation. Table 5.1 summarises the menstrual cycle.

Actions of the ovarian hormones

Most of the organs and tissues of the body are normally mature and functioning at birth or soon after, and they continue in their job until death or just before. The reproductive system and its associated structures do not follow this pattern. They do not reach maturity until they are stimulated by the appropriate hormones; they do not function if the source of these hormones is removed or disturbed in some way, and they are considerably affected by the processes of aging and childbearing.

The principal hormones which affect the reproductive system are oestrogen and progesterone, produced mainly by the ovaries, and, in a lesser proportion, by the adrenal glands. Disturbances of ovarian hormone production may thereby result in an outpouring of androgens in an attempt to keep up the oestrogen and progesterone levels in the bloodstream.

Oestrogen is inactivated by the liver; if there is a failure in liver function, the oestrogen activity may be greatly increased.

The actions of the ovarian hormones upon their various target organs, that is those organs which are especially designed to respond to these hormones, are shown in Table 5.2.

Oestrogen brings about the body changes of puberty. Together with androgens, it is responsible for the growth and pattern of pubic and axillary hair. In addition, there is some evidence to suggest that oestrogen plays a part in the retention of calcium in the bones.

Table 5.1 The menstrual cycle can be divided into four phases: menstrual phase of 4 days; proliferative phase of 10 days; secretory phase of 11 days; regressive phase of 3 days

Pituitary gland	Ovary	Uterus (endometrium)
Menstrual phase FSH released	follicles start to ripen	endometrium is shed, except for the basal layer
Proliferative phase FSH continues to be released; level of FSH drops 24 hours before ovulation; LH is released—the LH 'surge'	follicles continue to ripen, one much more than the others—the graafian follicle; produces oestrogen and some progesterone; graafian follicle grows, distends ovarian capsule, and it ruptures, releasing its ovum—ovulation	repair and rebuilding of the endometrium
Secretory phase LH continues to be released for a few days then level drops rapidly	corpus luteum develops from ruptured follicle and produces progesterone and some oestrogen	endometrium thick and highly vascular. Glands of endometrium become enlarged; secrete and store glycogen, mucus and other substances which can nourish a fertilised ovum
Regressive (or premenstrual) phase Low levels of oestrogen stimulate production of FSH	corpus luteum degenerates (limited life span); therefore levels of progesterone and oestrogen fall	endometrial growth and secretion ceases → ischaemia of surface layers → cells die → bleeding below surface → gradual stripping off of whole functional surface → menstruation

Table 5.2 Actions of the ovarian hormones

Oestrogen	'Target organ'	Progesterone
Proliferation of endometrium stimulates growth of myometrium	uterus	enlargement of stromal cells and glands; mucus and glycogen secretion
Growth of cervical glands; abundant secretion of clear thin mucus	cervix	change of secretion to scant amount of thick mucus
Growth of cells of vaginal epithelium; glycogen appears in cells	vagina	maturation of cells of epithelium ceases. Surface cells degenerate and are shed → release of glycogen
Growth and health of vulval tissues	vulva	
Growth of duct system; enlargement and pigmentation of nipple and areola	breasts	growth of the alveoli

Progesterone acts upon all the organs of the reproductive tract but only if they are being, or have been, acted upon by oestrogen. With oestrogen, it causes fluid retention in the tissues. Progesterone also affects other body tissues, leading to the deposition of fat, and is thermogenic, ie it raises the basal body temperature by about 0·5°C.

Changes due to aging and childbearing

So far the structures of the reproductive system have been discussed only as they are during the phase of maturity. Many differences arise as the hormonal influences begin to take effect, and as they are withdrawn. Many structural changes are due to the processes of pregnancy and childbearing. These will now be considered because many of the gynaecological disorders arise as a result of these factors.

Infancy

The reproductive organs of a newborn baby are of course very tiny. But a week or two later they have become even smaller. At birth, the baby girl has the same hormones (oestrogen, progesterone, placental lactogenic hormone) in her bloodstream that her mother has. Her 'target' organs have, therefore, responded to their stimulation. The endometrium has been built up, the vagina is exfoliating cells and its reaction is acidic, and there is some breast development. The vulva may seem large, and the labia prominent. When the source of the hormones (the placenta) is removed, the effects of their sudden withdrawal may show in the baby as it does in the mother. The functional layer of the baby's endometrium is shed, perhaps giving rise to a minute display of blood; the breasts may swell and 'lactate' before subsiding.

In structure, there are many differences to be noted. The ovaries are not scarred, never having ovulated. The cervix of the uterus is longer than the body of the uterus. The labia remain prominent until growth of the surrounding tissues makes them assume more normal proportions.

Childhood

In childhood, there is a very gradual maturation of the organs until the time of puberty. The various changes which occur then are discussed in the next chapter.

Reproductive years—before bearing children

Once ovulation has occurred (see page 32), scarring is apparent on the ovarian capsule. The uterus has grown so that the corpus is twice the length of the cervix, and it has turned forwards to an anteverted position. The oviducts extend to, and their fimbriae almost embrace, the ovaries. The cervix is tightly closed with a pinpoint opening only. The endometrium is thick and spongy in its cyclic preparation for pregnancy. The vaginal walls are firm and arranged in rugae (folds). Normal flora and acidic vaginal secretions are present. The vulva is healthy—the labia majora and mons pubis are well endowed with subcutaneous fat and covered by public hair.

At the climacteric, and after bearing children

The stock of hormone-responsive ovarian follicles diminishes gradually through the reproductive years. By the age of forty-five to fifty, most of the potent follicles have been used. As there are very few follicles ripening, a much smaller amount of ovarian hormone stimulation reaches the target organs. To add to this, there has been considerable stretching of, and weight bearing by, the uterus, vagina and vulva. The breasts begin to show signs of atrophy. The ovaries show a lot of scarring and are smaller in size. The oviducts start to shrink a little and separate away from the ovaries. The uterus is about the same size, the slight atrophy caused by less hormonal stimulation being balanced by the stretching caused by pregnancy. The fibres of the muscle wall, however, are beginning to be replaced by fibrous tissue and the endometrium is thinner. The cervix, having dilated to allow the passage of a child, never completely closes off again. The external os has a more oval-shaped opening instead of its tightly closed pinpoint opening.

The vaginal walls lose some tone and may no longer properly support the bladder or the rectum; prolapse may occur. The rugae are less evident. The vaginal secretions diminish and the pH changes from acid to neutral to alkaline. The vaginal orifice may gape slightly. The vulva also loses some of its tone and its subcutaneous padding may start to disappear. There may be scarring due to episiotomies or perineal tears from childbirth. The hair on the mons and outer labia becomes more sparse and the Bartholin's glands are less active.

After the climacteric—progression towards old age

The changes which occur at the climacteric are now simply exaggerated. The ovaries are inactive; the ovaries, the oviducts and the uterus are shrunken and fibrosed. The vagina is small and the rugae have disappeared; there are no vaginal secretions, and the vulva has atrophied.

It would not be fair to leave this picture as dismal as it appears at first glance. The reproductive system is designed to function during those years when a woman is likely to be physically and mentally capable of bearing children; when she is going to have the energy to cope with them. As the body ages, some of that energy is needed to keep the woman functioning well enough to live and enjoy living.

Other aspects of these changes in the reproductive organs and their effects will be discussed in the next chapter.

6 Changes in the life of a woman

All people experience changes as they grow through life. Maturation, both physical and mental, occurs from childhood through to old age. Specific changes affect both males and females as they enter, and then leave behind, their years of reproductive potential. Adapting to these changes and emerging unscathed, healthy in body and mind, is the ideal eventual outcome, but in our complex society it can be, all too often, a difficult process.

The purely anatomical and functional effects of the extremes of the reproductive years—adolescence and the climacteric—have been discussed in the previous chapter. There is, however, far more involved in these processes than just the growth or atrophy of the reproductive organs. The body alters and so does its owner's image of it. Responsibilities change and so too does daily life. Abilities and opportunities are increased or decreased and others take their place. These events are all normal in themselves but require adjustment and readjustment, and in some cases the adjusting is the difficult part.

Much has been written about these stages of adjustment and much of it is very good. Writers of medical and nursing publications see the need to give attention to the problems of adolescence and the climacteric, and they are producing some excellent material on the subject. The lay press is also responding to the demand for knowledge in these areas. Magazines aimed at the teenage market have a lot to say about sexuality and gynaecology. The matter aimed at their mothers has just as much to say about this and adds, as well, a lot relating to the menopause and climacteric. Most of this material is accurate and well written. Indeed, for some, it answers those little problems that arise from time to time that are slightly annoying but nothing more. But the correspondence columns still show evidence of innocence, ignorance and confusion. Perhaps this is due to misinterpretation of the material read; perhaps it is because the material fitted some, but not all, aspects of one reader's particular situation. Maybe the information presented does not tally with what her doctor said, or it may differ from the advice and experience of her mother, her sister or her friends.

Who does she ask then? If she is lucky she feels free to ask her doctor or some other person who has specialised knowledge, knows *her*, and will give her time. Failing that, she is open to the influence of either remote or misinformed, but enthusiastic, sources; sources that are potentially more harmful than good. One response to this need for accurate informed knowledge has been the establishment of women's health centres. These centres aim at providing both preventive and therapeutic care and education for women, and they are succeeding in their objectives.

Nurses have close contact with people, and at certain times, and in certain situations, can have a signifcant influence. Their approach to and feelings about their own adolescence and climacteric will be individual. They cannot, however, base their nursing judgments and actions on their own experiences or feelings. They have a responsibility to be alert, and to be eager to learn about the important aspects of these matters, to read carefully both professional and lay journals and to avoid at all times any tendency to label people because these people are experiencing, or are at the age of, particular and profound changes in their lives.

Adolescence

Adolescence is the period between childhood and maturity, and biologically extends from ten to nineteen years of age. Two other words must be defined at this stage. *Menarche* is the first episode of menstrual bleeding, the first menstruation; this, like the menopause, is a single, once-only event. *Puberty* is the stage of life at which a person's reproductive organs mature, and at which he or she is potentially able to reproduce.

Adolescence in the female, therefore, includes puberty, which in turn includes the menarche. Puberty is the stage at which the obvious secondary sex characteristics, breast development, public and axillary hair and the female contour, appear. These changes are gradual, extending over a period of up to five years. The menarche may occur at any time between the ages of ten and sixteen, the average age now being thirteen years.

Physical changes in adolescence

The complex hormonal interplay which awakens ovarian hormone production has been discussed on page 32. Puberty is usually preceded by a sudden growth in height of five to ten centimetres when the girl is about ten years old. Then the following changes take place:

ages 10–11 breast and nipple development commences; pubic hair starts to appear ages 11–14 skeletal growth slows down; the breasts continue to develop and the genitalia grow; the vaginal epithelium grows and acid secretions appear; the menarche occurs

ages 15–18 axillary and pubic hair fully develops; acne appears in 60 per cent; breasts have reached full (nulliparous) development, and skeletal growth ceases.

Puberty is said to be precocious when the menarche occurs before the girl is nine years old. It is said to be delayed when there is little evidence of oestrogen activity by the age of sixteen, although specific investigations are not usually commenced until she is eighteen.

Psychological changes in adolescence

Adolescence has been described as a time of turmoil, a time wherein the young person pining for individuality has to sort out what will be his or her future. It is, indeed, a time for making important decisions and the conflicting pressures from every side make these decisions very difficult. The obvious physical changes, seen in the mirror and felt within, create in many teenage girls a preoccupation and anxiety about themselves. They may feel secure only when they appear externally (to the *tiniest* detail) in looks and behaviour exactly as every other girl in their circle. Ill-timed criticism from parents or other older people will reinforce their intention to be like their peer group and at the same time be an individual. Criticism can have far more potent adverse effects. When it comes from people who have the responsibility of guiding adolescents towards important and far-reaching decisions, the serious and sensible matters will be overshadowed by resentment about the little things.

The whole area of sexuality—the significance of being female, coping with menstruation and discomfort and awareness of the opposite sex—opens up with a rush. It is almost impossible for a girl to ignore the flood of messages aimed at her; to consume, wear, wash with, or experience, whatever the advertisers have to offer. These messages are, almost without exception, full of subtle or overt hints that the most important thing in life at the moment is to be a sexual success. How does a girl, striving for excellence in a chosen area (or even struggling desperately to achieve enough to prevent later unemployment) cope with this continuous input of the glories of sex? When she cannot foresee that she will be free for several years to accept the responsibilities and emotional involvement that sexual activity involves, what does she do with her body that is already set to go?

Decisions about sexual activity are not the only distractions during adolescence. Pressure from the peer group is heavy; if those with whom the girl *can* relax and *can* communicate are involved with drugs and/or alcohol why should she not join them? If they leave school early or leave home early, why should she stay bound to convention or parental ties? Why should she receive the education that her parents did not have, just so that they can remind her that she owes them everything?

Adolescence is usually the last major period of influence in a person's life. The preparation for this period is vitally important. The need for this has been recognised. From the first day at kindergarten children are now encouraged to be active in making decisions that will affect their own welfare. Discussion and explanation have replaced direct commands. The birds and the bees have flown; in their place is a carefully-structured informative sex education programme, led by school counsellors, teachers, doctors, nurses and other specially trained people. No longer are the boys in a co-educational school sent home an hour early on the day that the sanitary-pad and tampon people show their film. Nor do the girls receive threats, even of expulsion, should they open the plain brown envelope and look at the little booklet before they reach the privacy of their bedrooms. Now they learn together from a very young age. They learn the right words, not euphemisms. They experience lecture demonstrations from members of groups such as the Nursing Mothers Association. They rightly learn so much about how lovely and natural the whole reproductive process is, that it is so unfair when their bodies are ready before their life situations allow them to go ahead. Add to this the enormous energy that has to be suppressed by being confined to a classroom or other space, the weariness at other times caused simply by the demands of a growing body, the financial or other dependence on adults, and the pressure to conform to their peer group and to their parents. Is it any wonder that this age group is often labelled moody, morose, 'revolting adolescents'?

Gynaecological problems in adolescence

No normal girl while going through the physiological and psychological adjustments of the puberty process will welcome gynaecological problems. Sensitive about her body and not wanting to be different, she may have more anxiety than her particular gynaecological condition normally merits. The two factors which emerge at this time, the onset of menstruation and the awareness of sexual potential (and for some the beginning of sexual activity), are the main problems that bring the girl to the doctor or other adviser. She could be worried about:

Amenorrhoea: every other girl in the class has started her periods. Or her mother or sister had started them when they were younger than she is now; or maybe the menarche has occurred but the periods stopped. A very real fear of something being very wrong.

Irregular periods: 'We were taught that they come every month. Am I abnormal?'
Dysmenorrhoea: that everybody tells her to be 'sensible' about, but it's bad.
Vaginal discharge: that she read about in the poster about cancer in the tram. Or saw something about in the VD booklet.
Early sexual problems: '*It* was awful and *he* was awful. And it hurt and I bled. He says he's got to study now but I know he just doesn't want me any more. Is there something wrong with me down there?'
'Cystitis': 'It's agony but I can't tell my mum. And she asks me all the time.'
Contraception: 'He says that girls always look after themselves now and that I wouldn't like it if he wore anything. But you get a bad name if you go prepared don't you? It's like asking for it, isn't it?'

And, 'I think I'm pregnant. What am I going to do?'

One extreme and complex condition that may partly be caused by a reluctance to assume womanhood and its implications, is *anorexia nervosa*. This condition is managed by the psychiatrist, but the girl may first go to a doctor complaining of absence of menstruation, which always accompanies true anorexia nervosa.

Other gynaecological conditions occurring in this age group are less common, but include ovarian cysts, late-manifesting intersex conditions and developmental disorders.

Nursing the adolescent girl

Very few young nurses are completely at ease when looking after adolescent girls. Their own problems may be too recent, perhaps not yet fully resolved. Nursing involves close personal encounters, embarrassing procedures, body exposure and establishment of a caring attitude within a clearly-defined nurse-patient relationship. It is difficult for the nurse who has not become used to nursing to deal with intense, personal questions such as, 'Do *you* think I'm a bad person?'. The nurse has to be so careful in her response. If the nurse has the slightest idea of the influence that nurses can have when people want reassurance, she will know that her answer may not only be interpreted to mean something quite different altogether, but will be repeated everywhere as well. Thus, the young girl in hospital with acute salpingitis (*possibly* contracted through promiscuous intercourse) can inform the world that nurses approve of the whole thing or 'they' at 'X' hospital are all very morally lax and no better than the rest of the people around. Of course, the nurse's answer could come out the other way—giving the girl the impression that the staff were censuring, making her feel guilty, 'nobody there cares, and it's a horrible place'.

Young nurses have difficulties because they may be too close to the situation. Older nurses may have difficulties because the years and changes in the world have set them too far apart. The restrictions and restraints of their own youth may have caused an intolerance to the seemingly unnecessary fuss about the 'youth of today'. There can be an element of jealousy felt towards those who still have lovely skin, shining hair and the joy of anticipating the years ahead. The noise, the mess, the number of visitors surrounding the adolescent patient upset the rest of their orderly wards. The way they get better and go home after being 'such a bother' may be considered unfair when old Mrs 'X' is not progressing at all and she has been so 'co-operative'. And the girl's parents may be at the desk or on the phone all the time worrying about her when she (the nurse) could tell them that if they had shown enough interest in their daughter before this, they would not have this worry now.

This bad picture of the nursing profession is, of course, not typical, but it is something about which a nurse has to be wary; her own experiences clouding her professional attitude and thus affecting the quality of her care for people. In a situation such as the reception and care of a girl who has been raped, all such judgments and attitudes are flung aside, but they can creep back again when dealing with the less dramatic and more mundane situations.

As well as this most important consideration of attitude towards the adolescent girl, the utmost should be done to make her hospitalisation as pleasant as possible. Whether she is brash or shy, she is still likely to be sensitive. If she is lonely, occupation or company must be provided. If her company is unsuitable it should be changed. It is unlikely that a teenage girl will be delighted by detailed descriptions of her room-mate's gynaecological history, especially if the room-mate has undergone a few horrific operations. Some hospitals have now established units for adolescents only; in the absence of such a unit nurses are aware that adolescents have special needs, and one of those needs is the preservation of an intact ego and, at times, protection from people with too much experience. Changing beds can usually be accomplished without embarrassment or annoyance to either party. A nurse may say, for example, that they always like to keep Dr X's patients together (or apart!) if possible, or they want to fill up a different part of the ward. This simple measure can have very positive effects.

Nursing the adolescent patient can be a very rewarding experience. It can be a give and take effort; a two-way learning situation. The problems encountered and overcome aid the nurse's appreciation of people in this age group. The opportunities for enlightenment, preventive care and education are there for the alert nurse to give, but to do this she must have adequate knowledge herself and be able to transmit it.

Climacteric

The climacteric is the 'change of life'. The word comes from the Greek word *klimacter*, a step, and that is what this life phase is, a step from the long period of reproductive potential into a period, almost as long, of life when it is no longer possible to become pregnant.

It is important to distinguish between two words here: *climacteric* and *menopause*. Climacteric refers to the cessation of ovarian function. The specific symptoms that occur at this time due to the lowering of oestrogen levels are the climacteric symptoms. The cessation of periods is one of the most significant symptoms. The menopause is the cessation of menstruation, ie the last menstrual period. It is, therefore, not realised until some months after it has occurred, unless it has been artificially induced for some reason.

The climacteric occurs during the three or four years before the age of fifty in most women. It is rare for menstruation to continue much beyond this. The process is usually gradual, with the body adjusting slowly to the decreased ouput of oestrogen. Over half of all women manage to go through this period with no real symptoms at all. Some others, despite their intentions not to be bothered by the climacteric, experience a number of physical and emotional difficulties at this time which they can only ascribe to this phase. Other women *expect* problems; they have been warned of this dreadful 'change of life' from adolescence onwards and so they may experience most of the symptoms, feel them more strongly and seem to have the whole process for an interminably long time.

Physical changes at the climacteric

The mechanism that operates in the transition from ovarian activity to inactivity is not fully known. The chapter on physiology described the complex hypothalamic-pituitary-ovarian relationship, and the way these structures respond to the circulating levels of the specific hormones. It is believed that the ovary simply ages; in other words, at a certain stage in life its remaining ova no longer respond properly to the stimulation of the pituitary hormones. Because there is little ovarian response to FSH, there is insufficient oestrogen released into the bloodstream. The low oestrogen levels in turn create a response in the pituitary gland, which sends forth far more FSH to try to stimulate the ovary. While doing this, other anterior pituitary secretions may be overproduced and this overproduction may continue for some years until it settles back to normal. The result then, of the ovary having aged, is a marked *lowering of oestrogen production* and a marked *increase in pituitary activity*. It is these two factors that cause the physical changes and symptoms associated with the climacteric.

Menopause

The cessation of menstruation is due to oestrogen withdrawal. The menstrual periods prior to the menopause are often irregular and may be either heavier or lighter than usual. Ovulation itself is irregular and less and less frequent at this stage. The follicle may try to respond to stimulation, it may try to develop to the stage of ovulation, but because of its age be unable to reach that point. Meanwhile, it is releasing quantities of oestrogen which cause the endometrium to proliferate. If the attempt to reach ovulation is prolonged, the endometrium proliferates to a greater degree than normally. When the follicle regresses and ceases to secrete oestrogen the endometrium breaks down, and the loss is heavier than normal. Later, the ovarian response is even less, producing minimal amounts of oestrogen, and so the endometrial proliferation and its subsequent shedding is much less than normal. Eventually there will be no ovarian response, no endometrial proliferation and no menstrual loss—the menopause will have occurred. Occasionally it is an abrupt process, the regular and normal periods simply ceasing.

Atrophy of the reproductive organs

The reproductive organs and the secondary sex characteristics are target tissues for oestrogen and progesterone; just as they developed when these hormones arrived in significant amounts at puberty, so the process is reversed when the hormone levels fall (the tissue cells contain specific hormone receptors). These atrophic changes have already been described in detail; it is sufficient here to repeat that the organs all undergo a very gradual but marked reduction in size and elasticity, and the natural defences against ascending infection are considerably weakened.

Bone changes

Osteoporosis, a condition in which there is a reduction in the total amount of bone material in the bones, is an associated effect of oestrogen withdrawal. Its incidence is higher in women who have had an early cessation of ovarian activity without oestrogen replacement therapy and in those who smoke. It causes the characteristic 'widows hump' seen in many old ladies who have no other orthopaedic disease. It can cause backache and, in severe and prolonged cases, lower vertebral fractures can occur following minor strains or exertions. Oesteoarthritis may appear for the first time.

Hot flushes

Flushing is probably the most common and well known of the climacteric symptoms. It is distressing to the woman when she thinks it is obvious, and even when it is not evident to the observer she still feels flushed. The flushing affects mainly the face and neck, but it makes her feel hot all over. She may take her jacket off and put it on again several times within the space of an hour, and be conscious of doing so. When night sweats occur as well, she loses sleep and so is tired during the day. She may disturb her partner's sleep, or may soak their sheets and so have to move to a separate bed.

The hot flushes are caused by vasomotor instability due to a high level of unopposed gonadotrophin. They rarely last for more than half a minute, but at their peak can occur up to forty times a day. They occur particularly when the woman is excited or fatigued, or after hot or spicy food or alcoholic drinks.

Virilising changes

Many women approaching the menopause fear that they will lose their femininity. Virilising changes do occur but they are rarely obvious. The increased pituitary activity results in increased stimulation of the adrenal cortex and therefore more androgens are produced. Unwanted hair sometimes grows on the upper lip, the chin, and down the arms, and the skin may become coarser.

Psychological changes at the climacteric

In addition to the purely physical manifestations of ovarian withdrawal and pituitary overactivity, the time of life itself in which this period occurs is one of unsettlement. It is important, however, to note that *no permanent psychological change will arise solely as a result of the climacteric.*

The physical changes produce anxiety. They may arise in loss of sleep, dizziness, inability to concentrate, and a preoccupation with the body and its functioning. The conditioned expectation of problems at this time will help to produce such problems. There may be anxiety about sexual functioning, about the possibility of pregnancy, or about the non-possibility of pregnancy again, ever.

There may be significant changes happening around the woman at this time. If she is a mother her role may have changed to that of grandmother—from an accepted adviser to a sometimes resented adviser. She has to cope with the departure of at least some of her children, giving them up to the demands of the work they have chosen or to the care of spouses that she may not have chosen had she had the choice. She may have to learn again to live with her husband, without (what may have been their major or only topic of conversation for several years) the children. She may notice for the first time that her husband is getting older too, and so fear for his future and for her own. Financial insecurity may be present in many situations, and this will further strain interpersonal relationships.

The woman who is alone at this phase in life, whether she is single, divorced, or widowed, will have other difficulties in adjustment.

The psychological adaptation to the climacteric is usually achieved within the space of one year. By then, some of the *advantages* of the menopause will be evident. The woman will be free of the tiring and messy business associated with menstruation. Once she is sure that her periods have finally ceased, she is freed from the fear of pregnancy so late in her life. Human beings were not made exclusively to reproduce and care for their young; after they have done this, they are usually then given about another twenty or more years of life to carry out the other aspects of their function in the world, and to share their experience and wisdom with others.

Gynaecological problems at, and beyond, the climacteric

Menstruation is often a source of uncertainty. It can be irregular, scanty or heavy. Periods are more difficult to manage. Premenstrual tension may be troublesome. Menstrual migraine headaches may appear for the first time.

Menopause may be premature or delayed; either is usually a source of concern to the woman. 'Spotting' may occur after the menopause. The informed woman will report this immediately. The semi-informed or anxious woman may worry about cancer while she might be leaving it to spread.

Sexual matters can bring a woman to seek advice. Dysparunia may have resulted from atrophic changes. Her sexual response may have changed; her interest in intercourse almost gone or alternatively suddenly awakened. She may want to know if intercourse is approved of after this period in life. Contraception can be a difficult problem at this time. Formerly used methods may be unsafe or unsuitable now. But there still may be some time left before she can be assured that she is no longer fertile.

New growths may arise. Even if they are proved to be benign they will have caused anxiety and possibly frightening symptoms.

Pruritus and *vaginitis* may occur in a woman who, because of her age and generation, regards these symptoms with shame as well as suffering their discomfort.

Displacements of the pelvic organs may come as a result of the general atrophy of the pelvic structures.

Incontinence of urine may complicate the matter, and add to the discomfort and annoyance caused by the prolapse.

Other physical conditions will emerge at this time. Those disorders associated with the reproductive system may be overshadowing important aspects of other medical conditions.

Management of the climacteric symptoms

The climacteric is, in effect, a hormone deficiency state. The line of management has, therefore, two main aspects—the restoration or replacement of the deficient hormone or the individual treatment of specific associated symptoms.

Hormone replacement therapy

Oestrogen given in small doses will prevent or subdue pituitary overactivity. It will prevent or reverse genital atrophy, and it will control hot flushes. It may prevent osteoporosis.

Oestrogen therapy is balanced by the administration of progestogens for ten days of every month. This prevents excessive endometrial build-up by causing withdrawal bleeding a few days after each course of progestogen is finished.

The woman receiving hormone replacement therapy during the climacteric is less likely to experience or be affected by depression or other psychological problems. Hormonal replacement will not, however, automatically correct pre-existing emotional disturbances. But it does often result in a feeling of well-being and the change of life assumes its positive aspect as a transitional but necessary phase.

Hormone replacement therapy has, also, a very positive effect in the prevention of osteoporosis, but this is considerably reduced in women who smoke. The woman's individual dosage of oestrogen is adjusted in relation to its effect and control of the symptoms that brought her to the doctor in the first place. The minimum effective dose is used at all times, and this is gradually tapered until the woman can stop taking the hormones without the risk of reappearance of oestrogen withdrawal symptoms. The therapy is usually necessary for a short period only, rarely lasting for more than one year. Long-term hormone therapy is given when an artificial climacteric has been produced by surgery or irradiation, but is usually withheld where malignancy of any of the genital organs was the indication for the procedure.

There are some problems associated with hormone replacement therapy. Nausea, headaches, skin changes, and breast tenderness occasionally occur, and these may be more unpleasant to some women than the climacteric symptoms themselves. Irregular bleeding may occur from the oestrogen-primed endometrium and this bleeding cannot be distinguished from that due to malignancy without obtaining and examining the endometrium to make sure. Oestrogens also affect blood clotting factors, glucose metabolism and liver function. They are, therefore, given with great caution, if at all, to women with a history of thrombosis, diabetes, and liver disorders. As well, hypertension and hyperlipidaemia have to be watched for carefully in the woman receiving this therapy. If uterine fibroids are present, their growth may be reactivated. Migraines may be intensified. The major risk feared is that of hormone replacement therapy causing carcinoma of the endometrium. There is statistical evidence of this in the case of *long-term therapy*, but none, so far, when oestrogen replacement is used on a short-term basis only.

All women should have regular gynaecological examinations in the years surrounding the climacteric. It is especially important when this therapy, with such potentially good and bad effects, is used and six monthly check-ups are recommended for the first two years at least.

Treatment of individual symptoms

Hot flushes

An alternative method of controlling hot flushes during the climacteric, where hormone replacement therapy cannot be used, is the administration of the drug, clonidine. Clonidine, which acts by altering vascular response, is used widely in the treatment of migraine. It is given in small doses at first and is then increased until either the flushing is controlled or drowsiness becomes a problem.

Local conditions

Local conditions resulting from pelvic atrophy, such as dyspareunia, vulvitis, vaginitis and urethritis, may be treated by the local administration of oestrogen in the form of creams or vaginal pessaries. Pelvic floor weakness can be improved by surgery or, to a certain degree, by physiotherapy.

Psychological symptoms

Psychological symptoms related entirely to the climacteric are, in many cases, reduced when the physical symptoms are made less severe. They are also made less when the woman is given attention and time from someone who is able to show understanding of the particular crises which can arise at the same age as the climacteric.

Common sense therapy includes education about the physical symptoms and appreciation of the psychological symptoms. It includes emphasising the temporary nature of these symptoms and the need for planning for the years ahead, after the symptoms have passed. In some cases where things really are difficult, sedatives are useful to overcome insomnia. In others, tranquillisers in small doses may be indicated as a help for the woman over the worst period. They are valuable in selected cases, but their abuse has led to a certain stigma being associated with their use. The fact that she has been prescribed such drugs may be more depressing or upsetting to the woman than her original emotional problems.

Postmenopausal bleeding

Vaginal blood loss should not occur after the menopause itself has been confirmed. Any blood or blood-like substance passed from the genital tract is treated as an indication of malignancy until it has been proven to be otherwise. *Immediate* investigation of postmenopausal bleeding is therefore of the utmost importance as malignancy may spread beyond the curable stage very rapidly.

Causes of postmenopausal bleeding

Vulval: inflammation, fissures, ulceration, carcinoma, urethral caruncle or eversion.
Vaginal: senile or other vaginitis, foreign bodies such as a retained supporting pessary, carcinoma.
Cervical: cervicitis, erosion, polyps, carcinoma.
Uterine: following hormonal stimulation, polyps, endometritis, carcinoma.
Tubal: carcinoma.
Ovarian: hormone-producing growths, carcinoma.
Other: blood diseases, pernicious anaemia, leukaemia or other haemorrhagic problems, liver disease resulting in altered oestrogen metabolism, hypertension.

Investigations

A careful visual examination and palpation of the vulva, vagina, cervix and pelvis is performed. Unless the cause of the bleeding is obvious and insignificant, the uterus is always curetted as well.

Treatment

The appropriate treatment for each cause of postmenopausal bleeding is described under the specific headings.

Vaginal bleeding may not be expected in the postmenopausal years, and thus may be confused with bleeding from the urethra or the rectum. Even so, these structures are not meant to be passing blood and the woman who notices even the slightest evidence of bleeding on her linen, clothing, underwear or toilet paper should be urged to seek medical advice, if for nothing but her own peace of mind.

Part II
The gynaecological examination

7 'What we are here for'

Doctors, nurses, and prospective patients cannot usually approach the subject of the gynaecological examination in an absolutely straightforward and dispassionate way. So it cannot be presented here simply as a description of a procedure and a list of equipment. (These facts certainly have to be included, but only within the context of the whole approach.) If it was as simple as this for the woman, there would be considerably fewer problems in gynaecological treatment and care. The number of reasons for delay would be halved; disorders would be discovered and treated when they are easy to treat. But what happens is that many a woman finds herself having to undergo the examination, having to discuss her menstrual, reproductive and sexual histories, and having to do it all by herself, and it is not simple.

Approaching the gynaecological examination

No two women feel the same way about going to the doctor for a gynaecological examination, nor do they behave predictably when they get there. Nor do any two doctors work (or listen to people) in exactly the same way. The examination done in the privacy of the specialist's or doctor's rooms will have a very different aspect from one carried out in an outpatient's department by a doctor who is probably a total stranger to the woman, and who is likely to have a number of medical students with him. Some women may prefer the impersonality of the hospital-stranger setting; others would never go to anybody but their own doctor, who is well known to them and who is trusted. Many are not given the choice.

Part II of this book takes a comprehensive view of all that the gynaecological examination might mean to the person who has to have one. It cannot include every reaction or emotion ever experienced and parts of it may well apply to physical examinations of other types. But it does include some of the reasons why the examination needs to be done, and it gives the more common reasons for delay in having it carried out. It looks at some of the feelings and fears that a woman may have about the examination; feelings that we must understand in order to understand her.

Part II also looks at what we as nurses often expect in the way of 'proper patient behaviour'. It describes specifically the things that a nurse can do, if necessary, to help a woman before, during and after the physical examination. It is hoped that it will ultimately add to the nurse's awareness of the fact that, in many cases, she has a complementary role at these examinations. It will be approached from the viewpoint of one who is working with outpatients in a large public hospital, but it can be modified and applied to include what goes on in both the ward setting and at the doctor's private rooms. One further word: no matter what the approach of the individual doctor to the gynaecological examination, there *is* a complementary role for the nurse to adopt and it is all aimed at making the experience as tolerable for the woman as possible.

Reasons for attending

Routine gynaecological examinations are often done in the absence of symptoms. These examinations are important for preventing problems and disease later on. Common indications include:

- the pre-marriage 'check-up'
- pregnancy diagnosis and postnatal examination
- contraceptive advice
- regular screening to exclude carcinoma of the cervix.

Other reasons for the examination, usually because there have been symptoms of malfunctioning, are:

- menstrual disorders of any sort
- urinary problems during and after the reproductive years
- vaginal discharge and unusual bleeding
- unexplained pelvic or abdominal pain, or low backache
- dyspareunia
- infertility
- undefined worry about the reproductive system.

Unfortunately there are some gynaecological disorders that are virtually symptom-free, hence the need for all women to have regular, routine physical examinations.

Reasons for delay

The factors which cause women to delay having gynaecological examinations are many and varied. They range from simply 'not getting around to it' to the woman having a real fear of the procedure itself. They cannot be listed in any order of importance because they each hold different significance for different people. Cultural attitudes, especially those held by Moslems and, in a different way, by some Southern European people, may forbid these women to undergo a vaginal examination before marriage, because of the importance of physical virginity, and may considerably restrict it afterwards. Perhaps the bridegroom or husband may not be able to entertain the thought of another man touching his wife and so may not allow her to attend. These attitudes are held in a different light in Australia today, but this does not allow us to dismiss them as unimportant; there are people from many different backgrounds living in this country and their difficulties with language and adjustment to our form of living do not need to be compounded by our lack of understanding in this sphere.

The more common reasons for delay are given below, in one or two cases exactly as they were told by women when they eventually arrived for a gynaecological interview and examination.

First, *embarrassment*. This is a big and understandable problem. Mixed up with embarrassment are the emotions of shame and guilt. All three are different but, according to their degree, they all affect one another. Embarrassment may result from a puritanical upbringing that treated sexual matters with secrecy and considered sexual activity only as a woman's duty; to be endured by a woman but never actually enjoyed. There are still a lot of people in Australia who think this way. If the interview should lead to questions about sexual intercourse, some women may not even want to admit to having done such a thing; such women certainly will not find it easy to introduce the subject themselves.

The *exposure* associated with the business of examination is another factor to be considered. The woman may never have been seen 'like that', even by her husband; then, when she gets to the clinic, she is expected to take off her clothes, climb up on to a couch, lie down and open her legs. No amount of draping can cover her feelings at a time like this. If she has a nurse there with her (not fiddling with equipment at the other end of the couch) she may be able to at least share those feelings.

'This is awful, dear. Fancy having to be like this'. A response like, 'Yes, I know (implying "I know how you must feel") but *you* know that it is important for the doctor to make sure that everything is normal' can lessen the embarrassment level and reinforce the fact that she has done the right thing. Embarrassment about having a particular symptom, for example pruritus or vaginal discharge, may make a woman decide not to go to the doctor: 'What would he think of me?'. Other minor factors may be involved; silly things like ugly toenails, or unsightly hairs on legs—things that she will get round to fixing up eventually—*then* she will think about going for the check-up. If a woman is embarrassed by the thought of exposure or of other people's opinion of her, or by anything at all to do with sex, she will probably decide that she does not really need to go to the doctor right away after all.

Fear that something else will be discovered is another reason for delay. The greatest fear is, understandably, that of cancer. After a routine cervical smear test, a common question is 'When will I know if it's cancer?'. Many women think that because the smear test is done, they must have cancer. They think like this because we don't inform them of the aims of preventive medicine. Following on from the fear of cancer is the fear of the treatment that will follow diagnosis of a condition, and the consequent disruption to living that could result. One woman stated, 'I know that I should have come here a year ago, but my daughter was getting married and I knew that there would be so much to do. Anyway, I wouldn't have spoiled her day for anything in the world'. The fact that a year ago she might have just had a simple diathermy, or a cone biopsy or excision at the most, whereas now she faces irradiation treatment and radical surgery, would be a cruel thing to point out. Another common fear arises because her problems might be directly related to her sexual activity. The vaginal discharge could be 'VD'. If so, who will have to be told about it? What if anyone from the hospital staff knows her and could see her records? It is easier to hope that it will clear up by itself.

On top of these fears there may be a *fear of the examination itself*. Because of a previous bad experience at a gynaecological examination, the woman may have determined never to come again, no matter what goes wrong in the future. The examination may have hurt, and nobody was there to help her through it. Memories of an ill-managed confinement may make her wary of all doctors, and particularly of those who practise obstetrics and gynaecology. Intercourse or tampons may have hurt her, so she fears that the instruments and the 'feeling around inside' will also hurt. She may never have had this examination before, but she may have been so frightened and misinformed about it that the thought of it all horrifies her. So she does not go, or she delays her going for very much longer than she should.

There are other reasons why a woman might delay. The sheer physical business of getting there on her own may be a problem. She may not be able to leave her job during working hours when the doctor is available. Even if she does not have outside employment, she may not be able to leave her children and she dreads taking them. She may not know how to get a referral to the gynaecologist or to the outpatients' department. Even if she does know how, she may be reluctant to go to the casualty section of the hospital to get the referral; what if she arrived when they were having a big emergency? If she goes to her local doctor she may be too shy to ask him, in case *he* thinks that *she* thinks that he is not good enough. She likes him, but wants to keep this particular area separate. She may worry that he might not refer her to the hospital, but instead to a 'friend of his' thus making her a private patient with all that that can entail in the way of bills for consultations, investigations, medications, and possibly hospitalisation. (But what woman is brave enough to challenge her local doctor about this?) One woman told what had happened to her:

> It was silly of me not to have told somebody right at the start. The fact was that we had not really got around to taking out extra private insurance for hospital benefits. What with three children at school, needing shoes and swimming lessons, and everything, it all meant that we had to watch the finances a bit more carefully—so we let the hospital benefits slide. When my periods kept on being so heavy, and I just had to see about them, the doctor sent me to a very good specialist. I never dreamt it would mean any more than just one or two visits, but as it turned out he decided that I would need to have my uterus out. He said that it was very straightforward and not to worry. The hospital that I went to was lovely, and the nurses were very kind, but they had only private rooms there, and I was in there for over two weeks, because I had trouble with the waterworks, and then started to bleed again, just as I was ready to go home. The bill was incredible; every single thing that had happened to me seemed to be written on the account! We paid it, of course, but it really hit us. I don't know what to do about the children's school trip that's coming up soon, and the thought of Christmas on top of that is appalling. Look, if I had anything else the matter down there, *I'd just put up with it.*

This kind of situation happens often enough; we just do not hear about it often enough. The resulting determination to 'just put up with' any further problems is what leads to such things as *dys*-pareunia becoming *ap*areunia, and is what allows pruritus to become chronic, leading to epithelial change and possibly carcinoma.

Whatever the reason for the delay, whether it be embarrassment, fear, finance, her own 'busy-ness', a feeling that the doctor is too busy to listen to her little problems, or just plain igorance (or innocence) of the necessity or procedure of having gynaecological check-ups from time to time, there is a need for us to understand these reasons. There is an answer for every one of them; in many cases it is a simple answer. It is up to us as nurses to find the opportunities to inform and convince those in the community, by health education, and by setting an example ourselves.

The nurse's expectation of the patient and vice versa

> Mrs Whatname is coming in again this afternoon. Do you know her? You soon will! She takes absolutely hours to get undressed, and will want to go to the toilet at least three times in the process. Then when you finally get her up on to the couch, she goes on and on about how she hates 'being like this'. You would think that she would be used to it by now!

This is the way one nurse might prepare another for Mrs Whatname's approach to a gynaecological examination. Most likely the second nurse will be prejudiced about Mrs W before she meets her and will find it hard to be anything but defensive with her.

Think of the effect of putting the information another way:

> Mrs Whatname will be here again this afternoon. Do you know her? Well, she will probably need a bit of help getting undressed. She's a bit slow, but I think it's because she's nervous and gets flustered. She keeps on wanting to empty her bladder and that's also because she's nervous. She'll need some help getting on to the couch so just see that she's right and try to remember to keep her covered. She's been coming to us for quite a while but still gets very embarrassed. Just give her a little bit more of your time and she'll be all right.

What *do* nurses expect of patients in the gynaecological clinic or rooms? Firstly, co-operation. A good patient does what she is told and she also knows to do what we may forget to tell her.

When she is asked to get undressed, she takes off her pants as well, so that we will not get annoyed and say, 'How do you suppose the doctor is going to be able to examine you with those on?'. It sounds cruel but it has been said. She is also submissive, she is quiet and she does not ask questions that we don't like or cannot answer. She does not complain about the time or tell you that she has been waiting longer than people who went in before her. (We know the time and we haven't been to afternoon tea yet!)

She is expected to be reasonably modest or else we view her with suspicion. But if she is too modest, she might be regarded as silly (and unco-operative). She is supposed to be reasonably well informed about how her body should function; but if she should show signs of wanting to know more than we are willing or can be bothered to tell her, or if she dares to use 'our' medical terms, we often react suspiciously (she is not being submissive enough). It feels ridiculous sometimes for us to be standing there (in our starched neatness, decorated with the buckles and badges that tell the world that we know such a lot), saying words like 'womb' and 'front passage'. But if these are the words that she knows and uses, then we have to use them too. We can use the alternatives as well, but we must not show off our knowledge; doing that will only make her feel uncomfortable and inferior.

One doctor with a lot of experience in this field has described nurses themselves as being possibly the most difficult group of women with whom to conduct gynaecological interviews and examinations. As nurses we probably have the knowledge, we know the right words to use and we know what is desired in the way of behaviour during the examination. But somewhere in our heads a fight goes on between the nurse-person and the patient-person. We do not want to show off, and we certainly do not want the doctor to discover that we don't have the right knowledge or that we have misinterpreted facts. The usual result is a very unsure manner and a dim recollection of facts on our part.

With regard to the expectations that nurses and patients hold towards each other, another question to answer is: 'What do *they* expect of *us*?'. The expectations of patients will, in many cases, have been formed from previous experience with the nursing profession. If nurses have been observed doing little else but calling out names and talking on the telephone, the woman probably wonders why they are there at all (especially if there has been a recent public outcry about nurses' awards and conditions). If the nurse has only been seen as a doctor's handmaiden, efficiently handing things and attending to the doctor's every need, once again the patient will have no personal expectations of the nurse. In fact, the woman may even feel that it is a case of two against one and she may even wish that the nurse would go away. Her previous experience, however, may have been one in which a nurse welcomed and assisted her, explained things and reassured her. So this woman will have expectations of such nursing care again, and she has every right to have those expectations. It is up to us to meet them.

A woman's expectations of nurses, if she has had no previous personal contact with the nursing profession, may result from whatever image has been built by the public media.

The image of 'hospital romance' given by the still-popular short novels and afternoon television shows, may be all that many people get. These books and programmes have entertainment value for many people, but the impressions gained by people who are fascinated by the world of white coats and pretty hairstyles, have little in common with what the nurse's job really entails. If this sort of preconceived image of nurses is in the minds of our patients, are they going to expect us to be of any real use to them when they come to discuss their very important and private worries?

Not all portrayals of nurses are quite like this; the big authority figure (all starch and enormous hat, disapproving and barking out orders), that used to be met in films and books, may still be in the memories of many people. If so, these people could be frightened of us. Few nurses like either of these concepts of themselves; we can, however, by our attention and kindness help to change both of them.

The position that nursing as an occupation may hold in a particular culture may also influence a woman's expectations.

We may not always comprehend the status that nursing holds in the eyes of people from other cultures or social groups. To some people nursing is a socially acceptable and respected profession; a full secondary education is now required before a student can begin the general nursing course. Those people who for one reason or another have been unable to reach this level of education may feel inferior to one who has succeeded in this field. Others, while appreciating the value of a full education, may regard nursing as a wasteful use of that education. Nurses do a lot of physical 'slushy' work—they don't need all those years of expensive schooling to do maid's work! The daughters of these people very rarely take on general nursing as a career. Their education is directed towards a more financially rewarding and (to them) a more socially respected goal. Thus, cultural and sociological factors may make a woman look up to, or down on, the nurse as she performs her work. It is to be hoped that we will consider the background of every patient in our care before we label her as 'difficult'. She is not difficult; we simply do not know her.

8 The gynaecological examination

When possible, the gynaecological examination is best carried out when the woman is about halfway through her menstrual cycle. This should avoid the time of menstrual bleeding with its resultant embarrassment for the woman. Also, although the taking of smears for cytological examination is possible, swabs for certain other investigations may not be satisfactory when taken during menstruation.

Nurses and receptionists in gynaecologists' rooms usually ask the woman the date of her last menstrual period and when the next period is expected before making an appointment for a consultation which is likely to involve a pelvic examination.

In general practitioners' rooms and, even more so, in large hospitals, the receptionist or appointment clerk may not be thinking along these lines. If the onset of a menstrual period coincides with the date of the appointment, the woman might cancel the appointment and so delay having a gynaecological examination which perhaps should not be delayed. One important point should be emphasised here. *If there is continuous bleeding or spotting involved, the woman should be seen as soon as possible, regardless of her menstrual dates.*

The time and the atmosphere before the examination can be very important. What does a woman think when she sees a very busy (and probably very efficient) office staff? Possibly that they are all in a hurry and that no-one is going to give her time to tell her story. Her symptoms are slight, and she is not really sick—maybe she should not have come! She may sit there thinking of the reasons for her visit to the gynaecologist. These reasons may seem less and less important when weighed against the anxieties about the examination itself. Will it hurt? How much clothing will have to come off? Other problems may be running through her mind. She may have to collect the children from school. The car may be parked at a meter. What will she do if the doctor is running late or if he has to go off to deliver a baby? She may have to go back to work and her boss wasn't keen on her having any time off. Possibly she has had to bring small children with her. Are they disturbing other people in the waiting room?

The nurse is a very important member of the office or outpatient staff. If she considers each patient as a person who has probably at least some of these thoughts and preoccupations, she is able to help her more. It is not difficult to announce to those waiting if the doctor is behind time. It will give them an opportunity to move the car, to make telephone calls if necessary, or to take the children for a short walk to fill in the time. It also shows a concern for them as people with lives to lead rather than as just 'patients', or, even worse, as 'this afternoon's list'.

Preparing for the examination

The nurse's role in the preparation of the patient for gynaecological examination will vary depending on the routine of the doctor or hospital.[1] One doctor might like to meet his patient and hear her story before she undresses for the physical examination. This doctor may feel that the psychological benefit to the woman of talking face to face with the doctor is of great value in achieving relaxation and trust on her part. Another doctor, probably because of a rushed time schedule, may prefer to have his patient made ready for the physical examination so that they can proceed without any delay.

Whatever the routine we can adapt our way of helping so that the woman knows what to expect and why. We should greet her by name and tell her who we are and what to call us. A quick look at her card to tell us her name, address, age, marital status and religion, may help us to understand her and her situation better.

We can tell her what clothes to take off and show her how to put on the hospital gown if one is used. We can ask her if she would like to empty her bladder or go to the toilet first 'because it is more comfortable for you and better for an accurate examination'.[2] We can ask her if she would like some help undressing; even if she declines, we can be close by and, after a little while, ask how she is getting on.

When she is ready we can show her where to sit down if she has not yet spoken with the doctor. If there is a delay at this stage, she may want to talk about herself, her symptoms, her fears of the examination, her children, other nurses, other doctors or the weather. Often what is said at this stage is told to us in the hope that

---

[1]This chapter, particularly the section dealing with pelvic examinations, has been written assuming that the procedures will be carried out by a doctor. For students of general nursing, such an approach is considered most appropriate, and most likely to match clinical experience. Of course, nurses do conduct full gynaecological examinations, especially in country areas and at specialised centres, such as Family Planning Centres. Postgraduate courses in gynaecology and midwifery provide more detail on the conduct of gynaecological examinations than this book can.

[2]The bladder should be empty for most pelvic examinations, but occasionally the doctor may need to check for stress incontinence; it is wise to find out if this is likely.

we will tell the relevant parts to the doctor. This important time slot is not for us to tell her our problems.

At this point we should find out what the woman knows about having a pelvic examination. This could be worded fairly simply—Have you had a gynaecological/pelvic/internal/woman's examination before?' 'Do you know what to expect?' If she says yes she has, yes she does, the nurse can still add the assurance that the woman can ask if she's unsure about anything as the procedure is going on, and that 'of course the doctor always tries to be very gentle'. If the woman does not know what to expect, a simple description of the routine as it is described in the next few pages may be of help to her. We should always warn that the examination will probably be uncomfortable but not painful, and that either the doctor or the nurse will say when the taking of deep breaths would be helpful'

When the doctor arrives we should introduce the woman to the doctor and him to her. This is another little courtesy that is so often neglected (because we are embarrassed?) resulting in the woman wondering who on earth she is about to tell her story to. After the introduction we should move away from the scene. If it is the practice of the hospital or individual doctor to have a nurse present throughout the interview, then the nurse must stay, but she must stand away from the scene, at the edge of the cubicle, but ready to respond to whatever the woman or the doctor might require of her. Sometimes if the woman is having difficulty telling her story, the nurse may contribute what she thinks is relevant. This may be appropriate if the woman has mentioned to the nurse certain facts relating to her home and family life as an explanation for visiting the doctor. But, apart from contributing when it really would seem to be useful, we stand away and look as though we are not listening to the conversation; in fact if we sense that it is unfair to the woman, we deliberately do *not* listen.

The gynaecological history

Taking a gynaecological history of a woman who is visiting the doctor for the first time, or after a long absence, is a comprehensive task. It will include her:

- age and occupation
- marital status and if she has regular sexual activity
- obstetric history and its outcomes
- menstrual history, menarche, menopause
- general medical history including operations
- significant personal events
- present symptoms.

Many doctors work through things that are easy for the woman to answer before they get to areas that may be the cause of problems.

By the time the doctor has completed the history taking and is ready to proceed with the physical examination, we should have assembled everything that is likely to be required, and labelled the slides and test-tubes if necessary. If we have done all this, we will not have to run in and out continually fetching things, and we will be able to stay with the woman.

The physical examination

What we need to have ready.

For a routine pelvic examination, a tray containing:

- gloves
- gown
- lubricant, water soluble
- sponge-holding forceps
- specula (Figure 8.1) (warmed)—Sims' / —bivalve } of a size suitable for this patient
- cotton-wool swabs.

It is also usual to prepare (preferably on a separate tray):

- glass slides and pencil
- wooden (Ayre's) spatula for cervical smears
- fixing solution
- sterile swab sticks
- labels and request forms.

Figure 8.1
The Sims' speculum (above) and the bivalve speculum (below)

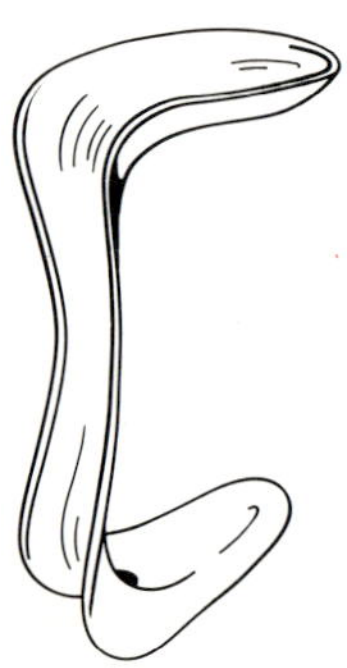

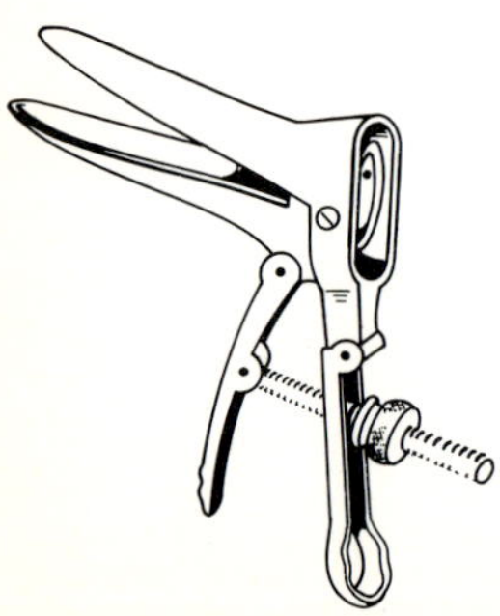

We should also have ready any special items that may be required for this patient, such as:

- pessaries (range of sizes)
- creams
- paints
- cauterising or cryosurgery equipment.

The room or cubicle should have:

- an examination couch or bed of suitable height
- a lamp that may be directed at the area (preferably one that will stay where it is put and not need to be held by the nurse)
- a footstool
- a supply of sheets and drapes
- a supply of perineal pads and paper tissues.

The tray of equipment used for the examination should be covered by a cloth to protect it from dust and to prevent the woman from having to stare at it. She may be frightened by the sight of it and by the thought of its possible use on her. Nothing could be more disconcerting than a display of gynaecological hardware set up to greet a woman as she walks into the room.

Handling the equipment

The routine examination is, because of the location of the area examined, not usually done as a sterile procedure. However, it does aim not to introduce infection and so any non-disposable equipment is sterilised before and after use, and careful handwashing is essential as some of the organisms encountered are extremely infectious. We know this, and quite often the patient knows it too. By washing our hands, and being seen to do so, we are both protecting ourselves (and our patients) and we are reassuring our patients.

A protective gown should cover our usual dress when we have to handle contaminated articles. The articles should be handled in a way that avoids directly touching that part which has been in contact with any potential source of infection. We do this as discreetly as possible. Disposable items should be placed directly into a lined, covered container. Non-disposable items should be rinsed immediately under *running* water. If this is not possible they should be submerged in an effective antiseptic solution which should be renewed frequently.

The washing of articles is done under running water using a scrubbing brush and soap. The articles are then dried and sterilised by autoclaving. Linen, including gowns that have been used by nurses or patients, sheets and any cloths used to dry equipment, is placed into a linen bag that can be closed at the top. If the linen has been contaminated by discharge, it should be put into a separate bag and labelled 'contaminated—possibly infectious'. Many centres now use disposable sheets for the examination couch; if so this is excellent, but even then we still need to be aware that the gowns and towels may be a source of infection (unless they too are disposable).

Positions used for the pelvic examination

Dorsal

The woman lies on her back with her legs drawn up and feet almost together. If a small pillow is placed under the woman's buttocks, the examination may be made much more comfortable for the woman and easier for the doctor (especially if the vagina has a posterior inclination). She then flops her knees open. The dorsal position is used for the whole of the examination by some doctors; by others it is used only for the bimanual examination, after the vulva, vagina and cervix have been examined with the woman in the Sims' position.

Sims'

This is an exaggeration of the left lateral position. The woman lies on her left side with her buttocks close to the edge of the couch and her back to the examiner (Figure 8.2). Her upper knee (the right knee) is flexed, perhaps resting on a small pillow, while her left leg is straight. We must be careful in making sure her left arm is not pinned underneath her body; it is better for her to have this arm behind her back. Some doctors ask the woman to lift up her right buttock with her right hand, thus helping to expose the vulva (and giving her something to do). The Sims' position is used for the

Figure 8.2
Sims' position

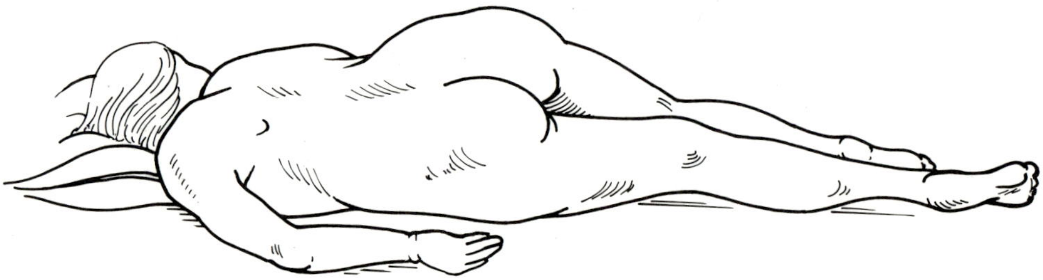

examination of the vulva, vagina and cervix. It enables a particularly good visualisation of the anterior vaginal wall because gravity causes the abdominal contents to fall away with a resultant 'ballooning' of the vagina.[3]

Lithotomy

In this position the woman lies on her back with her legs elevated in supports or stirrups. Her buttocks are brought close to the edge of the couch. Her legs should always be lifted up to the stirrups simultaneously to prevent back strain. The same applies when bringing her legs down again after the examination. This position leaves the woman feeling *very* exposed and the draping should be attended to most carefully and promptly.

Procedure of the routine gynaecological examination

Examination of the breasts and abdomen

This is done first, with the woman in the recumbent dorsal position with her arms down by her side. The doctor notes if there are any departures from normal in the development and shape of the breasts and nipples. He is able to see if there are any breast changes which could mean that the woman is pregnant. He will examine for lumps

[3]The Sims' position (and also the Sims' speculum) was named after a 19th century gynaecologist, James Marion Sims. There is a story told about his discovery of this position. A woman had fallen from a horse and had landed on her side, just as described above. Sims was the first doctor 'on the scene'. He started to examine her for injuries. As there was bleeding, he had to remove some of her clothing, but he did not disturb her position. He then realised that this would be a perfect position for exposing the anterior vaginal wall, and for examining and repairing vesicovaginal fistulae, which were common in those days of uncertain obstetric care.

Figure 8.3
Breast examination (left)

Figure 8.4
Abdominal examination (below)

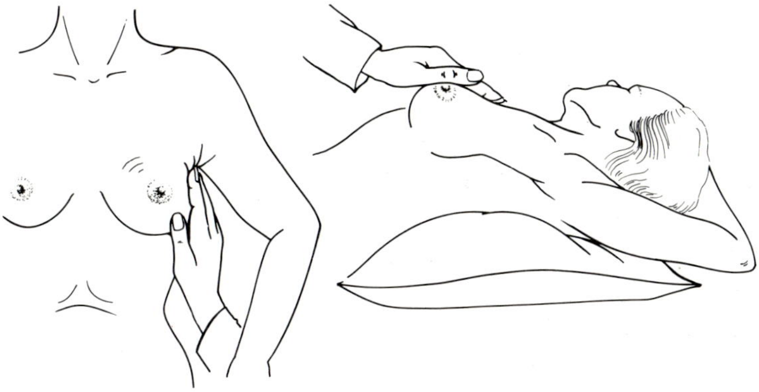

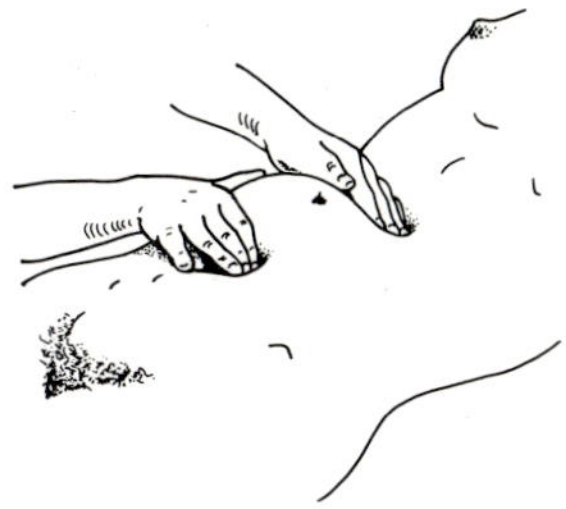

(Figure 8.3) and, if necessary, teach the woman to do this for herself (see page 74 for breast self-examination). He next palpates and percusses the abdomen (Figure 8.4), noting first its size and shape and any scarring present. He is looking for areas of special tenderness, and any tumours. Here, a full bladder could lead to a mistaken diagnosis.

Examination of the vulva, vagina and cervix

This is done with the woman in either the dorsal or the Sims' position. Good lighting is an absolute necessity for this. The doctor will observe for normal development of the vulva and for the presence of swelling, inflammation, discharge, evidence of mutilation of tissue by scratching or chafing, tenderness, lumps, warts or sores. He will feel to see that there is no enlargement of the Bartholin's glands. The entrance to the vagina will be examined for any unusual tightness, as this may be an indication for the use of a small speculum for the vaginal examination.

The next step is to insert a lubricated speculum,[4] by sliding it up and along the posterior vaginal wall, using a bivalve speculum (Figure 8.5) if the woman is in the dorsal position, or a Sims' speculum if she is on her side. In the latter case, the light should be directed not straight up the vaginal canal, but rather at an angle so that it is reflected from the Sims' speculum toward the anterior vaginal wall, which is the first portion of the vagina to be observed. Any loss of muscle tone, or prolapse is noted; if it is present or if there have been complaints or a history of stress incontinence, the woman

[4]Lubricant is used at the doctor's discretion. He does not use it when it may affect the result of the diagnostic smear, eg when vaginal discharge is present. Water would be a satisfactory substitute. He does use it (and uses it liberally) when the vagina is tight or painful, eg after vaginal or perineal operations, in a virgin or an elderly woman.

Figure 8.5
The bivalve speculum in position

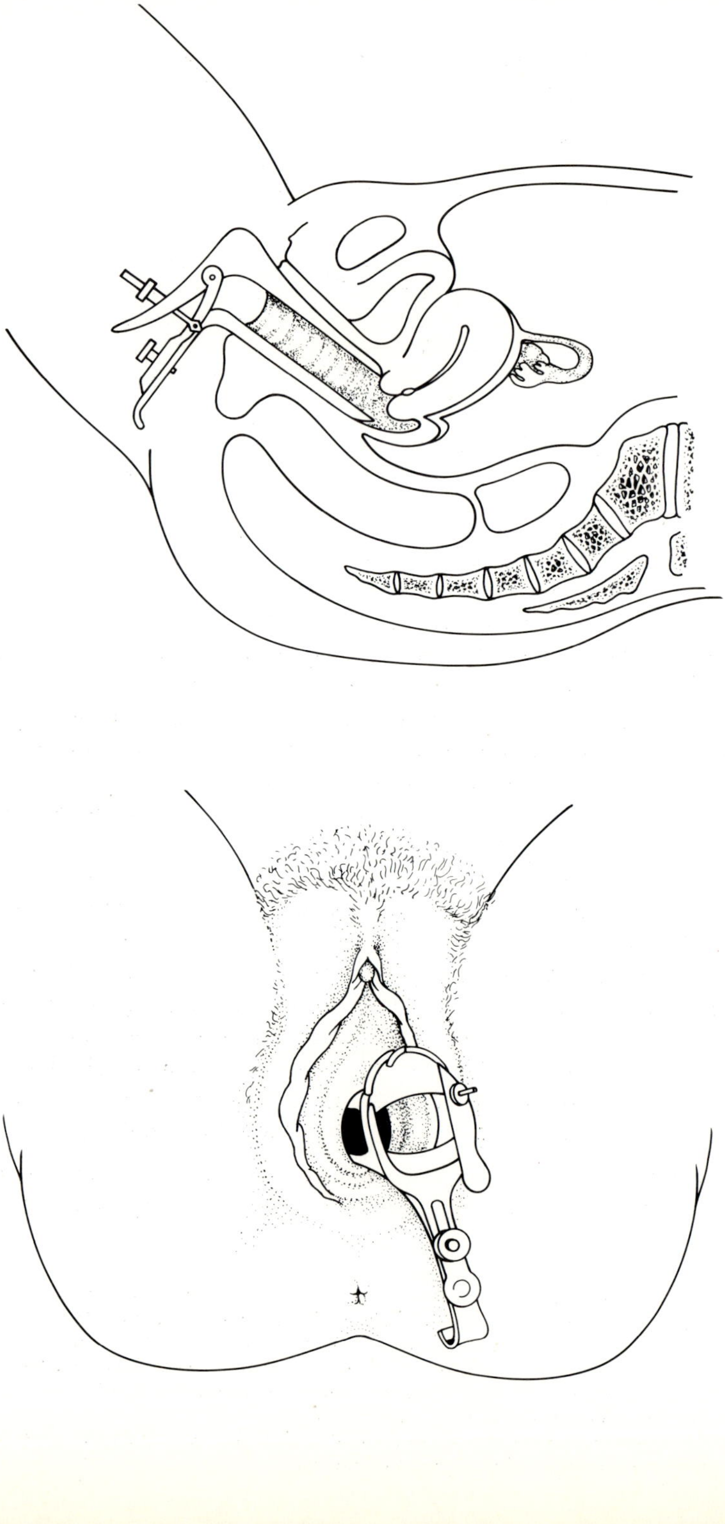

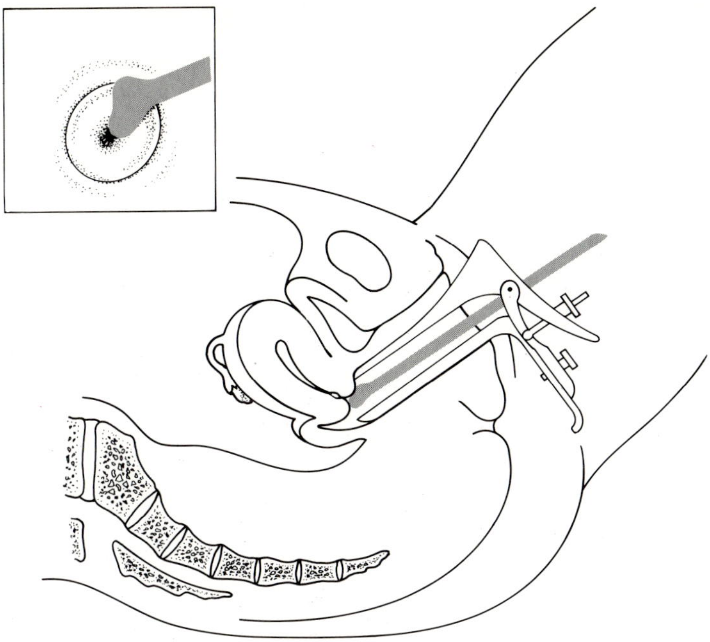

Figure 8.6
Cervical test being performed during speculum examination

may be asked to bear down or to cough to see if urine escapes. The bladder neck may be elevated (held up, supported with the sponge-holding forceps) to see if this makes any improvement.[5] The presence of discharge is noted, a sample taken for investigation if indicated, and, if the discharge is excessive, the vagina is cleared with swabs. The vaginal walls are observed for adhesions, redness, swelling and evidence of 'irritation'.

After this the cervix is visualised and the doctor notes its size and shape, and how far it extends into the vagina. (In other words, seeing if there is still the 'gutter' (fornix) as this tends to disappear in older women.) Any discharge from the cervix is noted and a swab for culture is taken if indicated. At this stage a 'scraping' of cells from the upper vagina and the external cervical os is usually done (the Papanicolaou smear, Figure 8.6) for examination of cell changes indicative of carcinoma.[6] The doctor will also be looking for signs of cervicitis, cervical erosion, polyps and Nabothian follicles.

The speculum will then be removed, the doctor observing the posterior vaginal wall, especially for prolapse, as the speculum slides out.

[5]Stress incontinence is rarely able to be demonstrated when the woman is lying down, because of the absence of the weight of the abdominal contents. Consequently the woman may have to stand up and, holding up her gown, attempt to cough or bear down to show stress incontinence. This can be extremely embarrassing for her. Some doctors may be reluctant to do this test, but as it may be the only way to give the true picture, it has to be done when indicated.

[6]The Papanicolaou smear can also show other abnormal cell changes, the woman's hormonal status, and if there is infection present.

Examination of the uterus and its appendages

At the completion of the speculum examination, the doctor will perform a bimanual examination (Figure 8.7). For this the woman will be in the dorsal position. The doctor will place one hand on the lower abdomen, just above the symphysis pubis and simultaneously with one or two fingers of the other hand, will feel from inside the vagina. In this way he can gain an impression of the shape and size of the uterus, its position, consistency and mobility. He may also observe tenderness of the uterus or ovary. If, at this stage, there is marked tenseness or inability to relax on the part of the woman, the doctor's impression may be clouded and the examination becomes of limited value. When the bimanual examination cannot be done easily because of this (or because the woman is extremely fat) it may have to be done while under general anaesthesia. This has one major disadvantage: the important sensation of pain cannot be taken into account.

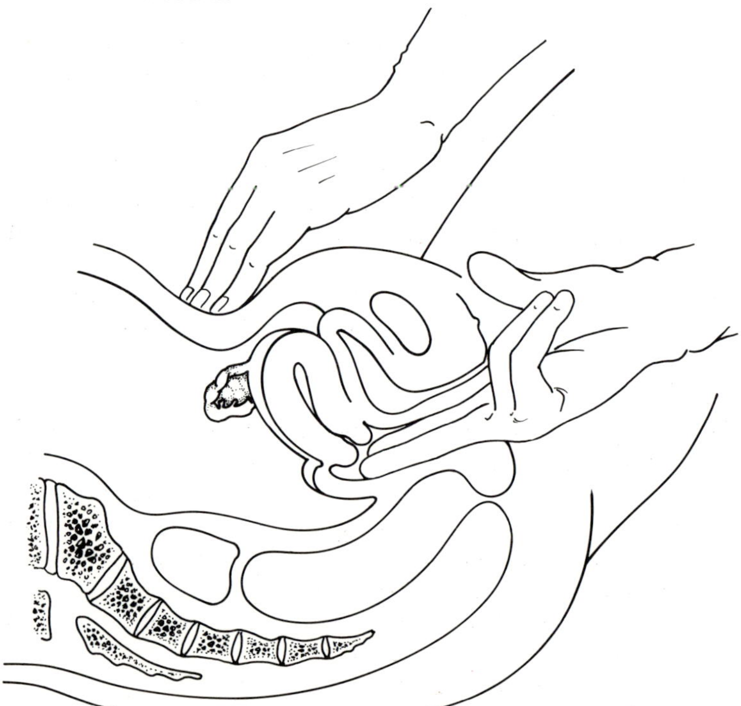

Figure 8.7
Bimanual pelvic examination

When indicated, a rectal or combined rectal and vaginal examination may be performed. A rectal examination only is done in preference to a vaginal examination for a young girl or a virgin.

Opportunities to help during the examination

The woman has to get up on to the examination couch. Couches are high up, so she may need a footstool in the right place. She may need help if she is old, or if she is very nervous, if she has arthritis or if there is some other reason that prevents her from 'jumping up' (as she is often told to do). Most women do not want help but it is a good idea for the nurse to stay somewhere close. She will need to be there as soon as the woman is up anyway to help to arrange the sheets and drapes. The nurse can then ensure that the woman is both comfortable and suitably positioned for the examination. When the doctor is ready to start the examination, the nurse can gently remove any sheets which may get in the way, taking care to uncover only as much as is necessary for adequate examination. If the next step involves the use of the Sims' position, the nurse can help the woman over on to her side. If the woman has done this before she will probably not want to be lifted and pulled; in most cases she will do this herself, much better. As long as we check that the position is right in the end (and that she is not uncomfortable), whether she has got herself up there alone or with assistance is of no matter. Once again the sheet is adjusted.

At this point we will often have to leave her, so that we can adjust the light and check that the necessary equipment is there and ready to use so that the doctor can manage single handed. Occasionally it might seem right to say to the woman 'I've just got to hold the lamp for a minute—will you be all right?'; even if she is very dependent upon the nurse and has asked her to 'stay with me, dear', she will want to co-operate and the nurse has just implied that she will return soon.

If the doctor does not say it himself and if it seems suitable in this particular case, the nurse may say something like, 'It will feel a bit uncomfortable now, but if you just stay relaxed it won't take very long at all'.

Once the doctor has all that he needs at hand and the light is directed in the right way, the nurse can return to the top end of the couch and stay there until the whole examination is finished. When the speculum has been removed the woman will be asked to turn over to lie on her back. Once again we can offer or give assistance if it seems suitable. We should then help her to assume the dorsal position or, if required, help her into stirrups, so that she is as relaxed as possible. The draping should be done carefully, considering both the woman's feelings of exposure and the doctor's need to have a clear field. If it can be arranged so that at least the upper thighs are covered, the woman is less likely to feel embarrassed. During the bimanual examination the doctor may suggest that she breathes up and down. If he doesn't, and it seems as though this breathing would be useful, the nurse can suggest it and may even do it with her. She may also (often with very good results) ask the woman if her legs are still relaxed. The nurse should stand close enough and have a hand ready if the woman wants to hold it, but she should never force this sort of contact upon her patients.

The woman may want to talk during the examination. If the doctor is concentrating on the size and shape and mobility of the uterus and many other things, he will probably not respond. Unless it is a direct plea for reassurance we are best advised to help her to tail off the conversation. One nursing sin sometimes committed is that in which a conversation arises between the doctor and the nurse while the woman is submitting her body to be handled. Always include the patient in the conversation. If this cannot be done then leave the conversation for another time.

After the examination

Usually a woman feels a bit 'strange inside' after having a pelvic examination. If we give her a short time to rest before she sits up it may help. If the doctor has not done so we should wipe away (from front to back) any lubricant, discharge, or blood that may be on the vulva; it is a horrible feeling to walk down the street feeling sticky and glued-up and thinking that everyone is staring at the way you are walking. We should give the woman a pad to wear if it seems necessary.

The woman who has not needed helping up onto the couch may need a little assistance in getting down. It is a good idea to let her sit up and get her balance before helping her down. The same applies to getting dressed. Once again we offer our assistance, but we do not hurry her, and she *does* have time to comb her hair if she would like to. We should endeavour to tidy up and remove any soiled linen and all the instruments before she reappears. Some women cannot feel at ease sitting there talking to the doctor if they feel that they have been the cause of the untidiness that the cubicle or room is now in.

After the doctor has completed the physical examination, he usually spends some time with the woman, telling her of his findings and giving her instructions in the management of any specific problems that she may have. He may write prescriptions or letters of referral. She will then be told when or if she needs to return. Some doctors do this talking while the woman is still on the examination couch; if so, the nurse can once again withdraw from the immediate area so that the woman and the doctor are able to have a few minutes together without a listener. Other doctors may decide to fill in time writing up the history until the woman has dressed and can speak with him in a more composed manner. In this case they will be face to face rather than having the woman lying down, looking up, in a position that is always to her disadvantage.

After the talk with the doctor, the woman will often want to see the nurse again. She may have questions that she 'didn't like to ask him'. She may not have understood his instructions about the treatment. She might not have received any instructions at all. She could be standing there holding a request form and wondering where she is supposed to take it, and what it will involve when she gets there. Sometimes the doctor has dismissed her with a cheerful, 'Well, I think that's about it', and then has disappeared. What does she do next?' (Figure 8.8.)

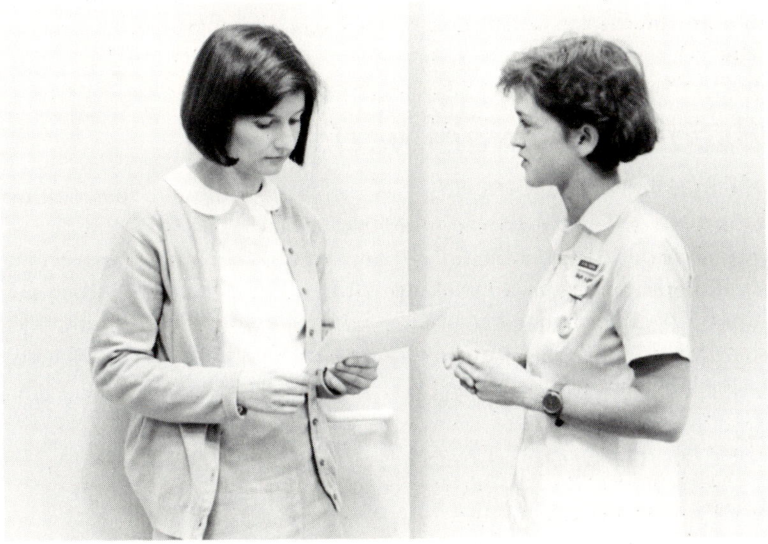

Figure 8.8
It is important to make sure that the woman understands all instructions before she leaves

We should always check that the woman knows exactly what to do—even if she is a doctor or a qualified nurse! Appointment slips, prescription slips and request forms should not go straight into handbags (at times it may be wise to put them in an envelope). She should hold on to them until she has delivered all of them. An important investigation or medication, forgotten, could delay effective treatment for weeks. We should refer any worries that we cannot honestly and safely handle ourselves, back to the doctor; it is not fair to send her off with doubts and unsolved problems when a few extra words would help.

Sometimes the doctor will ask us to explain something to the woman. If this happens it may be as well to reinforce our spoken words by writing them down. This is particularly helpful where there are specific instructions regarding medications, hygiene or symptoms to be watched for. The reinforcing effect is even stronger if we can use 'official' paper.

The post-examination time can provide a very valuable opportunity for education and for interpreting and underlining the doctor's instructions. It goes very quickly, so full use must be made of it.

Despite the length of this description of the gynaecological examination, the procedure itself, when performed by a competent doctor and when there are no complications, is relatively quick. It is over in a few minutes; it rarely takes any longer.

The woman's impression, however, of the duration of the examination (and of the exposure) will depend upon the consideration and the skill of both the doctor and the nurse as they attend her. The woman's decision to return to this doctor or to this hospital, or to any doctor or any hospital, for any gynaecological symptom, at any time in the future, will be based on her experiences with us, here, now.

Breast self-examination

No book on women's health is complete, without a description of simple *self-examination* of the breasts (see page 67 for breast examination as part of the full gynaecological check-up). No woman should go home from a check-up without being asked whether she knows how to examine her breasts, when she should do it, and what she should look for. All nurses can teach this simple and extremely important routine.

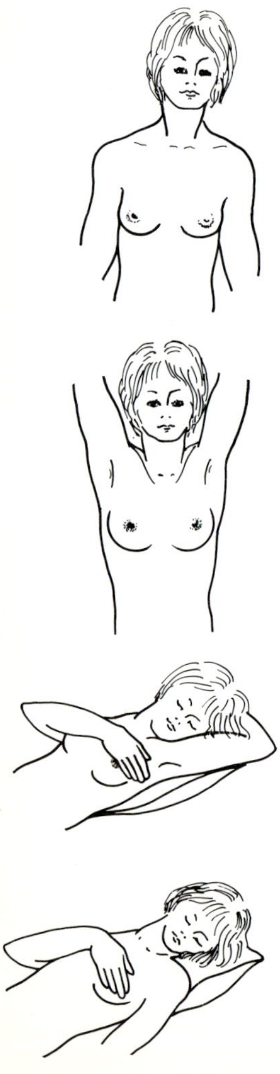

Technique of breast self-examination

Looking at the breasts (Figure 8.9):
- sit or stand in front of a mirror, in a good light
- keep the arms relaxed by the sides
- look for changes in the size and shape of the breasts and nipples
- look for dimpling or puckering of the skin, and for any discharge from the nipples
- raise the arms above the head and look at the breasts and nipples again.

Feeling the breasts (Figure 8.9):
- lie down with a small pillow or folded towel under the left shoulder
- lift up the left arm
- using the right hand, examine the left breast
- using the flats (not the tips) of the fingers, work over the whole breast, starting at the armpit and working in vertical 'strips'
- lower the left arm and feel the armpit area again, with the arm lying alongside the body
- change the pillow or towel to the other shoulder, and examine the right breast with the left arm
- note anything unusual, any thickness or lumps, and go to the doctor straight away if there is anything at all abnormal.

Regular self-examination of the breasts should be performed by every woman over the age of twenty-five years. It should be done every month, in the week following menstruation. This time is best because then any pre-menstrual fullness and discomfort has settled. After the menopause, the woman should choose a date that is easy to remember, such as the first of each month, and continue with regular self-examinations.

Allay the woman's fears by telling her that most breast lumps are not cancer, and the ones that are can often be cured, but only if they are discovered and treated *early*. Stress how important it is that she immediately see a doctor if any lumps are found.

Breast cancer

Breast cancer is the most common cancer occurring in females. It is now believed that as many as one in thirteen women will be found to have breast cancer. It is the major cause of death in females in the 35–45 years age group. It is also common in the elderly.

Most at risk are those who:

- have a family history of breast cancer
- have not had a child, or had their first child after the age of thirty.

If simple signs are detected early there is a very good prognosis, but once the disease has spread, the cancer is difficult to treat.

The National Health and Medical Research Council of Australia recommended in 1984 that women in the high-risk groups undergo a regular mammography (X-ray of the breast tissues).

9 Common gynaecological treatments and investigations

Treatments

Creams, paints and (chemical) pessaries

Local medications for the vagina and the vulva are, in most cases, ordered or supplied by the doctor, and are usually accompanied by adequate instructions (including diagrams) for their use; the patient follows these instructions and applies or inserts the medications herself. Even so we should make sure that she knows exactly how to manage such things as applicators, that she understands the best times of day for doing the treatments, and that, unless told otherwise, she should continue with the treatment even if her period should arrive halfway through the course. It may be helpful for her to know that the warming and/or lubrication of nozzles, applicators and pessaries often make their insertion easier. We can also remind the woman to refrigerate vaginal suppositories in warm weather.

We should tell her that disposable gloves are readily available from the chemist (and are not very expensive). Their use will help to cut down the spread of infection via hand towels and other items which may be used by other people. They may also be a help to those women who are reluctant to touch the vulval and vaginal areas directly. It is important, when recommending that these gloves be used, to place some emphasis on the fact that they *are* disposable, and that they should be discarded immediately after use. At this stage, it is also wise to give a short but clear explanation of the best way to clean and store any nozzles or applicators after use (see next page).

If the local medication is not to be applied by the woman herself because it is very messy (eg gentian violet) or because it could damage or hurt the healthy tissues (eg podophyllin or silver nitrate), this will need to be done by the doctor or nurse.

An unfortunate incident occurred as a result of an attempt to save one woman the bother of going every other day to the doctor for applications of podophyllin paint to vulval warts. She was given the bottle of paint, and told verbally to apply it carefully with cotton buds. Her understanding of English was limited. She bought, and used once, cotton balls. Her agony was undescribable.

Figure 9.1
Insertion of vaginal cream

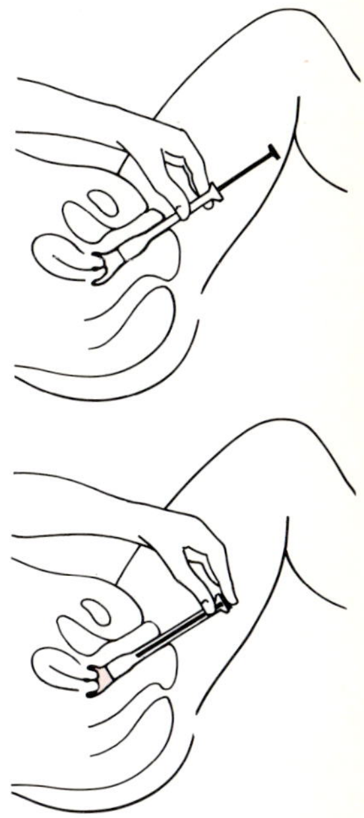

Vaginal creams and pessaries

The ideal time for doing these treatments is at the end of the day, after a bath or shower. The woman lies on her back in bed, with her legs drawn up. The labia are separated and the nozzle or applicator is inserted into the vagina and directed upwards and backwards so that the cream or pessary is deposited as high as possible without hurting (Figure 9.1). The applicator is then withdrawn slowly. (It may be useful to have a dish of water near the bed for soaking the applicator until it is convenient to wash it.) The cream or pessary will slowly dissolve overnight. A protective pad and cotton or disposable paper pants will prevent greasy stains from getting on the bed linen. The applicator should be washed first under cold, then warm to hot, running water, using soap, and dried with a paper tissue. It should be stored in a box kept solely for the purpose.

Paints

Paints for the vagina and vulva are usually applied by the nursing or medical staff. The area should be cleaned of any discharge and the paint applied carefully and only where necessary. A protective pad is always applied immediately. Many doctors advise the woman to shower about two hours later.

Figure 9.2
Diathermic cautery of the cervix

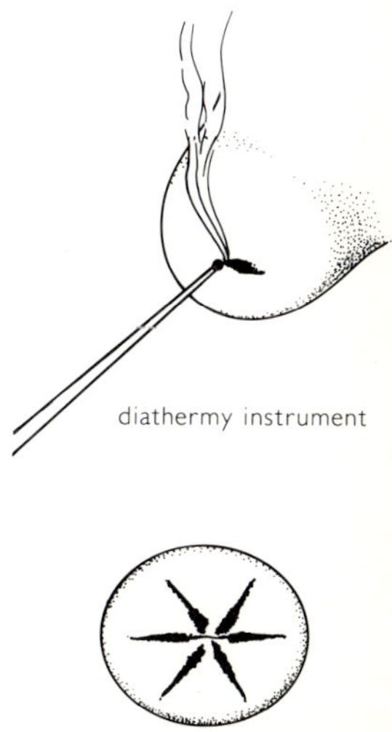

Diathermic cauterisation

Diathermic cauterisation is done occasionally as an outpatient procedure, for vulval warts, urethral caruncle or cervical erosion. Malignancy is always excluded first. Diathermic cauterisation of the cervix (Figure 9.2) is usually a painless procedure, the surface of the cervix being relatively free of pain fibres, but the woman may feel some discomfort or aching in the lower back. What does seem to be distressing to the woman about diathermy is the smell that arises, and the realisation that some part of her is being burnt. An explanation of the aim of the diathermy, emphasising the healthy tissue that will grow up under the cells that are being treated, may help. She should be warned about the smell before it is evident, and she should also be warned that there may be a little bleeding and an increase in discharge that may continue for another four to six weeks. (This may be one indication for douching, with saline, but this would be the doctor's decision.) She should not wear tampons, nor should she have intercourse until healing is complete.

Diathermy is never done in the premenstrual phase of the cycle because of the danger of infection ascending when the natural defences are lowered.

Complications of cervical diathermy are rare and usually occur only when there has been deep diathermy. They include cervical stricture, haemorrhage and infertility arising from the destruction of mucus-producing glands.

Cryosurgery

Figure 9.3 Cryosurgery of the cervix

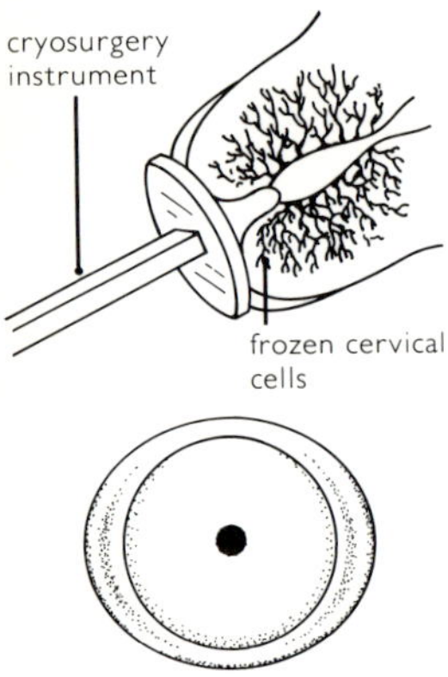

Cryosurgery—freezing or 'cold cauterisation'—is a newer technique that is beginning to replace diathermy. Nitrogen or carbon dioxide is used to freeze the affected areas in the same way that diathermy works by burning. It is reported to be less painful and appears to have a lower complication rate. (Cervical stenosis and infertility are uncommon.)

The instrument used resembles a small gun which is attatched to a supply of compressed gas. The tip of the gun is applied to the affected areas (Figure 9.3) for no more than two minutes. The woman may experience a feeling of intense cold and may become dizzy and light-headed for a short time. She should be allowed to rest and recover for at least fifteen minutes before getting up.

A profuse discharge will follow from about twenty-four hours after cryosurgery and will continue for up to two weeks. The discharge may be bloodstained, but should not become yellowish or foul-smelling.

Douching, intercourse and the use of tampons are not advised until the discharge has cleared completely—usually by two weeks after cryosurgery.

Vaginal douching

Vaginal douching is the irrigation of the vagina with fluid. The main medical indications for its use are to clean the vagina of excessive or infective discharge, to prevent the establishment of infection when a supporting pessary is in position, following the removal of a radioactive insertion and hot douching to help to arrest secondary vaginal haemorrhage post-operatively. It is also used as a routine hygienic measure in some societies, after intercourse as a contraceptive measure, and to protect against gonorrhoea. As well, when used before intercourse specifically to alter the pH of the vagina, it is believed, by some, to influence the sex of the baby conceived from that intercourse (alkaline douching if trying for a boy, weak acidic douching if trying for a girl).

Douching equipment consists of a bag or can to hold the fluid, a tube to convey the fluid and a specifically shaped nozzle (usually plastic) which can be comfortably inserted into the vagina. Solutions used include plain tap water, diluted antiseptic solutions, bicarbonate of soda (for alkaline douches), weak acids such as diluted vinegar, and many commercial preparations.

At home, the woman manages douching best if she lies in the bath for the procedure. After assembling the equipment, filling the can or bag with solution and allowing it to run through, testing the temperature, then clamping the tubing, she lubricates the nozzle with a bland jelly if necessary. She then lies down and inserts the nozzle gently into the vagina, in an upwards and backwards direction, then releases the clamp. The fluid will flow in and out again collecting discharge and debris on its way, until the container is empty. If she rotates the nozzle slightly, the fluid will reach a larger surface area. Pressure is controlled by the height of the container; 30 cm above the pelvis is usually the most satisfactory height. (Any higher than 30 cm could cause the water to enter the vagina forcefully and possibly injure the vaginal tissues or push bacteria or other organisms into the uterus and beyond.)

After the douching is over, the woman should stand up for a minute to allow fluid to drain from the vault before she dries the area. Sometimes she will need to wear a vulval pad to absorb any remaining fluid.

In hospital, or where the woman is unable to get into a bath, she will be helped on to a bed-pan, with her back well supported by pillows. Sterilised equipment is used and the amount of solution is generally 1200 mL. The return of fluid is observed and described. The woman is asked to cough to aid the expulsion of remaining fluid. This procedure can be both uncomfortable and embarrassing to the woman, so every effort should be taken to minimise these aspects of douching.

Douching is known to upset the natural defence mechanism of vaginal acidity if it is done too frequently. It is, therefore, inadvisable for a woman to douche her vagina without *specific* instructions for a medical indication. Any discharge or 'dirtiness' that she feels the need to clean away must first be examined for its cause, and the condition treated if the problem is to be controlled.

Vaginal packing

The vagina is sometimes packed to provide pressure to check post-operative bleeding. It may also be used pre-operatively to reduce oedema and aid in the healing of an ulcerated prolapsed uterus. Requirements for the sterile procedure are:

- large dressing tray
- warmed lotion for swabbing vulva
- 1 pair of long dissecting forceps
- 1 pair of sponge-holding forceps
- 2 rolls of sterile gauze (8–10 cm wide × 2 m long)
- sterile scissors
- Sims' or bivalve speculum
- sterile vulval pad.

The procedure is explained carefully, and the woman is asked to empty her bladder if possible. This is important because pressure from the pack will alter the position of the bladder neck and so may make voiding difficult afterwards. Adequate privacy is provided by screening and drapes. The patient is assisted into the left lateral or Sims' or dorsal position, whichever is more comfortable for her, while allowing sufficient access to and exposure of the area for the nurse or doctor. Good lighting is essential; a standard light is usually necessary.

The vulva is swabbed and the speculum inserted. Any clots in the vagina are removed with the sponge-holding forceps, and loose blood is mopped up with cotton-wool. The vagina is then packed firmly with the gauze, packing the posterior fornix first, then the anterior fornix, then the rest of the vagina. Remaining gauze is cut off with the sterile scissors. The vulval pad is applied, and held in place with a T-binder or stockingette. The amount of packing is recorded in the nursing notes, and a further note made when the packing is removed.

For aftercare treatment the woman is placed in a comfortable position and frequent observations of vaginal loss through the pack are made and recorded. Voiding must be observed; the usual nursing measures to assist voiding should be employed, but catheterisation may be necessary to empty the bladder and to maintain comfort.

Supporting pessaries

Sometimes when there is a contraindication or a disinclination to undergo surgery to repair a uterine displacement (see Chapter 18) the insertion of a supporting pessary will help to relieve symptoms. Modern pessaries are made of an inert, non-irritating material such as polythene, and therefore should not cause local reactions, as did the older pessaries. Once in position, the pessary cannot be felt (the upper vagina is insensitive), so the woman must be convinced of the necessity to return at least every six months for the doctor to check that no ulceration or necrosis of the vaginal walls has occurred.

The pessary is inserted following a careful vaginal examination. It is lubricated with water or water-soluble jelly, and is compressed between the fingers before being inserted and positioned, to rest first in the posterior vaginal fornix then in the anterior fornix. Several sizes may need to be tried before a suitable one is found. Sometimes the sight of the pessary may be frightening, as the following illustrates:

> On one occasion the seventeen-year-old granddaughter of a migrant woman was assisting by interpreting and translating for her grandmother. We showed her the ring pessary and explained how it worked

and how it would help to relieve the symptoms. She didn't hear us. All she could do was cry. 'Nobody is going to put something like that into my grandmother. It took us a long time to convince the girl of the benefits of this form of treatment. The old lady was lying on the couch with her eyes tightly shut through all of this. The proof came when we helped her to get down after the pessary had been inserted. Her face showed amazement and delight at the new feeling of freedom; freedom from the 'dragging' and 'falling out' sensations that she had experienced for many years. She kissed us all!

When a pessary is inserted, the doctor will usually explain how it works. If he doesn't, we can, by adapting our knowledge and terminology to the woman's understanding. A pessary does not cure the prolapse; it simply holds out the upper vaginal walls (Figure 9.4). This distending of the upper vagina means that the uterus cannot fall down (bringing the vaginal walls with it). Sometimes, because the pessary has stopped the continual strain on, and stretching of, the other uterine supports, these other supports regain some of their former tone.

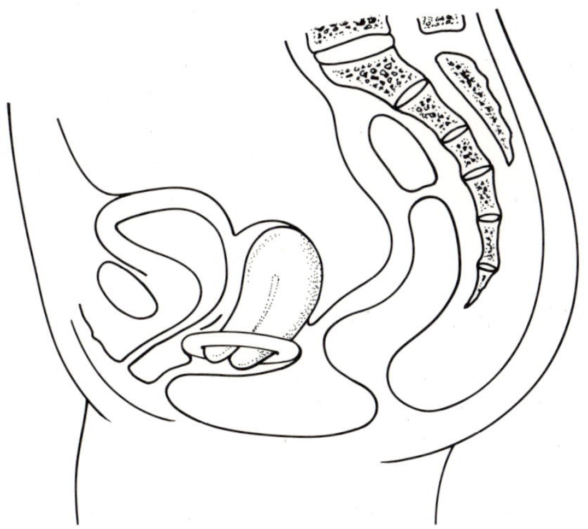

Figure 9.4
Supporting (ring) pessary in position

A few words of warning should be given to the woman before she goes home. She should come back to the doctor if she notices any discharge, bleeding or pain, or if the pessary slips, becomes noticeable or falls out. The problem may be a simple one—that the pessary was not quite the right size for her. But she should be seen, to make sure.

Investigations

Papanicolaou smear

The method of obtaining the smear has already been described, but a few words here about the preparation of the slides and their handling after use seem appropriate. The glass slides usually have a frosted strip at one end. On one side this strip has a rough texture; it is here that the necessary information for identification of the slide is written. The writing is done with a dark lead pencil, and while doing this we should be careful to handle the slide only by its edges or by its frosted end. The fixative solution should be prepared and the lid taken off the jar, so that as soon as the doctor has transferred the smear onto the slide, the slide can be put into the jar without delay. It is important that the surfaces of two slides in the jar do not come into contact with each other or the cells from one slide may adhere to the other, thus giving misleading results. A fixative spray is sometimes used (Figure 9.5).

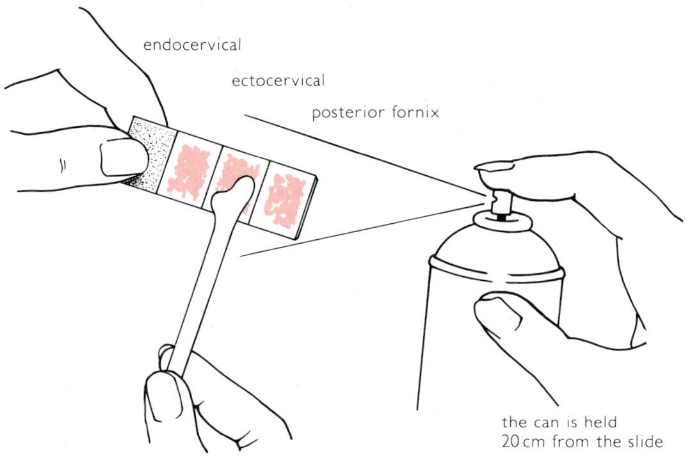

Figure 9.5
Spraying fixative onto the Papanicolaou smear slide

The woman may ask us when she will know if she is 'clear'. There is a different procedure adopted in each centre. If the policy of your particular centre is one of 'no news is good news', explain this to her. Emphasise that every result goes to the doctor before being filed away in her records. If the test was absolutely negative she will not hear about it, but she should still come back in a year's time for an examination, and possibly to have another smear done. However, she will hear very soon if there is any need to repeat the test, or if the results were not perfectly clear. 'This could be because the slide was contaminated or damaged or lost somewhere along the way, because the smear itself was insufficient in the number of cells on the slide, or for a variety of technical reasons. Of course, it *could* mean cancer so never delay coming for a repeat smear, but as you know there are these other reasons for having to have it repeated, don't be too worried at this stage.'

Colposcopy

This investigation (colposcopy: looking into the vagina) involves the use of a colposcope, an illuminated microscope designed specifically to examine the surface of the vaginal walls and cervix. It will magnify the area up to twenty times. It is often used when a smear test has shown suspicious or abnormal cells. It is also indicated for DES-exposed daughters.

The inspection is done slowly, with the woman in the lithotomy position, for quite a long time. If we are able to be with her, an understanding of her anxiety about the outcome of the investigation and of her embarrassment because of the prolonged exposure, must be shown.

The colposcope has given gynaecologists a great step ahead in the field of cervical and vaginal carcinoma investigation and treatment. It reveals if the tissues appear to be normal after all. It can indicate the exact sites for biopsy; random biopsy could miss the source of the 'suspicious' cells that showed in the smear. Colposcopy has in many cases reduced the necessity for the woman having to have a cone biopsy with its attendant dangers of infection, bleeding and cervical stenosis.

Culdoscopy

Culdoscopy is still performed in some centres, although the increasing use of laparoscopy has largely replaced it for diagnostic purposes (except where adhesions or infection are known or suspected). It enables a visualisation of the pelvic contents through an illuminated tube that has been passed into the uterorectal cul-de-sac (pouch of Douglas) from the posterior upper vaginal wall. The woman has to adopt the knee-chest position, which allows the abdominal contents to fall away and leave space in the pelvic cul-de-sac. The vagina must be meticulously prepared to prevent the introduction of organisms into the peritoneal cavity.

Culdoscopy is rarely done without some sort of anaesthesia; usually a general anaesthetic is given, and because of the position adopted, special attention to the maintenance of the airway is necessary. If a local or spinal anaesthetic is used the importance of the presence of the nurse as a supporter and friend need not be spelt out.

Posterior colpotomy

Posterior colpotomy involves entering the pouch of Douglas either by a small transverse incision or by the insertion of a needle, usually with the patient in the lithotomy position. The transverse incision is used to drain a pelvic abscess, the needle is used for diagnosis, especially to reveal blood in cases of tubal pregnancy.

Sterile vulval pads must be changed hourly after this procedure, and meticulous care must be taken in their handling and disposal.

Investigations for urinary symptoms

The 'mid-stream' specimen

Nurses early in their training are usually taught procedures for obtaining uncontaminated mid-stream specimens of urine, but they know that these specimens are not always easy to get. Sometimes it has to be remembered, that the outpatient, who has not 'submitted' herself in quite the same way that most inpatients can do, may find 'co-operating' to produce a specimen very difficult. If the procedure was requested straight after a pelvic examination, immediately before which she had emptied her bladder, there may be simply nothing to pass. She will then have to wait around, probably getting more anxious about her responsibilities at home or at work, and by the time there is some urine in the bladder, her mental state might not allow a proper relaxation of the right muscles and she might not be able to produce the specimen. Another factor that must be remembered is that an outpatient may have had to undress for an examination, then get dressed again, then get at least half-undressed once more to be swabbed down prior to the collection of the specimen. The inpatient, already in her nightgown, is saved all this. If the conventional methods of obtaining the specimen are not effective, the following may be worth some consideration:

After cleaning the vulva—the outer and inner labia, vestibule, and urethral orifice—with an appropriate agent (and also sealing off the vaginal orifice if necessary), the nurse will assist the woman to a commode chair, and will then cover her thighs with a small towel. With the usual catching receptacle removed, and when given the signal by the woman, the nurse, holding a bedpan or dish in one hand and the sterile receiver in the other, catches the first part of the stream in the pan or dish, then quickly slips the sterile receiver in to catch the 'mid-stream'. This system has one very great advantage; the sitting position is much more natural for voiding. It also has one disadvantage; not all commode chairs are built the same way. But if it can be done, and done carefully, the result will be what was ordered—an uncontaminated specimen of urine.

Micturating urethrocystogram

This investigation aims to demonstrate the efficiency (or otherwise) of the internal sphincter, and the angle of the posterior junction of the urethra and the bladder. The bladder is filled with a radio-opaque fluid and several X-ray photographs are taken with the bladder at rest, then while the woman is actually voiding, and then after she has voided.

Once again we have to remember how difficult it often is for any person to perform a private function like passing urine in front of other people. The procedure is not over quickly; even after it is all over she may have to stay until the films are checked before she can get dressed and leave. And her only preparation for the procedure may have been (from the doctor) 'I think we'll get an X-ray done on you'. If her only experience of X-rays is the routine chest X-ray, and for which she has only to take off her coat, why should she expect the undressing, the swabbing down, and everything else that is involved?

The woman must be given an explanation about this procedure. She should not be expected to go along without some idea in her mind of what it will entail. But that explanation should be given gently, and in the context of the contribution that this investigation will make in relation to the eventual relief from her particular symptom.

Ultrasound

Ultrasound is a method of visualising the interior of the body using high-frequency sound waves. It is a non-invasive method of diagnosing soft-tissue abnormalities, and is preferable to, and more informative than, X-rays, in most cases.

Ultrasound can show when ovulation is about to occur, the size and location of pregnancy sacs, pelvic tumours, fluid collections and other abnormalities in various parts of the body.

The woman having pelvic ultrasound investigation will be asked to drink a certain amount of water about one hour before the examination, and warned not to empty her bladder in that time. This is important because the bladder is used as a reference point and also elevates the uterus out of the pelvis.

Sound waves are directed from the machine through a microphone-type instrument towards the body. The sound waves bounce back to the microphone receiver and these echo patterns are translated into a picture.

Ultrasound is a simple and painless procedure, taking usually no more than twenty minutes.

Tubal patency tests

Hysterosalpingogram and tubal insufflation are procedures which are usually done at the outpatient level. These will both be discussed in the chapter on infertility for which condition they are most often performed.

Insertion of an intrauterine device

This procedure, along with other matter relating to contraception, is outlined in the chapter on family planning.

Part III
Diseases and disorders of the reproductive system

10 Intersex conditions

Sex determination

The genetic sex of an individual is determined at the time of conception. In the nucleus of each human cell are 46 chromosomes (arranged in 23 pairs), and this number (46) is retained in each new cell that is formed by cell division (mitosis).

Of the 46 chromosomes, 44 are called autosomes and are responsible for the characteristics of the person as whole; the hereditary physical and intellectual potential of the person is determined by these autosomes. (Greek: *soma*—the whole person.) The remaining two chromosomes are concerned with the sex of the individual. These sex chromosomes are not given a number but are called either X or Y. The female cells always contain two X chromosomes (XX) and the male cells contain one X and one Y chromosome (XY).

The division of the germ cells (the ovum and the spermatozoon) differs from mitosis, because when they ultimately conjoin to form a new combined cell or *zygote*, they bring only 23 chromosomes each. To achieve this, the germ cells undergo a form of reduction known as *meiosis* during the final maturation; half of the chromosomes (one from each pair) being retained and the other half becoming redundant. The ovum then will contribute one X chromosome at fertilisation. The sperm, however, will carry either an X or a Y chromosome, depending on which was retained at meiosis. If the sperm carries an X chromosome, its union with the ovum will produce a human cell containing 46 chromosomes—44 autosomic and two sex chromosomes, X plus X (46 XX)—a female zygote and a female individual. If the sperm contributes a Y chromosome, the result of the union will be 46 XY—a male zygote and a male individual (Figure 10.1).

The embryo develops initially as neuter or bipotential, with the rudimentary reproductive organs following the basic female pattern. It is the presence of the Y chromosome that stimulates the differentiation of the male gonads (testes) which produce androgens and thus cause the embryo to develop as a male. It is the absence of the Y chromosome which allows the female (XX) embryo to differentiate with female gonads (ovaries) and so develop along female lines.

As well as the genetic factors in the chromosomes, the final sexuality of the individual is dictated by four other contributing factors:

Gonadal sex: the development of the ovaries or testes in response to the absence or the presence of the Y chromosome.

External genital sex: the appearance of the external genital organs, stimulated by the presence of androgens.

Hormonal sex: the development, at puberty, of the secondary sex characteristics in response to hormone production by the differentiated gonads.

Psychological sex: this is usually developed in accordance with the obvious genital sex, but it is also greatly influenced by the social environment of the individual and by any close relationships which he or she may make with other people.

Figure 10.1
Sex determination at the time of conception

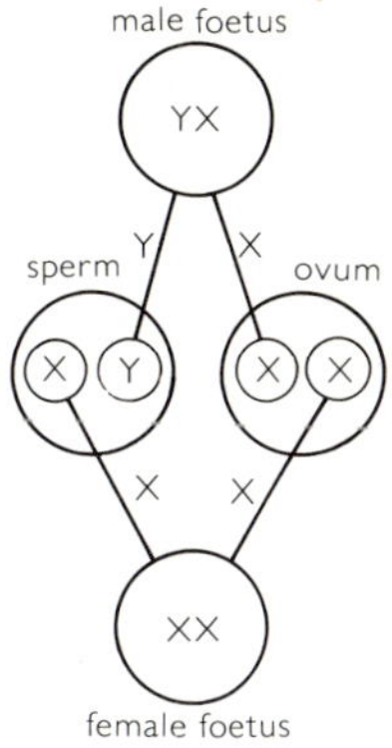

Conditions of intersex

Intersex may be defined as a condition in which there is imperfect or incomplete differentiation into male or female.

Hermaphrodites

The true hermaphrodite is a very rare being; one who possesses both ovarian and testicular tissues. The hormonal secretions of either may dominate, and so the external sexual characteristics may be either male or female. Individuals have been seen who produced normal, viable spermatozoa and also menstruated.

Pseudohermaphrodites are more common than true hermaphrodites. These people possess the gonads of one sex while exhibiting some of the external sexual characteristics of the opposite sex. Only the more common types of pseudohermaphrodite are mentioned here; a full discussion of the range of intersex conditions is provided in most of the books on gynaecology written for the medical profession.

Turner's syndrome

Turner's syndrome results from a chromosome deficiency which results in 45 chromosomes in a cell. The missing chromosome is a sex chromosome, either X or Y, and this leaves the cell chromosome make-up (or karyotype) as 45X0. As there is no Y chromosome, there is no male development, and the embryo will develop along female or neuter lines. At birth the infant will appear to be female, but as there is only one X chromosome the ovaries develop poorly ('streak' ovaries). Other common features of the syndrome include webbing of the neck and a short stature. The 'streak' ovaries do not function, neither ovulating nor producing the ovarian hormones (oestrogen and progesterone).

The first sign may be the failure of the girl to develop secondary sex characteristics at puberty (Figure 10.2). She may visit the doctor

Figure 10.2 (left) Turner's syndrome

Figure 10.3 (right) Klinefelter's syndrome

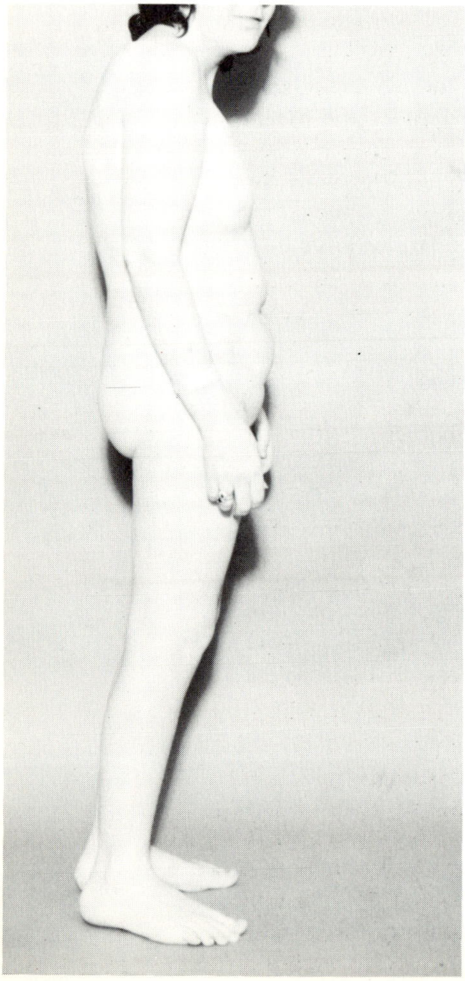

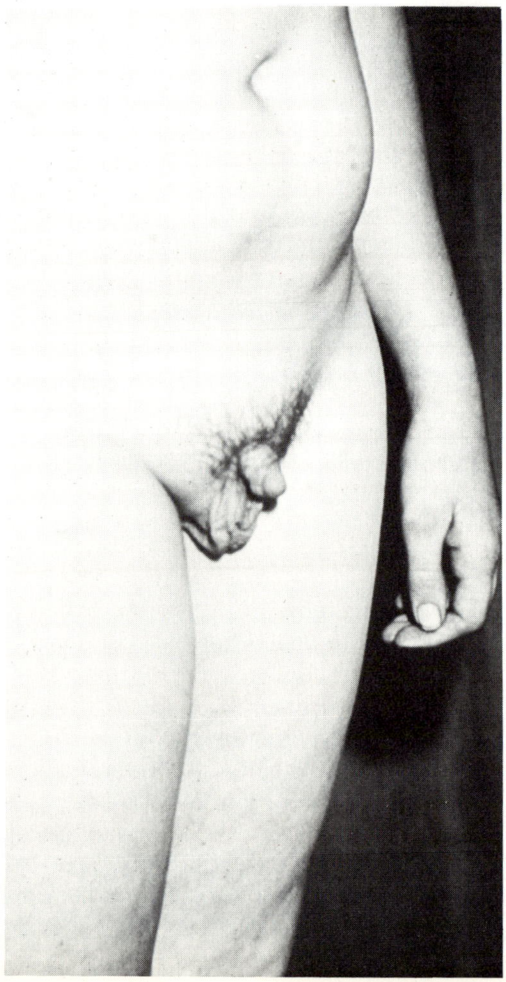

because of the absence of periods. The obvious lack of hormonal stimulation of the 'target' organs will lead the doctor to suspect an ovarian dysfunction.

The treatment of Turner's syndrome is usually based on the gradual introduction of oestrogen in tablet form, to allow development of the breasts, vagina and vulva. The uterus will be infantile, but under oestrogenic stimulation the endometrium can be built up. The management of the hormonal therapy needs to be under the careful supervision of an expert in this field. The treatment allows the woman to feel, and function as, a normal female except that she will be unable to produce her own children.

Klinefelter's syndrome

Klinefelter's syndrome is also a chromosome abnormality. In this condition there is an extra sex chromosome present (47XXY). The Y chromosome is present so there is some development of the male gonads, but the individual remains effeminate with a high voice, a clear skin and a tendency to obesity. The testes do not completely descend, and the external genitalia are small (Figure 10.3). Gynaecomastia (female-type breast development) may appear after puberty. There is a tendency for people with Klinefelter's syndrome to grow taller than average. Because of the limited development of the testes, sterility is a feature of this condition.

There is no specific treatment for this syndrome, but in selected cases testosterone replacement therapy may be helpful. Psychological support is indicated after the diagnosis has been made.

Adrenogenital syndrome

The adrenogenital syndrome results from an abnormality in foetal development, which leads to a basic absence of an enzyme essential for the synthesis of steroids in the adrenal cortex. Because of incomplete synthesis, intermediate products appear, and these are strongly androgenic.

In the female foetus, the androgens affect the external genitalia resulting in masculinisation; the labia fuse and the clitoris enlarges (Figure 10.4), thus resembling the male genitalia with hypospadias. A similar picture can result from the mother receiving hormonal treatment to prevent or arrest spontaneous abortion. These administered hormones have some androgenic activity.

After birth the female child undergoes an early physical and sexual development following the male pattern. The ovaries are present but do not function, and there is no menarche. The child is, in many cases, brought up as a boy and, if the condition is not discovered early, may be unable to adjust to living as a female.

In the male child, the excessive output of androgens can cause a great acceleration of physical and sexual growth and strength. The description 'Infant Hercules' has been used in reference to this syndrome.

Figure 10.4
Adrenogenital syndrome

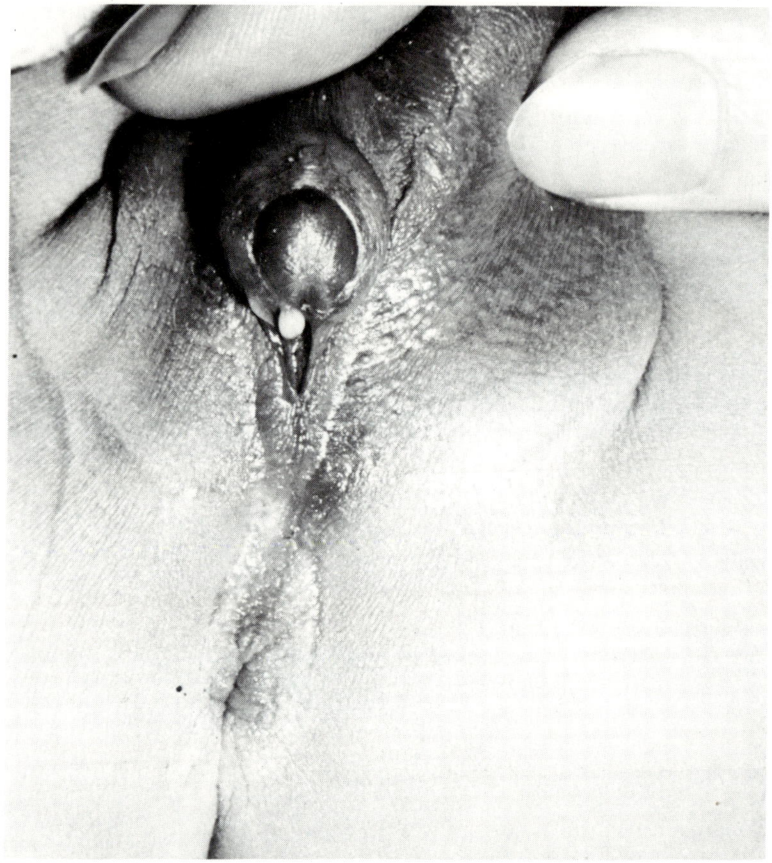

The treatment of the adrenogenital syndrome, if started early, can correct the condition. Corticosteroids are given to replace the deficiency. This treatment is continued for the rest of the person's life, but the doses are small and can be regulated by periodic assessment of the hormone breakdown products in the urine. The external genital abnormalities are corrected surgically; if possible this is done before the child starts school.

Feminism and virilism

Physical and behavioural traits which are inappropriate for the genetic or genital sex of the individual, and which do not come under the headings already discussed, are often described in medical works as 'feminism' (in a male) or 'virilism' (in a female). These states may begin before or after birth.

Feminism

The manifestations of feminism may include:

- often slight body build
- undescended testes, hypoplasia of penis
- development of breast tissue along female lines (gynaecomastia)
- smooth skin, weak hair growth
- high pitched voice
- behavioural patterns, preferences in lifestyle, dress and companions not in accordance with the usual or accepted male pattern.

The causes of feminism may include:

- *genetic:* masculine genes are present but weak
- *diseases or drugs:* affecting the hypothalamus, pituitary, adrenals, or testes
- *androgen deficiency*
- *psychological factors:* these are many and complex, but probably work through the hypothalamic-pituitary-sex hormone feedback system.

Virilism

Virilism in a female may be manifested by:

- heavy or stocky build and 'muscular' striding gait
- enlargement of the clitoris, male pubic hair pattern
- coarse skin, acne, hirsutism
- deeper than normal voice.

The causes of virilism may include:

- *genetic:* minor virilism may be an inherited trait
- *excessive androgens:*

  1 adrenal hyperplasia (Cushing's syndrome) which may be caused by (a) overstimulation of adrenal glands as a result of pituitary disorders, leading to overactivity of the adrenal cortices, or (b) benign or malignant growths of the adrenal glands

  2 ovarian malfunctions including the Stein-Leventhal syndrome (see page 99) and hormone-producing ovarian tumours

  3 androgen therapy

  4 in response to great stresses, eg burns
- *psychological:* as for the male.

It should be stated here that, as was described earlier in this chapter, a female is female because she is not a male. It is the relative lack of androgens which controls the obvious feminine characteristics. It is when the quantity of circulating androgens rises significantly above normal that the target tissues will respond more to androgens than to oestrogens.

11 Developmental disorders

Development of the reproductive system in the embryo

The gonads (ovaries or testes) develop initially as abdominal organs; the ovaries later descend towards the pelvis and the testes later descend through the inguinal ring to the scrotum.

The rest of the upper reproductive tract develops from a system of ducts, the *Wolffian* ducts and the *Mullerian* ducts. In the male, the Wolffian duct system grows and develops while the Mullerian system regresses. The opposite happens in the female (or in the absence of androgens). Vestigial remnants of the alternative duct system remain in both the male and female, and these are sometimes the site of cystic or other growths.

The urinary system is also developed from these ducts, and malformations of the upper genital tract are often associated with malformations of the renal tract.

The Mullerian ducts from which will be formed the upper female genital tract—the fallopian tubes, the uterus and most of the vaginal canal—grow from above downwards. Approximately half-way along their length they fuse together, then the fusion line is obliterated. The upper (separated) parts of the ducts will develop to become the fallopian tubes; from the point of fusion downwards, the uterus and vagina will form.

The lower part of the vagina is developed from the *urogenital sinus*, into which projects the fused Mullerian duct. The urogenital sinus has an external urogenital membrane that will become the hymen. The centre of this membrane normally breaks down while in the embryonic stage, thus allowing communication with the outside, while still affording some protection for the internal organs.

Disorders of development

Imperforate hymen

In this condition the hymen is completely blocking the vaginal orifice. It may not be noticed until puberty, when the girl is brought to the doctor because she has not begun to menstruate. There may have been other symptoms of menstruation present but no blood flow (cryptomenorrhoea). If the condition is not discovered early, the menstrual flow will accumulate, filling first the vagina (haematocolpos) and eventually the uterus (haematometra). Some of the fluid will be reabsorbed leaving a very thick, dark, bloody substance.

Treatment

The imperforate hymen is incised, usually with a cross-shaped cut, to allow the built-up menstrual flow to escape (Figure 11.1). Some doctors prefer to excise the membrane completely to allow better drainage. This procedure is done in hospital, usually under general anaesthetic, and the patient is kept in hospital until the resulting flow has stopped. Antibiotics are always prescribed because the bloody drainage is an ideal medium for the growth of infective organisms. Vulval washdowns using a mild antiseptic solution, eg chlorhexidine 1:5000, are performed four-hourly and are followed

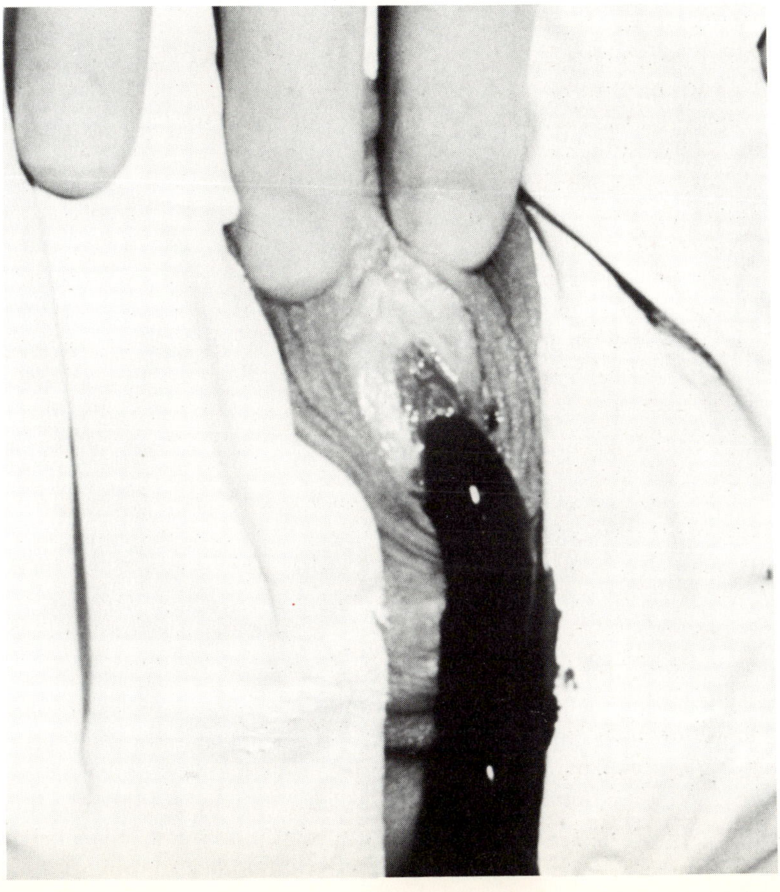

Figure 11.1
Release of menstrual blood following incision of imperforate hymen

by application of a sterile vulval pad. The patient should shower twice daily in preference to tub-bathing. Any procedures such as douching or pelvic examination, which might cause the drainage (or infection) to ascend higher in the genital tract, are avoided for some weeks.

The girl or woman who has this treatment for an imperforate hymen will be introduced to menstruation in a sudden and possibly unpleasant way. Our very special attention to her feelings during this experience is vital.

Malformations of the vagina

The vagina may be absent, hypoplastic, duplicated (Figure 11.2) or septate. Associated malformations of the uterus are sometimes, but not always, present. These conditions are caused by the failure of the lower parts of the Mullerian ducts to form or to fuse, or by the failure of the line of fusion to break down. Usually there is a small part of the lower vagina present; that part which has developed from the urogenital sinus.

Figure 11.2
Duplication of the vagina

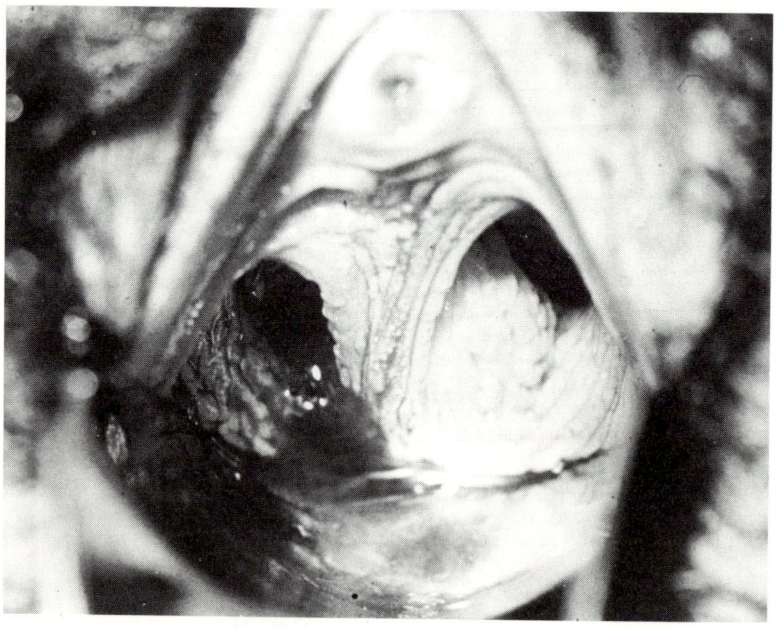

The presenting symptoms will vary according to the degree of malformation. Amenorrhoea will result from any obstruction to the blood flow as occurs when the vagina is absent or has a transverse septum, or when there is similar uterine or cervical maldevelopment. Vaginal malformations may also result in dyspareunia or apareunia. Infertility may be the complaint if intercourse has been occurring, but has taken place using the blind-ended side of a septate vagina. A septate vagina may also cause obstruction of the birth canal during labour.

Treatment

The treatment of vaginal malformations aims to create a functional vaginal canal as an outlet for the menstrual flow and to allow satisfactory sexual intercourse or to prevent difficulty during labour, as the case may be. If the vagina is absent or hypoplastic, an artificial vagina may be constructed using skin grafting followed by the regular and frequent insertion of vaginal dilators.

Malformations of the uterus

The uterus may be absent, hypoplastic or 'infantile', septate, single but with a depression of the fundus to give the appearance of two horns ie 'bicornuate', or completely duplicated. Some developmental disorders of the uterus and vagina are shown in Figures 11.3 and 11.4.

Amenorrhoea will result from absence or hypoplasia of the uterus.

Menorrhagia will often occur where there is an increased surface area of endometrium as in the septate, bicornuate or duplicated uterus.

Dysmenorrhoea may occur in these cases because the muscle fibres are not arranged in the usual pattern for efficient contraction and co-ordination.

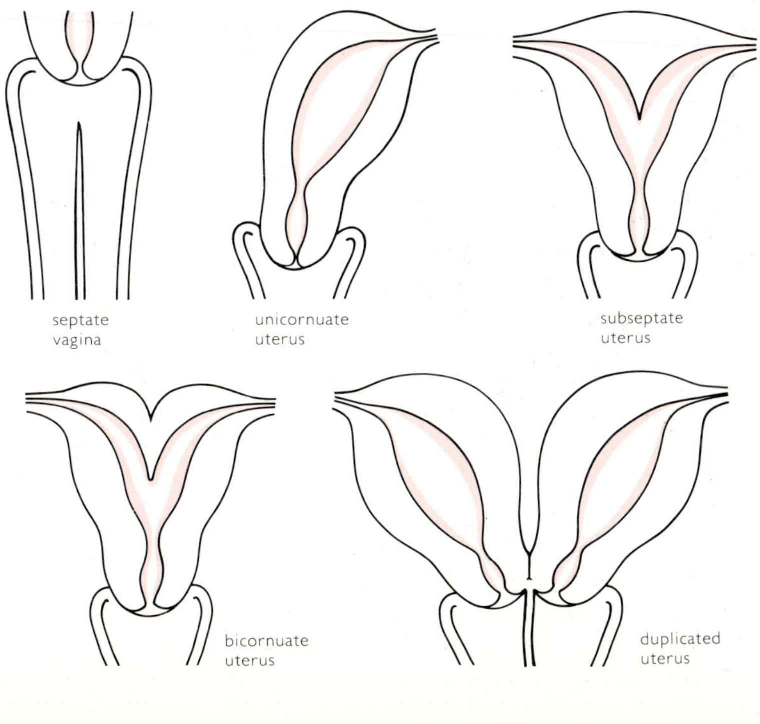

Figure 11.3
Developmental disorders of the uterus and vagina

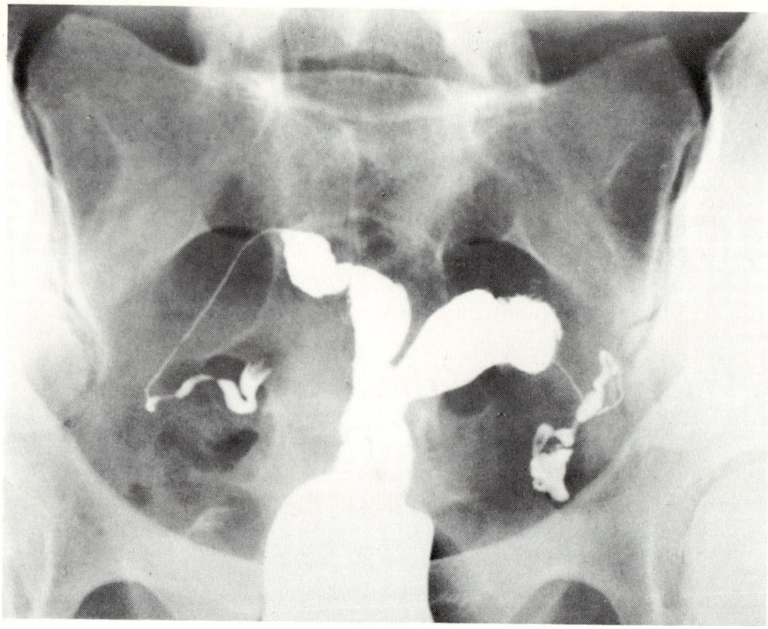

Figure 11.4 X-ray (hysterosalpingogram) showing duplication of the uterus (bicornuate)

Problems in labour may arise because of the abnormal muscle pattern or because the empty side of a bicornuate or duplicated uterus may cause a mechanical obstruction.

These conditions are treated, if possible, to prevent or relieve the symptoms they have caused. Any pregnancy following the surgical correction of a uterine malformation will probably be delivered by elective caesarean section, to prevent the possible rupture of the uterus during labour.

Malformations of the fallopian tubes

Absence of both of the tubes that convey ova from the ovaries to the uterus will, of course, result in infertility. If only one tube is absent and an ovum migrates across the peritoneal cavity, is fertilised and then enters the tube on the opposite side, the ovum may be ready to embed while still in the tube, and may thus become an ectopic pregnancy (see page 234).

Malformations of the ovaries

The ovaries develop separately from the rest of the reproductive system. The ovaries may be present and normal while the genital tract is absent or malformed. However, in the absence or maldevelopment of the ovaries, the genital tract will remain infantile because it is dependent upon the stimulation of the ovarian hormones to develop fully.

12 Disorders associated with menstruation

Menstruation has been defined as the periodic shedding of blood and the functional layer of endometrium from the non-pregnant uterus during the reproductive years. The menstrual loss should be moderate in amount, between 50–150 mL; it should not form into clots, and it should not cause too serious a disruption of normal activity.

The most common of the disorders associated with menstruation are:

- the absence of menstruation, ie amenorrhoea
- profuse or heavy loss with periods ie menorrhagia
- irregular or unusual bleeding, metrorrhagia
- painful periods, dysmenorrhoea
- the exaggeration of the general body changes which occur prior to menstruation, the premenstrual tension syndrome.

Amenorrhoea

Amenorrhoea may be defined simply as the absence of menstruation. For menstruation to occur and to be evident, there must be proper functioning of the hypothalamus, pituitary, ovary and endometrium, and there must be an escape route for the menstrual flow.

Amenorrhoea may be due to either physiological causes or to pathological disturbances of the normal menstrual functioning. As mentioned earlier (page 13), the psyche can also be an important influence. When the girl or woman has never menstruated, she is said to have primary amenorrhoea. Absence of menstruation after the menarche is termed secondary amenorrhoea, and is investigated usually when the woman has missed three cycles.

Physiological amenorrhoea

- primary before puberty
- secondary during pregnancy
  during lactation
  after the menopause

Pathological amenorrhoea

Causes of primary pathological amenorrhoea

At the hypothalamic or pituitary level: tumours or disturbances resulting in the non-release of FSH. General debilitating diseases and thyroid or adrenal disorders may affect the functioning of the pituitary gland.
At the ovarian level: absence of the ovaries or genetic faults resulting in the non-release of the ovarian hormones.
At the uterine level: absence or hypoplasia of the uterus, or an endometrium that does not respond to hormonal stimulation.
Obstructions to the outlet: absence or blockage of the vagina will prevent the escape of the menstrual flow (in the same way as an imperforate hymen).

Investigations

Investigations for the cause of primary amenorrhoea are not usually commenced until the girl has reached the age of eighteen years. They include:

- general physical examination with special observation of secondary sex characteristics, to assess whether development is present, ie evidence of oestrogen production
- gynaecological (pelvic) examination, to exclude obvious developmental defects such as imperforate hymen or absence of the vagina or uterus. Sometimes a rectal examination is performed in preference to a vaginal examination
- pregnancy (urine) test, to exclude pregnancy
- X-rays of the chest and skull, to exclude tuberculosis and pituitary growths
- retinal examination
- urinary glucose tests including glucose tolerance test
- blood tests—electrolytes, thyroid function tests
- chromosome analysis
- endometrial and vaginal smears, to see if these tissues have been influenced by oestrogen
- estimation of hormonal levels in urine excreted over a period of twenty-four hours
- laparoscopy or culdoscopy, to visualise the ovaries.

Treatment

The treatment of primary amenorrhoea will be directed towards the removal or correction of the cause. If no obvious cause is found the girl simply may be asked to wait longer for her periods to start. It would be explained to the girl (and to her mother) that although it is unusual for the menarche to be late, it is not unknown for it to occur at the age of nineteen or twenty in otherwise perfectly healthy girls, and that the condition itself is not harmful.

Appropriate advice about general health, diet and lifestyle is given as necessary. In some cases oestrogen therapy, given on a cyclic basis, is prescribed to stimulate endometrial growth and withdrawal bleeding, and to improve breast development. The oestrogen is introduced slowly, gradually increasing the dosage, otherwise nausea and soreness of the breasts might result. Hormones are only administered after thorough investigation of the condition, as they could mask the true cause of the amenorrhoea.

Causes of secondary pathological amenorrhoea

At the hypothalamic level resulting in the non-release of the releasing factors of the pituitary hormones:

- emotional stress or disturbances. An extreme desire for, or fear of, pregnancy, a change in environment or lifestyle, new responsibilities or loss of security, are all factors which may affect the functioning of the hypothalamus, but the woman may not be consciously aware of their effect. The absence of menstruation associated with the condition anorexia nervosa is probably due to the psychological factor as much as to the malnutrition
- tumours and diseases of the brain
- 'post-pill amenorrhoea': when there is continued suppression of the gonadotrophin releasing factors after their inhibition by the administration of oral contraceptives.

At the pituitary level resulting in the non-release of the gonadotrophins. Amenorrhoea caused by pituitary factors is often accompained by other signs of pituitary malfunctioning:

- tumours or disease of, or close to, the pituitary gland
- systemic diseases, especially those involving the thyroid or adrenal glands. Tuberculosis, diabetes, malnutrition, and almost any acute illness may upset the normal pituitary function
- excessive production of the pituitary hormone, prolactin. The amenorrhoea may be accompanied by milk formation in the breasts, the amenorrhoea-galactorrhoea syndrome. This condition is not fully understood; it may, in fact, be at the ovarian level that the excessive production of prolactin takes effect
- pituitary failure following great blood loss, eg post-partum haemorrhage (Sheehan's syndrome).

At the ovarian level resulting in the non-release of the ovarian hormones:

- removal of the ovaries
- irradiation of the pelvis, including the ovaries
- ovarian tumours
- polycystic ovaries, causing the Stein-Leventhal syndrome, in which the developing follicles do not mature enough to ovulate

but instead become cystic. This syndrome appears in the early reproductive years, between the ages of fifteen and thirty, and is associated with a higher than average production of androgens which may give rise to hirsutes
- chronic pelvic and ovarian inflammation.

At the uterine level resulting in the non-shedding of the endometrium:
- removal of the uterus
- damaged endometrium, following deep curettage (Asherman's syndrome) or radium therapy
- local infection—endometritis.

Obstructions to the outlet: cervical or vaginal stenosis, or adhesions following gross inflammation, burns, radiation or vaginal surgery.

Investigations

A careful physical examination is performed first, and a pregnancy test is done in every case. If there has been a recent episode of significant emotional stress, most doctors decide to wait one or two months before doing further investigations. These investigations are basically the same as those done for primary pathological amenorrhoea.

Treatment

If a definite cause is discovered, the treatment will be directed at that cause. The general health of the woman is assessed and steps taken to improve it if necessary.

Cyclical hormonal therapy (as with the contraceptive pill) or progestogen alone can be given to induce or test for withdrawal bleeding. If a pregnancy is desired, the administration of clomiphene citrate or gonadotrophins may induce ovulation (see page 245).

Scanty menstruation

Scanty menstruation or hypomenorrhoea refers to menstrual bleeding which is either short in duration (lasting less than two days) or small in amount. It may be normal for some women and in no way affect their reproductive functioning. In others it may be the result of hormonal or emotional disturbances similar to those causing amenorrhoea. Hypomenorrhoea could, in fact, lead on to amenorrhoea. Occasionally scanty menstruation is due to a decreased area of functional endometrium, eg following uterine surgery or deep curettage.

The investigations are the same as for amenorrhoea, and the treatment is that of the cause, if known. In other cases, explanation and reassurance that scanty menstruation is, in itself, not harmful, may be all that is required.

Menorrhagia

Menorrhagia is the term used to describe heavy or profuse menstrual bleeding; the flow usually occurs at normal intervals but is increased in amount or duration.

Polymenorrhoea refers to periods that are normal in amount but which occur too frequently, ie at intervals of less than twenty-one days. *Polymenorrhagia* refers to periods that are both heavy and frequent.

When a woman seeks medical help for excessive or abnormal periods, the doctor listens carefully to the words that she uses because, as mentioned in the chapter on the symptoms of gynaecology, there are several factors that may influence a woman's response to menstrual bleeding. The passage of clots is a significant sign; in this case, the menstrual flow must be well above normal if the usual anticlotting agents released by the endometrium are not able to cope with the volume or rate of blood flow.

Causes of menorrhagia

Hormonal imbalance

Any variation from the usual pattern of oestrogen and progesterone secretion could cause menorrhagia. The variation may be hypothalamic, pituitary or ovarian in origin. Emotional stress may be manifested by menorrhagia through hypothalamic influence in much the same way as it causes amenorrhoea. The pituitary gland, affected by pituitary, adrenal or thyroid disorders may respond by excessive secretion of gonadotrophins. Lesions of the ovaries such as cystic growths may disturb the normal output of the ovarian hormones, with the resultant effect of excessive endometrial growth.

Hormonal imbalance is especially likely to occur at the times of puberty and the climacteric. At these times, the ovarian follicles do not always mature sufficiently to result in ovulation, so the corpus luteum will not form, or if ovulation does occur the corpus luteum may not form properly. The result in either case will be a relative lack of progesterone. The action of oestrogen that is not balanced by adequate progesterone influence is likely to cause excessive proliferation of the endometrium as in endometrial hyperplasia.

Other causes

General body disorders, such as acute illnesses involving fevers, or blood diseases, eg thrombocytopenic purpura, leukaemia, pernicious anaemia. Anticoagulant therapy does not directly cause menorrhagia.

Other disorders causing menorrhagia are hypothyroid states and dietary deficiencies, fatigue, or emotional strain resulting in poor general health.

Uterine causes

Fibroids: the presence of fibroid growths in the uterus causes menorrhagia in two ways:

- by increasing the surface area of the endometrium; a larger surface is built up and the bleeding of this larger surface will result in a greater menstrual flow
- by restricting or interfering with effective uterine contractions, thus prolonging the menstrual flow.

Polyps increase the surface area of endometrium.

Infection: chronic low-grade endometritis, eg following miscarriage.

Adenomyosis interferes with uterine contraction.

Multiparity: after a number of pregnancies, significant amounts of the uterine muscle fibres may be replaced by fibrous tissue which will impede satisfactory contractions.

Developmental disorders which increase the endometrial surface area, eg bicornuate, septate or duplicated uterus; or which interfere with contractions, eg uterus unicollis with or without a rudimentary second horn.

Tumours and endometriosis causing an increased blood supply to the uterus.

Intrauterine contraceptive devices: for the first three months after insertion of one of these devices, menorrhagia is common and is probably due to irritation of the endometrium. In most cases this settles by itself without treatment, but in some cases it is necessary to remove the IUD.

Investigations

A thorough medical and pelvic (vaginal) examination is always done when a woman complains of menorrhagia. Some time is spent taking a history and special attention is given to any evidence of stress, worry or tension.

The pelvic examination will reveal any enlargement, irregularity and tenderness of the uterus or ovaries. If this examination shows no abnormalities, a provisional diagnosis of dysfunctional uterine bleeding is made.

Special investigations

These include:

- blood examination, for haemoglobin estimation and, if indicated, for white cell count and full blood examination
- examination under anaesthetic, followed by a diagnostic curettage, to show the endometrial response to hormones and to exclude carcinoma. The curettage may also reveal uterine polyps
- estimation of urinary gonadotrophins, oestrogens and progesterones as indications of hormonal activity.

Treatment of menorrhagia

If the blood loss is really heavy, bed rest is advised and sedation may be necessary. Anaemia is usually corrected with oral iron; at times, however, a blood transfusion may be necessary. Dilatation and curettage is often curative as well as diagnostic but many doctors prefer to wait until severe bleeding has passed before doing a curettage.

Hormone therapy is used to control heavy bleeding. Large doses of oestrogen will raise the level of this hormone to above the bleeding threshold and so will stop the bleeding temporarily. They will, however, cause further proliferation of the endometrium and so are only used as a first-aid measure. Following the control of a serious bleeding episode, treatment is aimed at restoring a balanced ratio of oestrogen and progesterone either by the administration of progestogens (in the case of unopposed oestrogen secretion) or by the suppression of ovarian hormone production using one of the combined or sequential types of oral contraceptive pills.

A hysterectomy is performed in those cases where hormone therapy is unsuitable or unsuccessful, or where large fibroids or endometriosis are present. If more children are desired, *myomectomy* will remove fibroids and still conserve the uterus for childbearing.

Careful attention to diet and lifestyle should be shown. The importance of sufficient rest must be emphasised, even to the extent of sitting down with the woman to write a list of her usual day's activities and so help her plan an alternative that allows time for physical and mental relaxation.

Metrorrhagia

Metrorrhagia refers to irregular or unusual bleeding from the vagina, occurring at times other than menstruation. It is a symptom never to be ignored; the discovery of abnormal vaginal blood loss must always be investigated.

Causes

- at ovulation, 'spotting' may occur. The loss is usually very small and is probably due to the slight drop in oestrogen level that occurs just prior to the formation of the corpus luteum
- cervical inflammation, erosion, polyps or carcinoma may cause slight bleeding, especially after intercourse or vaginal examination
- vaginal inflammation, ulceration and atrophy
- endometrial carcinoma
- complications of early pregnancy (see Part V)
- confusion with rectal bleeding from haemorrhoids.

Investigations

A careful visual examination of the vagina and cervix is done. A colposcopy may be indicated. A Papanicolaou smear is always taken. A dilatation and curettage is often performed and the endometrium examined for suspicious changes.

The woman may be asked to begin a chart of any bleeding and to see the doctor next time she has a bleeding episode.

Treatment

No treatment is begun until cervical and endometrial malignancy has been excluded; apart from the 'twisting-off' of any obvious cervical polyps.

If infection of the cervix or vagina is present, it is treated (as described in Chapter 13). Any malignant changes are treated by surgery or radiotherapy, according to the stage or spread of the growth.

Ovulation 'spotting' is managed by the administration of small quantities of oestrogen, just sufficient to keep the oestrogen levels above the bleeding threshold. The oestrogen is taken for six or seven days, beginning three or four days before the expected ovulation. This treatment is only given after all other causes have been excluded.

Dysmenorrhoea

Dysmenorrhoea is excessive pain associated with menstruation. There are very few women who do not experience some discomfort at the time of menstruation and the reaction to this discomfort depends on a great variety of factors. If the pain is severe enough to interfere with the woman's usual daily activity, especially when she wants to get on with it, her symptoms must not be ignored. There are two types of dysmenorrhoea: primary (spasmodic), in which the pain is due to menstruation itself, and secondary (congestive), in which there is usually associated organic pelvic disease. Figure 12.1 shows the different sides of pain in primary and secondary dysmenorrhoea.

Primary dysmenorrhoea

Primary dysmenorrhoea affects mainly girls in their mid to late teens and may persist until the late twenties after which it usually disappears. It only occurs after ovulation has been established, and so may come as a shock to a young girl who has experienced the relatively pain-free menstruation of anovulatory cycles for a while following the menarche. The pain does not arise until within twenty-four hours before the flow starts, after which severe colicky

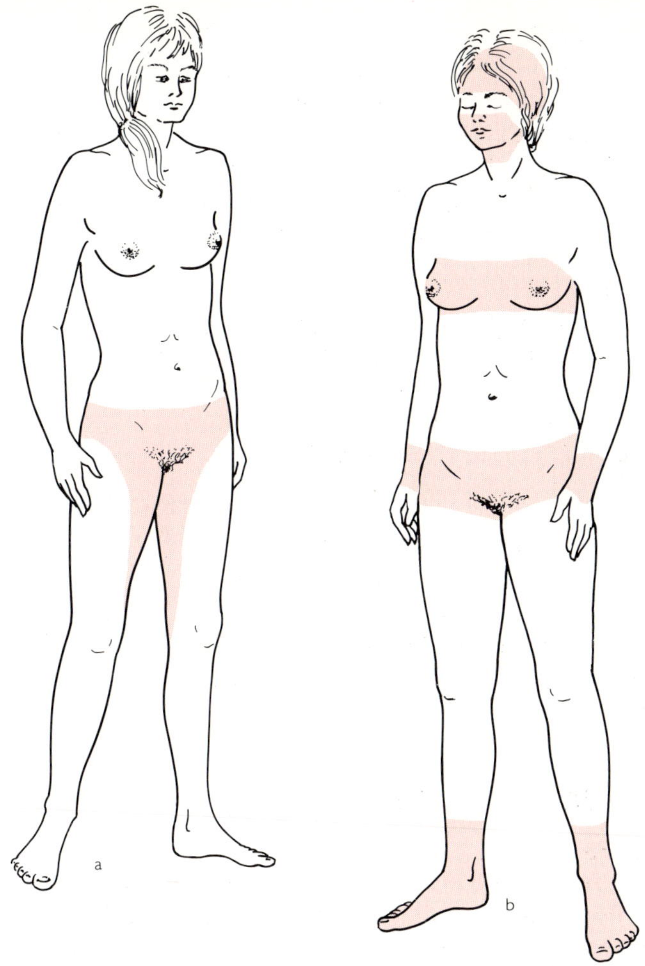

Figure 12.1
Sites of local and referred pain in (a) primary and (b) secondary dysmenorrhoea

pain is felt centrally in the lower abdomen and back. The pain is worst in the first twelve hours after the onset of the period, then it usually eases up and is generally quite bearable for the remainder of the flow. Nausea and diarrhoea may accompany the acute phase and there is often a drawn, tense facial expression.

Causes

General factors associated with primary dysmenorrhoea include a faulty attitude to menstruation and sexual matters, environmental and parental pressures and general ill-health. Specific causes include:

- the presence then withdrawal (as the corpus luteum degenerates) of significant levels of *progesterone*. The arterioles supplying the muscle layer of the uterus go into spasm and the ischaemia of the muscle produces a pain similar to angina
- progesterone is also believed to stimulate the production of

prostaglandins, which are found in high concentrations in the uterus. These substances are released just before and during menstruation and their function is to stimulate contractions and clear the uterus of blood and debris. They probably contribute to the associated symptoms, eg nausea, headache, fainting episodes and bowel and bladder irritability
- muscular inco-ordination—if there is improper functioning of the autonomic nervous system, spasm of muscles of the uterine isthmus and internal cervical os will arise. Developmental disorders will also cause muscle inco-ordination
- rarely, obstruction to the flow, because of an extremely narrow cervical canal or due to a clot lodged in the cervix, may cause dysmenorrhoea.

Investigations

The diagnosis is usually made after a full interview and a rectal or vaginal examination. The doctor will be careful to exclude organic disease and endometriosis. If the patient is a young girl and is accompanied by her mother, most doctors prefer to interview the mother and the daughter separately, and then together, so that an assessment of family attitudes to the subject can be made.

Treatment

Explanation and education about normal menstrual function is of great importance. If fear through ignorance is present, any pain will be exaggerated. Attitudes can be examined and old wives' tales dispelled.

During the acute phase, the pain is helped by rest with warmth to the lower abdomen and the administration of suitable non-habit forming analgesics.

Aspirin has an anti-prostaglandin effect and is a good analgesic for dysmenorrhoea. Ponstan (menefenaemic acid) tablets can also be very effective. In most cases, the period of rest should not be allowed to extend for too long or else the dysmenorrhoea may become a very good excuse for avoiding work or school. Multi-vitamin/calcium tablets taken in the week before menstruation have proved useful.

Exercise and the avoidance of constipation, coupled with prevention of worry and tension, are important at this time. Some doctors recommend a series of special exercises designed to aid in stretching the ligaments and relieving menstrual pain.

Antispasmodic drugs, such as hyoscine butylbromide, are often of use in reducing colicky contractions.

The suppression of ovulation by the administration of the contraceptive pill for six months will usually effectively relieve the dysmenorrhoea. When the course of treatment is completed the ovulatory cycles return, the periods are often less painful. As it is not always wise to give oestrogen to a young girl whose skeletal growth may not be completed, progestogens alone may be prescribed. The progestogens, taken from day 5 to day 25 of the cycle, will act to relax spasm of the arterioles in the myometrium without inhibiting ovulation, which makes it useful for those women who desire pregnancy but who suffer from spasmodic dysmenorrhoea.

Dilatation of the cervix to relieve cervical spasm and obstruction is done less frequently nowadays.

Pregnancy and the vaginal delivery of a baby almost always cause a great improvement and in most cases effect a cure of primary dysmenorrhoea.

Secondary dysmenorrhoea

Secondary dysmenorrhoea presents later in life, usually not beginning until after the mid-twenties. It presents as a 'dragging' pain in the lower abdomen, back and thighs, for some days prior to the onset of the flow and it may continue throughout the period, easing only at the end of the flow.

Causes

- pelvic inflammation
- endometriosis
- retroversion of the uterus
- 'pelvic congestion', in which there is an increased blood supply to the uterus. This type of dysmenorrhoea is often accompanied by menorrhagia, and psychological factors such as anxiety or depression may be present

Investigations

A detailed history is obtained, followed by a thorough physical examination. Special attention is paid to the coexistence of any other gynaecological symptoms, especially menorrhagia, dyspareunia, pruritus or premenstrual tension. A uterine curettage may be indicated. Laparoscopy may be performed in cases of suspected endometriosis or pelvic inflammation.

Treatment

As for primary dysmenorrhoea; rest, warmth, regular simple analgesics, attention to diet and exercise and the avoidance of constipation are all of benefit.

Psychological assessment and exploration of the woman's feelings about menstruation, sex and having children may be a necessary step before instituting further treatment.

The investigation and treatment of underlying causes such as endometriosis, pelvic inflammatory states, cervical stenosis and uterine displacement are discussed in the appropriate chapters.

Premenstrual tension syndrome

'Premenstrual tension' refers to a collection of symptoms occurring any time during the latter half of the menstrual cycle and in which there is an exaggeration of the normal physiological changes due to the presence of oestrogen and progesterone together in the circulation. The symptoms almost always subside at the onset of menstruation. The syndrome appears to be more common in women over the age of thirty years, and is often more marked in those who know that they have several more years of childbearing ability left, yet have as many children as they feel that they can mentally cope with or physically manage.

The features of this syndrome include:

- emotional instability, depression, headaches (often severe—menstrual migraine)
- constipation
- abdominal swelling and discomfort
- oedema of hands and feet
- breast sensitivity and enlargement.

In many cases of premenstrual tension the woman is aware of the changes that are happening but is unable to control her mental and nervous responses. Various studies have related the highest incidence of crime, suicides, and accidents caused by women to the times of their premenstrual phase. Simpler events like breaking dishes and general clumsiness are apparent to most people.

Causes

The exact cause is unknown, but the symptoms are thought to be due to either a hypersensitivity to oestrogen or to an abnormally high ratio of oestrogen to progesterone in the latter half of the menstrual cycle. The oestrogen dominance leads to sodium and water retention in the tissues, and the symptoms are all due to the oedema. Women who are of an anxious or unstable temperament are certainly prone to suffer from this syndrome, but in many well-adjusted, stable women, the symptoms appear with just as much force; so the syndrome should never be the reason for labelling a woman as neurotic.

Treatment

After taking a detailed history and conducting a pelvic examination to rule out any coexisting gynaecological problems, the doctor's first task is to explain how retention of fluid, caused by oestrogen, can give rise to the symptoms, emphasising the part that cerebral oedema plays in the manifestation of the nervous symptoms. Such an explanation is of tremendous help to the woman who is bewildered by herself, and her actions, and often this knowledge is sufficient for her to modify her social and intellectual activity during

days of cycle	month 1	2	3	4	5	6
1						
2						
3						
4						
5						
6						
7						
8						
9						
10						
11						
12						
13						
14						
15						
16						
17						
18						
19						
20						
21						
22						
23						
24						
25						
26						
27						
28						
29						
30						
31						
32						
33						
34						
total						

Figure 12.2
A menstrual chart for recording physical and emotional events in relation to the menstrual cycle. This can help a woman to plan her life so that it is not dominated by her cycle

Menstrual chart
Fill in this chart using the following codes. You may become aware that recurring physical states are connected with your menstrual cycle.

Code	
p	period
hp	heavy period
lp	light period
h	headache
m	migraine headaches
l	lethargy, loss of energy
w	water retention
b	backache
in	insomnia, difficulty sleeping
br	sore breasts
g	gain in weight
fc	food cravings (usually sweet)
c	constipation
cr	cramps
fl	flatulence, passing wind
dia	diarrhoea
sp	skin problems
ir	irritable
a	angry
d	depressed
s	sad
v	vulnerable
t	tearful
u/s+	unsociable/sociable
ta	tense and anxious
f	forgetful
dc	difficulty concentrating
cl	clumsy
p−/p+	less productive/more productive
cr	creative
e	energetic
sx	interested in sex, aroused
ha	happy

Note: Day 1 on this chart is the first day of bleeding, continue down the column until you get your next period, then start the second column etc.

those days. She may find it useful to keep a menstrual chart like that shown in Figure 12.2. This, along with limiting her fluid intake and the avoidance of extra salt and salty foods, should bring the effects of the syndrome to a more manageable state.

Exercise is extremely good therapy for the woman with PMT. Deliberate, relaxing, body movement (eg swimming breaststroke) will aid the whole vascular system by feeding oxygenated blood to the whole body, and thus will promote a feeling of well-being.

Eating wisely is also very important. The blood-sugar level should not become too low. Proteins and complex carbohydrates will provide blood sugar levels that remain sufficient for proper functioning from one meal to the next. Meals should not be skipped or headaches and irritability can result. Vitamin supplements may be of benefit, especially Vitamin B6, when taken during the second half of the cycle.

Diuretics are often of value where the above measures are insufficient. They are taken for the last ten days of each cycle or, preferably, commenced the day before the symptoms are likely to arise. If the cycle is irregular, knowledge of a method of determining the day of ovulation, such as by examination of the cervical mucus (see Chapter 22) will be of great help to the woman by giving her a date to calculate from. Where diuretics are used, the woman should be aware of the need to replace possible potassium loss. It is a good idea to specify the taking of a glass of orange juice or the eating of a banana with each diuretic tablet taken. Some women have found that half of the usual dose taken twice daily achieves a better management of their symptoms.

Sedatives or mild tranquilisers in small doses may be necessary in some women. They are usually prescribed for the latter half of the cycle.

Hormonal therapy is usually only given if the above measures are *not* successful, and consists of progestogens, eg duphaston, given from day 18 to day 25, to balance the dominant oestrogen. Progestogens may be taken orally or in suppository form. Some doctors prescribe bromocryptine. An alternative method is to temporarily suppress ovulation using oral contraceptive pills, as premenstrual tension is normally limited to ovulatory cycles.

Many doctors feel it well worthwhile arranging for the woman's partner to be present while the causes and management of the premenstrual tension syndrome are explained. It is far from easy for a woman to adapt her lifestyle and activity during the more difficult days without her partner's full understanding, co-operation and help.

13 Pelvic infections, sexually transmitted diseases

Natural defences against infection

Because there is a continuous open pathway allowing ascent of infection (via the vagina, uterus and fallopian tubes) from outside the body through to the peritoneal cavity, a natural system of defences against infection is necessary (Figure 13.1).

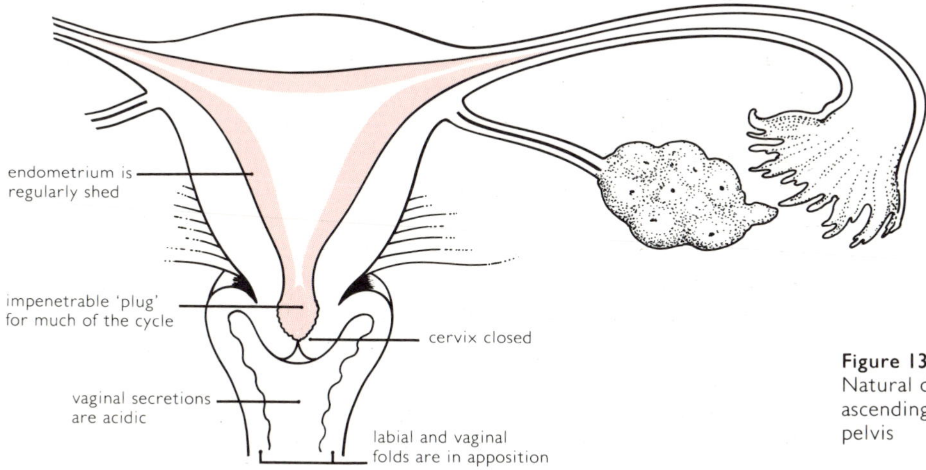

Figure 13.1
Natural defences against ascending infection in the pelvis

The *vulva* is arranged so that the labia are normally in contact, closing off the entrance to the vagina. In addition, the secretion of the apocrine glands is believed to act chemically against fungal organisms.

The *vagina* has an unbroken surface, without any glands opening on to it. The vaginal moisture is normally acid and the vaginal walls are in apposition.

The *cervical secretions*, for a large part of each menstrual cycle and for the whole duration of a pregnancy, form a plug of mucus that blocks off the entrance to the uterus.

The *uterus* regularly sheds its lining and, presumably, with it, many of the organisms which might have ascended from the lower genital tract. Thus they are unable to gain a hold for long in the uterus.

Weakening of the natural defences

These defence mechanisms may be affected or upset by a variety of factors.

Vulval closure is often less efficient after childbirth.

Before the onset of puberty and after the climacteric, when there is very little circulating oestrogen, the vaginal secretions are not acidic. Also the regular shedding of the endometrium is not occurring at these times in life.

Although menstruation is itself regarded as one of the natural defences, the absence of the cervical mucoid plug and the presence of blood may favour the establishment and ascent of vaginal infections during menstruation. For this reason, some doctors advise that women wear a diaphragm for intercourse at this time.

Following labour or abortion there is often a lowered general resistance to infection because of blood loss and weariness. At these times, infection can gain a hold in the uterus and quickly travel into the bloodstream because of the raw placental site. Retained products of conception provide an ideal breeding ground for organisms. The cervix and vagina may be lacerated or bruised. There is also the possibility of the introduction of infective organisms during procedures such as vaginal examination.

The excretory outlets of the bladder and bowel are very close to the vaginal entrance. Unless careful attention is given to the wiping of the vulval region, from the front towards the back, bowel organisms can be brought forward and, at times of lowered resistance, be a very real problem. This method of wiping is one that has to be learned; it does not usually come naturally. (An opportunity to teach this point may arise when demonstrating the correct way to apply or remove a vulval pad—'from front to back, you know, just as you wipe after using the toilet. That way means there's no chance of bringing any infection forward.')

Other points relating to genital or sexual hygiene should be mentioned whenever possible; very often our own embarrassment stops us from giving a small piece of information that might make a great difference to a woman's comfort, happiness and gynaecological health.

Vulvitis

Acute vulvitis

Acute vulvitis is often associated with vaginitis—vulvovaginitis—but sometimes it occurs without vaginal inflammation. In acute vulvitis the vulva is swollen, red and very uncomfortable, with pruritus and burning. If it is not cleared quickly secondary infection may occur.

Causes

- vaginal discharges, which may irritate the sensitive skin
- urine left on the skin. This may be seen when a woman who suffers from urinary incontinence wears protective pads held in by a waterproof garment of some sort. Plastic, nylon and other synthetics can create a 'hot-house' atmosphere which may worsen the problem
- chemical irritants can cause inflammatory reactions if the skin is unusually sensitive or if the woman is allergic to particular substances. Soaps, detergents, some talcum powders, coloured toilet papers, contraceptive creams and appliances, douching solutions and deodorants applied to the vulva have all been blamed for local reactions. Drugs which cause generalised skin erruptions often cause vulvitis as well
- diabetes—a higher than normal sugar content in both the urine and the vaginal secretions favours the growth of *Candida albicans*
- friction—tight underclothing or sanitary pads may abrade the skin, opening the way for infection. Friction may also occur during intercourse when there has been inadequate lubrication or stimulation
- poor hygiene—lack of regular washing may result in the collection of irritating discharge between the folds of the vulva. Incorrect wiping of the anus and perineum may bring bowel organisms forward

Treatment of acute vulvitis

The vulva is examined carefully under a good light. Swabs of any discharge are collected for culture and antibiotic sensitivity testing. A thorough history is taken and matters involving hygiene, underclothing and possible causes or allergy are discussed. The urine is tested for sugar and, if indicated, arrangements will be made for a glucose tolerance test.

Specific treatment will be instituted after the cause has been found; in the meantime, soothing lotions and ointments, especially those with an anti-inflammatory and anti-allergic action, will be used. The management of any associated pruritus is discussed on page 139.

Specific vulval infections

Folliculitis and furunculosis

Folliculitis occurs when staphylococcal organisms infect the openings of the hair follicles of the mons and labia. The small abscesses are very painful and the condition is hard to clear.

Furunculosis is a deeper extension of folliculitis, resulting in a large, extremely painful pus-filled swelling.

Treatment

Attention to vulval hygiene and careful education of the patient is of great importance. Exposure to air and also to ultraviolet light is helpful. The area should be washed with antiseptic soap, followed by the application of a weak anti-infective lotion such as chlorhexidine. Any infected hairs are removed. Antibiotics are usually given systemically, and suitable analgesics are necessary until the antibiotic therapy has controlled the condition.

Bartholinitis

Inflammation of the Bartholin's glands may be due to infection by staphylococci, streptococci, *E coli*, gonococci and other organisms. Acute bartholinitis, presenting as a very painful red swelling on the labia, is treated with antibiotics, analgesics and rest. A swab is taken to exclude gonorrhoea. If there is abscess formation the abscess is drained rather than allowing it to burst, but a better method of treatment is *marsupialisation*—the formation of the gland into a pouch which opens into the vaginal entrance.

Bartholin's cyst (Figure 13.2) may occur when the duct of the gland has become fibrosed from chronic or repeated infection, or when it has been damaged by an episiotomy or perineal repair. With the gland unable to drain, cystic formation occurs, with loss of function of the gland. This condition is treated by marsupialisation (Figure 13.3) or by excision of the whole gland.

Figure 13.2
Bartholin's cyst

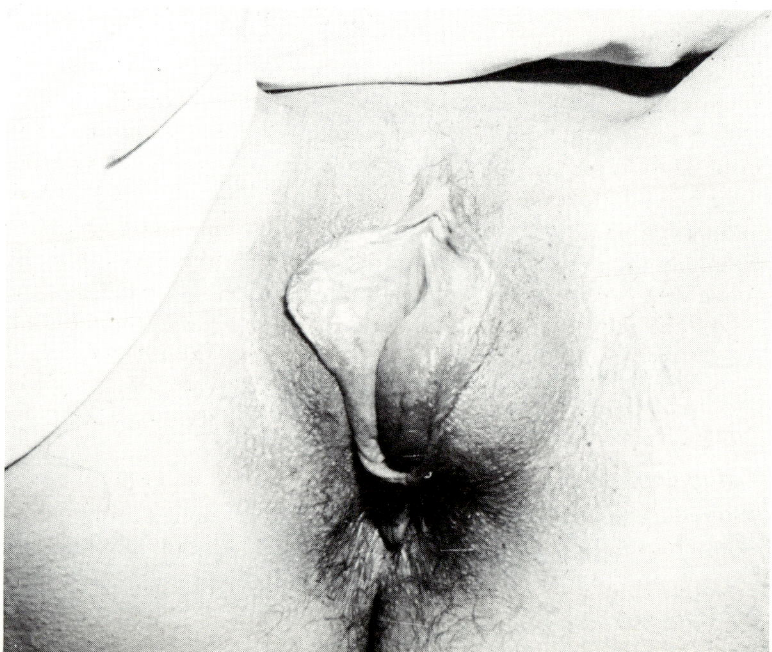

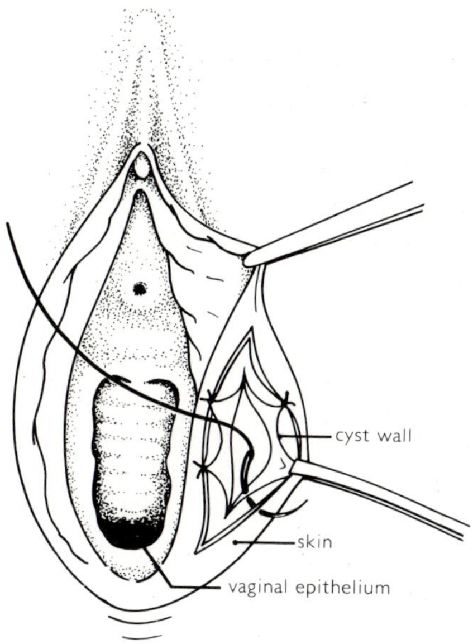

Figure 13.3
Marsupialisation of Bartholin's cyst

Pediculosis pubis

These tiny mites may infest the pubic region and cause intense irritation and scratching. The mites can be seen as small (1 mm) insects crawling around in the pubic and perianal hair. They are white when hungry and red-black after they have bitten. The scalp and axillary hair may also be infested and so these areas should be examined when the mites have been found in the pubic region.

Treatment

The pubic area is shaved and a specific lotion, usually benzyl benzoate, is applied, immediately after a hot bath. (The bath will open up the burrows.) Benzyl benzoate should never be applied directly after shaving as it would then cause intense irritation and burning. In some cases, a 1 per cent malathion shampoo lotion followed by careful combing with a fine-toothed metal comb will be just as effective.

Instruction in maintaining good hygiene and preventing spread of the condition is an important part of the treatment. Some clinics recommend that all clothing and bed-linen be disinfected by boiling or dry-cleaning. Mattresses should be aired in sunlight for a full day, and not used for at least a week afterwards.

Sexual contacts should be followed up and treated as well.

Venereal warts

Condylomata acuminata are caused by a papilloma virus, and are spread both venereally and by self-inoculation. These cauliflower-like warts proliferate easily around the vulva and the perianal area.

Bleeding and discomfort may occur on defaecation. Podophyllin paint is applied to the warts every two to four days until the condition has cleared. Diathermy and cryosurgery are also effective and are used in some centres, and liquid nitrogen has proved most useful as an office procedure. Diathermy or cryosurgery under general anaesthetic is usually recommended where there are more than ten warts. Sexual contacts will also need treatment.

Chronic vulvitis

Acute vulvitis, if not cleared by treatment or if prolonged by scratching, may develop into a chronic state. In a number of cases, the woman will have tried self-medication for a long time, perhaps to avoid the embarrassment and shame of having to say that she has been scratching that area. Senile (atrophic) vulvitis commonly arises after the menopause when the normal resistance provided by the ovarian hormone activity is lowered. There is usually a slight yellowish vaginal discharge which is very irritating to the vulval tissues.

Pruritus is the main symptom of chronic vulvitis. If the condition is not treated, hypertrophy of the surface epithelium may occur, as the body attempts to replace the damaged cells quickly. Areas of the vulva become thick and keratinised, and are whiter than the surrounding tissues. These areas are collectively termed chronic epithelial dystrophies (formerly termed leukoplakia: the term leukoplakia is now restricted to one specific condition). They are always examined closely, and a smear or scraping taken for cytological examination, as squamous cell carcinoma of the vulva is preceded by one of the chronic epithelial dystrophies in about 50 per cent of cases. (See Figure 13.4.)

Treatment of chronic vulvitis

Local or general causes are excluded or treated. In senile vaginitis, oestrogen creams and vaginal pessaries, or systemic oestrogen therapy in suitable cases, will restore the normal tissue resistance to infection. They are very effective in controlling the condition, after which they are gradually withdrawn. If leukoplakia is present a simple vulvectomy *may* be performed; if malignant cells are discovered, the vulvectomy is radical, involving a wide excision of skin and lymph nodes.

Vaginitis

Inflammation of the vagina may occur at any age and be due to a number of causes, but the pH of the vagina is the regulating factor. In an acid environment the growth of many organisms is inhibited. If the pH balance is disturbed, infecting organisms may multiply rapidly. There are various causes of vaginitis and it is not uncommon for more than one to be present at one time.

Oestrogen deficiency vaginitis

In childhood, before oestrogen stimulation has caused the formation of an acid vaginal fluid, vaginitis may occur with discomfort and an irritating, perhaps burning discharge. It is usually associated with poor hygiene but occasionally is caused by self-exploration or the insertion of foreign bodies. An examination under anaesthetic may be necessary to exclude the presence of foreign bodies.

If no previous specific cause is found, education in full personal hygiene may be all that is necessary. As well as special attention to the washing and drying of the vulva, handwashing and the provision of separate towels for each member of the family should be emphasised. Relief of the associated pruritus is described on page 136.

After the menopause, the vaginal epithelium becomes thin and dry and, as it is no longer protected by the acidic vaginal secretions, organisms may grow and cause inflammation and discharge—senile

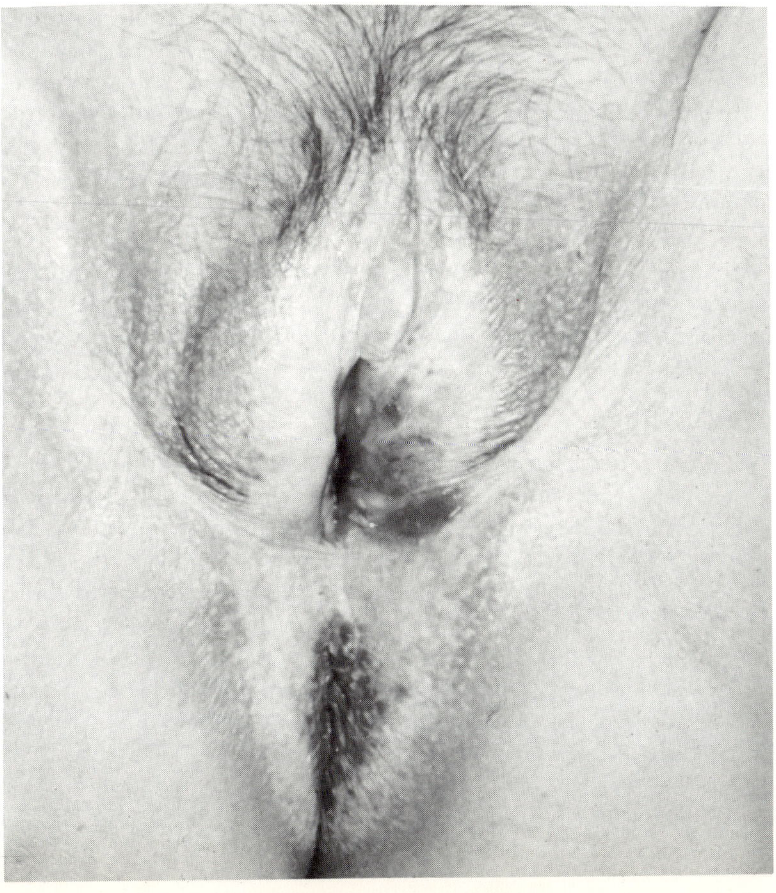

Figure 13.4
White areas of the vulva (leukoplakia): vulval dystrophy. The woman (aged 84) had suffered from pruritus for 20 years

vaginitis. The vaginal walls are red and sore, and may bleed easily. If not treated, the infection may ascend to cause endometritis. Senile vulvitis is commonly present as well, with pruritus, and burning on micturition.

Before any treatment for senile vaginitis is begun, the possibility of malignancy must be excluded, as the discharge, if blood-stained, could mask bleeding due to carcinoma of the cervix or endometrium. In the absence of any serious lesions, the doctor will usually order oestrogen, either locally in the form of pessaries or creams, or orally. The oestrogen will improve the resistance of the vaginal epithelium and should clear the condition. Acidic vaginal jelly (applied each night into the vagina) would be used instead of oestrogen in those cases where hormonal therapy is contraindicated.

Trichomonal vaginitis

This relatively common condition is caused by a protozoal organism, *Trichomonas vaginalis*. It causes a thick, profuse, frothy, irritating, foul-smelling discharge which may be white, yellow or green in colour. Trichomonal vaginitis is usually spread by sexual intercourse but not in every case; it may be spread by the common use of towels and other toilet articles and it is occasionally found in the vaginal secretions of children who have had no sexual experience. The organisms may lie dormant in the vagina and bowel for long periods and only become pathogenic at times of low resistance. Vitamin deficiency is known to predispose to the onset of trichomonal vaginitis.

Diagnosis is made by examining a fresh saline suspension of the discharge through a microscope. If trichomonads are present they are seen to be moving amongst pus cells. Vaginal examination may reveal small red spots on the vaginal walls. A smear is usually taken to culture for the presence of gonorrhoea.

Treatment

The specific treatment is metronidazole 200 mg three times daily after meals for one week, or a single 2 g dose of tinidazole. (Pregnancy and breastfeeding are contraindications to these treatments; nausea and alcohol intolerance are common with their use.)

To avoid reinfection, her sexual partner must be treated simultaneously, and intercourse should be avoided until they are both free of infection. A follow-up smear is usually taken two months later and the treatment repeated if necessary. Vaginal pessaries containing natamycin may be used as a supplementary treatment. Instruction in hygiene measures may be necessary and will include at least daily showers or baths, frequent changes and correct laundering of underpants, and care in handling clothing and linen. A course of multi-vitamin or Vitamin C tablets is often recommended.

Monilial vaginitis

This condition, also known as candidiasis or 'vaginal thrush', is caused by the fungus *Candida albicans*, and is the most common type of vaginitis. The fungus is a normal inhabitant of the vagina but causes symptoms only when the vaginal environment is so altered that the fungi are able to multiply greatly. The altered conditions include higher levels of glycogen in the vagina due to the elevation of the levels of either oestrogen or glucose in the bloodstream. As a result, monilial vaginitis is particularly common during pregnancy, in women taking oral contraceptives, and in diabetic women. With the alteration of the normal vaginal bacterial levels, as occurs during a course of antibiotics (especially the broad-spectrum type), the fungal growth may not be kept in check. If tight synthetic underclothing is worn and genital hygiene is neglected as well, only a very slight change in vaginal environment is needed to bring on the condition. Thrush can be spread by sexual contact.

The main symptom is extreme pruritus. Discharge is often scant but it is thick, white and cheesy. Raw areas may be seen on the vaginal walls.

Treatment

A vaginal swab will be taken. The predisposing cause or causes should be investigated and corrected if possible. If diabetes is suspected, full investigation is necessary. Oral contraceptives are usually discontinued, temporarily at least. (Alternative measures are offered if necessary.) Attention is paid to the personal hygiene and type of underclothing usually worn. Local treatment consists of the insertion of nystatin pessaries morning and night for at least two weeks, possibly longer. The patient must be told to continue the treatment during menstruation if it should occur, and to finish the course as prescribed even though the symptoms will improve. The treatment is difficult for some women to accept so the last point must be stressed. Painting the vagina with aqueous gentian violet solution (1 per cent) is an effective treatment but has the disadvantage of staining any material that the paint touches. Care taken in the application of the paint and in the protection of clothing and linen by the use of large vulval pads should overcome this problem. Reinfection from the bowel is not uncommon so oral nystatin may be prescribed to inhibit the growth of bowel fungi. Male sexual partners are also treated and uncircumcised men must be sure to apply the (nystatin) cream under the foreskin.

Natural unpasteurised yoghurt inserted into the vagina is useful as a first-aid measure for restoring an acid environment. Cold yoghurt can be very soothing when applied to a burning irritated vulva and vagina.

Gardnerella vaginalis

Formerly known as *haemophilus vaginalis*, gardnerella can be a normal inhabitant of the vagina. Its overgrowth can cause vaginitis, the symptoms being a grey discharge with an unpleasant odour. It is a common condition and often coexists with other organisms.

Other causes of vaginitis

Allergic reaction to locally applied chemicals such as those in contraceptive agents, vaginal deodorants or douche preparations are possible causes. Hypersensitivity to prescribed vaginal creams and pessaries sometimes occurs. The cause is eliminated and oral antihistamines are prescribed.

Foreign bodies such as forgotten tampons and trauma or burns to the vagina may also cause an inflammatory reaction.

Cervicitis

Acute cervicitis

This usually only occurs in gonorrhoea or during the puerperium but sometimes occurs with the use of intrauterine devices. Acute vaginitis is often present as well.

The cervix appears red and swollen and is tender. The treatment is to correct the infection which caused the condition. Exclusion of malignant change is always necessary.

Chronic cervicitis and cervical erosion

Chronic cervicitis (endocervicitis) may follow acute cervicitis or may appear as a chronic change following cervical laceration during childbirth. It is believed to arise to some degree in at least 20 per cent of parous women.

Endocervicitis is caused by a variety of non-specific organisms. Inflammatory changes occur, usually above the junction of the columnar and squamous epithelia (the transformation zone). The mucus-secreting columnar epithelium of the cervical canal is able to heal more quickly than the thicker squamous epithelium which covers the cervix projecting into the vagina: the columnar epithelium, there, spreads out beyond the external os and appears to evert or 'pout'. The surface area is healed but appears red (through the thinner covering) and there is a greatly increased production of cervical mucus. Previously, this situation was referred to as 'cervical erosion'. Small retention cysts (Nabothian follicles) caused by blockage of some of the mucus ducts may be seen on the surface of the cervix.

Symptoms

In addition to the increased production of cervical mucus and its resultant discharge, there may be complaints of low backache, deep dyspareunia, dysmenorrhoea, and menorrhagia due to pelvic congestion.

Treatment

After investigation for, and exclusion of cervical malignancy, the erosion is treated by diathermic cautery or by cryosurgery (a freezing method using solid carbon dioxide). This will destroy the chronically infected surface tissue, and after it has sloughed off new growth of normal tissue should occur from underneath. A cone excision is done when there is any possibility of malignancy.

Cervical ectropion

Ectropion is a condition in which laceration of the external os and chronic cervicitis have caused the edges of the endocervix to turn outwards. The exposed columnar epithelium is likely to become infected and give rise to discharge and slight bleeding.

After investigation to exclude the presence of malignant changes, the ectropion is treated by diathermic cauterisation or cryosurgery.

Endometritis

During the reproductive years, with the regular shedding of the endometrium, infections are not usually able to become established, and so are rare.

Acute endometritis may be caused by the introduction of infection during uterine operations or procedures, by gonococcal infection, by the retention of products of conception (usually dead placental tissue) or foreign material within the uterus.

Chronic endometritis may be due to malignancy, infected polyps, tuberculosis, cervical stricture, or lack of resistance because of senile atrophy.

The treatment of endometritis consists of the administration of antibiotics, drainage of the uterus by cervical dilatation if necessary and, when the infection has cleared, the examination of endometrial tissue for malignant or tuberculous change.

Salpingitis and salpingo-oophoritis

Acute salpingitis

This is usually accompanied by inflammation of the ovaries and quite often both tubes are affected.

Causes

The causes include:

Gonorrhoea: ascending organisms affect the lining of the tube.

Septic abortion and puerperal sepsis: the organisms spread via the bloodstream (locally) and tend to attack the outer covering of the tube.

Tuberculosis: spread via the bloodstream, and affecting both the lining and the outer coat of the tube (Figure 13.5).

Appendicitis: with the inflammation spread across the peritoneum. In this case, generalised pelvic peritonitis is usually present.

Figure 13.5
Tuberculous salpingitis

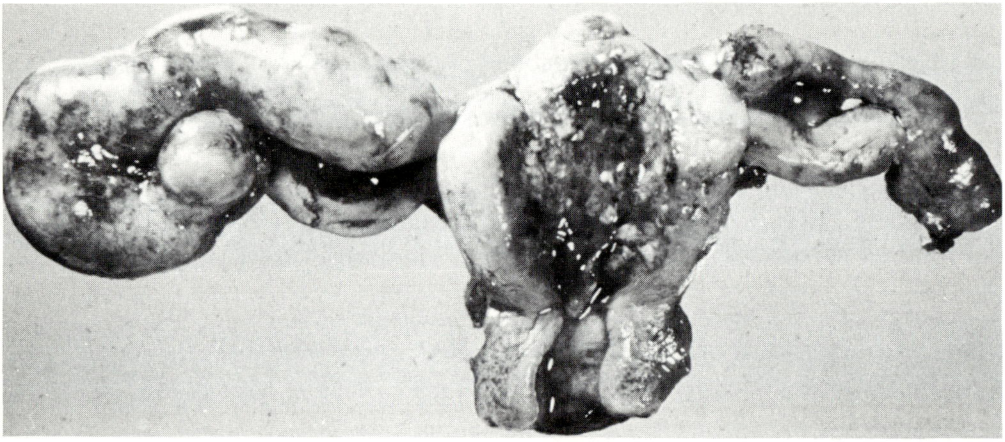

Symptoms

Salpingitis often has a sudden onset although it may sometimes be preceded by a vaginal discharge, or an abnormally heavy menstrual period. Severe pain is felt in both iliac fossae. High fever, tachycardia, nausea and malaise are present. Pelvic examination is extremely painful.

Treatment

The patient is admitted to hospital and is allowed only very limited activity until the temperature and pulse have shown normal readings for *seven days*. Swabs of cervical and vaginal discharge are sent immediately for culture and sensitivity. Blood cultures may be indicated. Until the results of these smears are known it is wise to 'barrier' nurse the patient. Frequent careful observations of vital signs are essential.

Pain is relieved by the administration of effective analgesics, usually a suitable narcotic by injection, progressing to milder, oral analgesics as the condition improves. Extra relief may be obtained by the use of well-protected hot-water bags applied to the abdomen.

Antibiotics are given immediately, in large doses, either by the intravenous or intramuscular route. After the initial course, the antibiotics may be continued orally for some weeks, to ensure complete control of the infection and to prevent a renewal of infection.

Diet on admission will be restricted to fluids only for the first day or two, followed by the gradual introduction of a light, nourishing diet.

Full nursing care including special attention to vulval hygiene is necessary.

Following discharge from hospital, intercourse should be avoided for at least six weeks or until the inflammation has completely cleared.

Consequences of acute salpingitis

Where the inner lining of the tubes has been inflamed, occlusion of the fimbrial ends by adhesions may result in a hydrosalpinx or a pyosalpinx. Occlusion of the lumen of the tubes will result in infertility. Where the lumen is constricted but not completely closed, the woman is more prone to subsequent ectopic pregnancy.

Where the outer coats of the tubes are inflamed, peritubal and periovarian adhesions may occur and these ultimately give rise to the symptoms of chronic salpingitis.

Chronic salpingitis

If acute salpingitis does not completely resolve, the tubes are likely to remain chronically inflamed. Sometimes salpingitis may occur without an acute attack. The symptoms may include dysmenorrhoea, menorrhagia, dyspareunia and attacks of pain and pyrexia especially at the time of menstruation. If pus has collected in the tubes, bilateral tender masses may be felt on bimanual pelvic examination. The woman's general health is affected; malaise and lethargy are common.

Treatment

The patient is encouraged to rest as completely as possible and advised against having intercourse until the condition is completely healed. Antibiotics may be given if bacteriological investigations have shown an active infection. Usually, however, the symptoms have arisen because of adhesions and pelvic congestion and so will only be relieved by surgical intervention. The doctor will usually wait until the woman's health has improved somewhat by conservative treatment, before doing a laparotomy. He may remove the tubes only but this is rare because there is usually associated chronic inflammation of the rest of the pelvic organs and salpingectomy on its own will not relieve the symptoms. For this reason, a hysterectomy and bilateral salpingo-oophorectomy is usually done, although an attempt to conserve some ovarian tissue is made, if possible, in a younger woman.

Pelvic peritonitis

Pelvic peritonitis may follow acute salpingitis or any severe infection of the genital tract. It may spread from appendicitis or diverticulitis, or be a part of general peritonitis. Ruptured ectopic pregnancy or other pelvic bleeding may give rise to an infected haematoma. Chemical irritation from douching fluids, ruptured dermoid cysts or vernix and meconium (after caesarian section) may cause pelvic peritonitis. Drainage and pus collects in the pouch of Douglas, often causing a pelvic abscess.

The woman is ill with acute pain, a high swinging temperature and usually she has diarrhoea.

Treatment

The treatment is the same as for acute salpingitis plus the removal of the cause if known. Pelvic abscesses are drained through the posterior vaginal fornix (posterior culdotomy) and pus is sent for examination. Sterile vulval pads must be changed hourly after this procedure, and carefully handled and disposed.

Toxic shock syndrome

Toxic shock syndrome (TSS) is a severe poisoning of the body by an unidentified toxin produced by the bacterium, *Staphylococcus aureus*, an organism which is found on the skin and in the nose of about half of the population. It is also normally found in the vagina of some women. Under certain conditions this bacterium multiplies in the vagina. The main effect of the released toxin seems to be the *suppression of the body's immune system.*

About one thousand cases of TSS have been reported worldwide since 1975, and more than half of these have been in the USA. There have been several cases of TSS reported in Australia. Most victims are menstruating women, but 5 per cent have been men or children. The disease may exist in a milder form, and its incidence may, in fact, be far greater.

Symptoms

A combination of one or more of these symptoms will be present:

- a sudden onset of high fever—more than 38·9°C
- bloodshot eyes
- vomiting, diarrhoea
- extreme muscle pain and abdominal pain
- body rash with shedding of skin scales later.

TSS is more likely to occur during menstruation and when tampons are used.

Causes

The toxin produced by *Staphylococcus aureus* is the cause of the illness. Associated factors are:

- the onset of TSS seems to occur during menstruation and is associated with the use of tampons
- *Staphylococcus aureus* has been shown to multiply in tampons under simulated menstrual conditions
- super-absorbent tampons affect vaginal lining by drying it out too much and thus leading to microscopic ulcers. These ulcers may provide a port of entry for toxins into the body
- body changes during menstruation may provide an environment where *Staphylococcus aureus* multiplies readily.

Prevention

The risk of TSS could be significantly reduced by not using tampons. The role of tampons in the disease is still not known, but there is a definite association. Those who do choose to wear tampons should be aware of the symptoms of TSS. A woman, becoming ill during a period, should remove the tampon and seek medical advice immediately. A vaginal swab should then be taken to test for *Staphylococcus aureus*.

Sensible precautions for the use of tampons

- wash hands before changing tampons
- avoid handling tampons unnecessarily
- change tampons at least once every four hours during the day
- use a pad instead of a tampon if bleeding is slight, or to prevent drying out of the vagina
- avoid the use of tampons if they cause pain or discomfort
- use a pad instead of a tampon at night

The use of sea sponges instead of tampons is not recommended. Although they do not appear to cause the same degree of vaginal dryness as tampons, they have been found to contain chemical pollutants from the sea.

Further research is being conducted into the problem of toxic shock syndrome, and warnings about health risks are now to be included in all tampon packaging.

Sexually transmitted diseases

The incidence of sexually transmitted (venereal) diseases has risen in recent years and they have become the commonest communicable diseases in the world today. Misconceptions about these diseases still exist despite attempts at widespread public education. Many people still assume that protection from pregnancy bestows automatic protection against venereal disease. There was some degree of truth in this when contraceptive methods were limited to physical barriers (eg the condom) or to the immediate washing out of the vagina after intercourse by douching or spraying. Now that contraception can be practised by remote control, as it were, that 'protection' has gone. The contraceptive pill, intrauterine devices and sterilising operations for the male or female have no effect in the prevention of venereal diseases. In fact, their widespread use, removing the fear of pregnancy from promiscuous sexual intercourse, combined with the emergence of different attitudes towards sexual morality, are probably the main reasons for the resurgence of these diseases. Other misconceptions about these diseases are that you 'can't get it again' and that it is 'incurable'. Contamination from towels and toilet seats is often blamed; it does happen, but very rarely. The organisms usually require a moist, warm location for survival. Exposure to cold air, water or soap will almost always cause their rapid destruction. In western countries, the most prevalent sexually transmitted diseases are chlamydia, gonorrhoea and syphilis. Several other diseases, however, can be transmitted through sexual contact. In all cases the woman's sexual partner will need treatment to prevent the recurrence or spread of the disease.

Gonorrhoea

Gonorrhoea, the second most common and widespread of the notifiable sexually transmitted diseases, is a bacterial infection. It enters the body via the genital tract, from where it may spread to other parts. The organism responsible is the gram-negative *Neiserria gonorrhoeae*. Natural immunity is *not* acquired after having had the infection. The incubation period is from two days to two weeks in most cases. The bacteria first attack those tissues which are not covered by squamous epithelium—the urethra and the paraurethral (Skene's) ducts, and the ducts of the Bartholin's glands. The disease then spreads to the cervix causing acute cervicitis.

Symptoms

The early symptoms of gonorrhoea are localised, and include dysuria—frequency and burning on micturition, a purulent discharge (which may be slight and so go unnoticed), vulval soreness but not pruritus unless a trichomonal infection is also present. Sometimes these symptoms are mild and may be mistaken for a simple bladder irritation.

Occasionally gonorrhoea is first suspected postnatally, when a newborn baby's eyes are grossly infected from contact with the organism in the birth canal.

If untreated, the inflammation spreads to the uterus and fallopian tubes, and thick pus completely fills the lumen causing acute salpingitis, eventually resulting in strictures, fibrosis and, finally, infertility. Adhesions cause pain, disturb menstruation and, if they spread to the area of the rectum, cause chronic constipation.

In many women, the symptoms are slight, even absent. The condition may settle into a carrier state where the woman is able to infect other people for many weeks.

Diagnosis

All females with dysuria and a history of recent sexual contact should be screened. Smears are taken from the urethra (by 'milking' the urethra and Skene's glands), the Bartholin's ducts and the endocervix, and are sent for examination and culture. Because people who present with gonorrhoea could have syphilis as well, blood is taken for syphilitic studies before treatment for gonorrhoea is begun.

Treatment

Admission to hospital is not usually necessary unless there are acute or serious complications, eg salpingitis. The medications given to treat gonorrhoea differ at each hospital and clinic, but many still use large single doses of procaine penicillin (3×10^6 units initially, and $1{\cdot}5 \times 10^6$ next day) preceded and followed by oral probenecid to delay the excretion of the penicillin. Alternatives to penicillin are spectinomycin, cotrimoxazole, and doxycycline. Tetracycline may be given as well.

Because gonorrhoea responds so well to antibiotics and because of their easy availability, a new problem has arisen in the management of venereal diseases—that of self-medication. Self-medication may be sufficient to control the symptoms but not always to eradicate the condition, and rarely are the sexual partners treated as they should.

Advice must be given regarding personal hygiene and abstinence from sexual intercourse to avoid infecting others or being reinfected.

Chlamydia

Chlamydia is caused by the organism *Chlamydia trachomatis*, which is the causal organism of non-specific urethritis in the male. It can be readily sexually transmitted, and its clinical manifestations are identical with those of gonorrhoea. Chlamydial pelvic infection is now shown to be more common than gonococcal.

The infection is suspected when ordinary cultures are negative. Chlamydia lacks an essential ingredient of cell metabolism, ATP. It is dependent on living cells for this, so it is truly intracellular and very difficult to grow except by tissue culture. This fact also accounts for its general resistance to common antibiotics.

The use of (oral) doxycycline is at present believed to offer the best chance of controlling the infection.

Syphilis

Syphilis is caused by a corkscrew-shaped organism, *Treponema pallidum* (spirochaete). It is spread by direct contact, the organisms entering the body by burrowing through cracks and abrasions. Although sexual intercourse is the usual means of transmission, any contact with the organism may, if conditions are suitable, result in its spread. Lesions can occur on almost any part of the body, but the vulva and cervix and the mouth are the commonest sites.

Primary syphilis

The incubation period averages about three weeks but may be shorter—ten days, or longer—up to three months. One or more lesions or chancres appear, as painless shallow ulcers about 1 cm in diameter. The sores may not be noticed, especially if on the inner aspect of one of the labia, or on the cervix. Figure 13.6 shows *extensive* syphilitic ulceration. The sores usually close over after a few weeks and remain as just hardenings. The inguinal lymph nodes enlarge and become hard but are not painful. During this stage, blood tests for syphilis will remain negative, and the patient usually has no idea that she is infected.

Secondary syphilis

About two months later, the spirochaetes invade the bloodstream and a generalised rash may appear. The rash is not itchy and is usually copper coloured, but in some cases may be so mild that it goes unnoticed. Mouth lesions may occur, with a sore throat, glossitis, and small white linear ulcers. Syphilitic alopecia may occur. There is often generalised lymphadenitis and the constitutional symptoms of (mild) fever. The only genital manifestation that arises, and then not always, is the appearance of multiple flat vulval and perineal warts—condylomata lata.

The disease is highly infectious during the primary and secondary stages, that is, when the skin lesions, chancre, rash or warts, are present. These stages can last for up to two years.

Tertiary syphilis

If the symptoms of secondary syphilis are not treated or pass unnoticed, the disease can remain quiescent and not manifest itself for periods varying from ten to thirty years. It is during this period that the millions of spirochaetes in the bloodstream attack various organs and structures in the body, especially the heart, brain, ears, eyes, joints and bones, ultimately causing severe degenerative changes, generalised paralysis and often insanity.

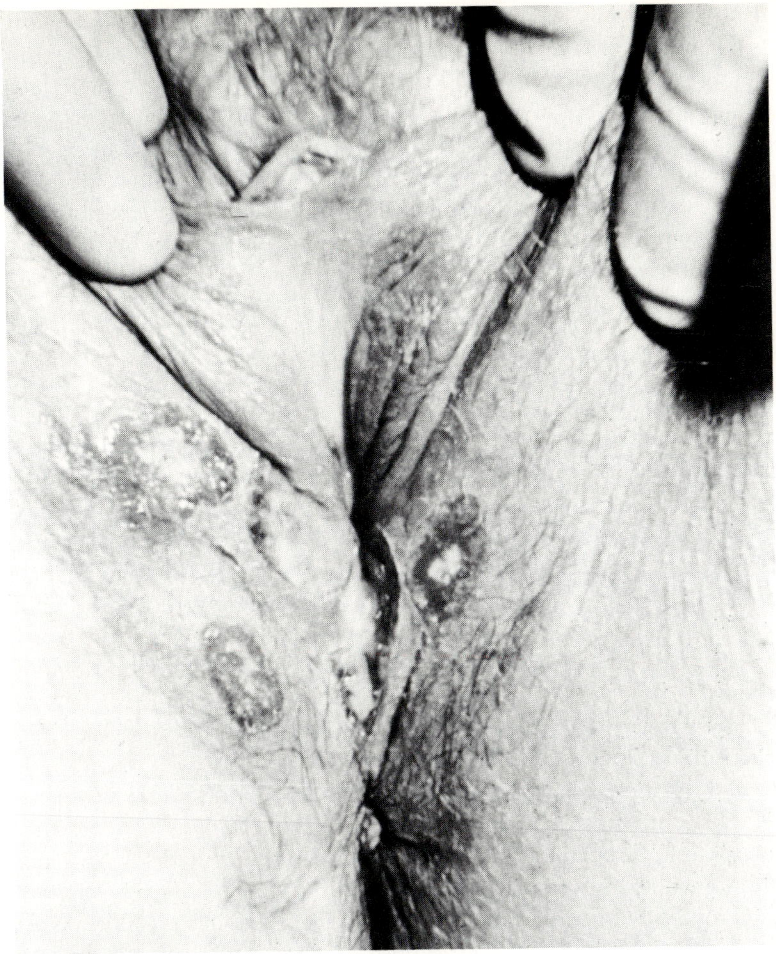

Figure 13.6
Extensive syphilitic ulceration

Investigations

Examination of a scraping taken from the chancre is the only definite means of diagnosis of syphilis in the early weeks. Blood tests are commenced six weeks after possible infection and, if negative, repeated six weeks later. Sexual intercourse should be avoided until a diagnosis has been made and, if necessary, until treatment has been completed. A number of blood tests are performed, including Wassermann reaction (WR) and venereal disease reference laboratory (VDRL), and will usually be positive at six weeks. Fluorescent treponemal antibody (FTA) test or treponemal immobilisation (TPI) test is often done as an extra check as they are specific for syphilis and are very accurate.

Treatment

Penicillin is still the treatment of choice for early syphilis. Large doses are given, for example IM procaine penicillin, 1·5 million units daily for ten consecutive days or LPG (long-acting penicillin G) 1 vial IM weekly for three weeks. This will completely cure the condition but will not provide protection against future reinfection. In the later stages of syphilis, the doses may have to be very much higher. Tetracyclines are given in cases of penicillin sensitivity but are less effective. Routine blood tests are continued at intervals over the next two years and if a pregnancy occurs during that time, an extra course of penicillin may be advised to protect the foetus from congenital syphilis.

Herpes simplex virus: genital herpes

There are two types of herpes simplex virus (HSV)—type I, which causes common cold sores on the lips, and type II, which causes lesions in the lower genital tract. They can, however, both be found in the opposite sites. Although they are microscopically different, both types produce very similar effects. As with other viruses, HSV are able to remain alive in the body indefinitely after the first infection, travelling along the nerves to a ganglion near the spinal cord where they survive in a dormant state. They may be reactivated at times of physical or emotional stress (or for no obvious reason).

Recurrences are generally, although not always, less severe than the initial attack.

Genital herpes infections are becoming a widespread problem. Although not yet a notifiable disease, their incidence is certainly increasing. They are the subject of many magazine articles, and self-help groups have formed in an attempt to pool the experience of sufferers, provide emotional support, referral when necessary, assist research and perhaps come up with ideas to relieve symptoms and possibly prevent attacks.

Herpes genitalis is highly infectious and is spread by direct contact with the lesion, ie by sexual intercourse and orogenital contact. It has an incubation period of two to seven days, possibly longer, from the time of contact.

Significance of genital herpes

- it can recur at any time, with distressing symptoms and disruption of sexual activity
- its possible association with cervical malignancy
- its danger to the newborn baby if active during pregnancy

Genital herpes and cervical carcinoma

Although the cause of cervical cancer, like most other cancers, is unknown there appears to be an increased risk of it arising in women who have had genital herpes. (Sexual activity, specifically intercourse, is the common factor.) It is particularly important for these women to have a Papanicolaou smear at least every twelve months.

Genital herpes and pregnancy

Recurrences may occur more frequently and are sometimes a little more severe during pregnancy. Because the herpes virus is a comparatively large virus it does not cross the placental barrier and so the foetus is not affected. But herpes is significant when it is active at the time of delivery; the baby can be affected as it comes down the birth canal. Newborn infants are particularly susceptible to serious and sometimes fatal infections with either HSV-I or HSV-II.

Obstetricians are careful to exclude active herpes in the three to six weeks before delivery in a woman who has a history of genital herpes. If viral cultures taken during this period are negative and if there are no active lesions at the time of labour then vaginal delivery is safe, but if there is any doubt the baby would be delivered by Caesarian section.

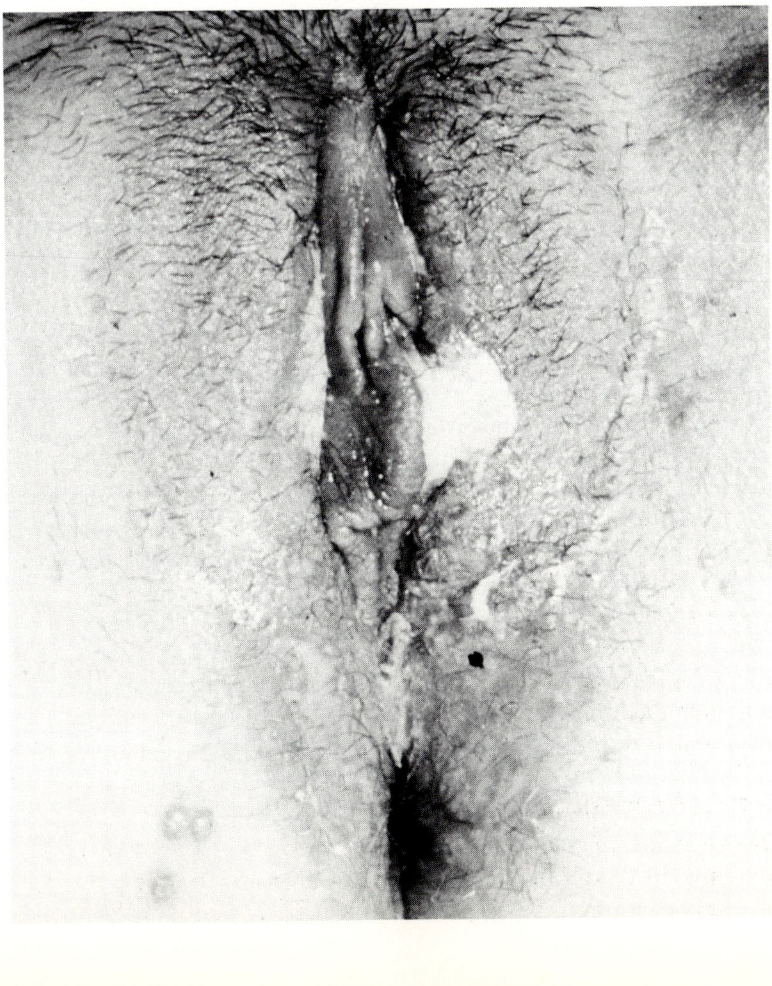

Figure 13.7
Herpes genitalis (blisters)

Symptoms

As with oral herpes, there is a prodrome of tingling and irritation before the lesions appear. Features *may* include:

- small red raised spots on the vulva, vagina and cervix
- blister development, then:
- shallow ulcers (Figure 13.7) which are extremely sore
- pain when passing urine
- flu-type symptoms: malaise, depression, slight fever
- discharge (yellow, green and watery)
- intense pain on intercourse
- rectal pain
- associated vaginal thrush infection
- '*cystitis*'—this can be so severe that natural voiding becomes impossible. Admission to hospital and the insertion of an indwelling (supra-pubic) catheter may be the only means of relief, especially in a first attack.

These symptoms may be present for four to eight days, after which the lesions will heal and the other symptoms subside.

Diagnosis

Diagnosis is made on the history of symptoms, by examining the lesions, by fresh cervical–vaginal smear and culture, and possibly by blood examination for antibody titre. Syphilis has to be excluded.

Management

Herpes, like many viral infections, is 'incurable', but it is usually self-limiting. Much research is being conducted into a cure for the condition and also for a vaccine which may eventually prevent genital herpes. The most promising specific treatment so far is a topical preparation—acyclovir, which is non-toxic and produces relief from discomfort and promotes more rapid healing. Acyclovir may also be given parenterally, when its use has been shown to shorten the natural history of an acute infection but does not clear the virus from the nerve sheath. The use of interferon for the treatment of herpes is also under investigation. *Symptomatic relief* during attacks includes:

- ice applied to the area twenty to thirty minutes at the first sign of an attack (may shorten the attack or make it less severe)
- simple hygienic measures—keeping the lesions clean and dry
- frequent salt or sodium bicarbonate solution baths
- local skin disinfection, eg using povidone iodine
- local anaesthetic ointment
- avoidance of irritants: soaps, underclothes etc.

General measures include:

- treatment of associated conditions, eg thrush
- attention to diet

- rest, and removal of stress if possible
- abstinence from sexual activity, especially intercourse, during an attack and for a short time after the lesions have healed.

Nursing management in relation to 'barrier' nursing, the disposal of linen and disinfection of baths and so on, will follow the guidelines as issued by each hospital or institution. Where there is a possibility of active herpes, every precaution should be taken, particularly when dealing with the vulva or perineum, eg disposable gloves would be worn for perineal shaves or toilets, urethral catheters would not be used.

Emotional implications

The woman (or man) who has contracted genital herpes will need to re-evaluate her whole attitude towards sexual activity and the conduct of her sex life. To be responsible she must tell prospective sexual partners, as cervical lesions may be present (and not realised) at almost any time. She could (although she should not) feel stigmatised, guilty or self-conscious about this condition.

During pregnancy those who have had genital herpes *must* inform the doctor so that a careful watch can be kept for any recurrence, especially as the pregnancy nears term.

Acquired immune deficiency syndrome

Acquired immune deficiency syndrome (AIDS) is a relatively recently discovered, but much-publicised condition, with severe and frightening effects and implications. It is believed to be carried by the human lymphotrophic retrovirus, HLTV-III and is transmitted specifically in seminal fluid, but also in rectal mucus, vaginal mucus, via the placenta, and in blood transfusions and blood products.

AIDS was at first linked almost exclusively to male homosexuals, but there have now been a number of cases among female prostitutes who have been sexual partners to bisexual males. It has also been reported in heterosexual men who have had sexual contact with prostitutes. AIDS is also appearing among intravenous drug users. Recipients of blood containing the virus have contracted and died from the disease. Babies are particularly at risk in this way, as are haemophiliacs.

The signs of AIDS may not appear until three to four years after the disease has been contracted. The first sign is generalised lymphadenopathy. About 20 per cent of those with this symptom, and who have been in contact with the virus, will develop the condition. They gradually lose their immunity to organisms (including the commensal organisms which become pathogenic to them).

Investigation of the syndrome is being treated as a matter of urgency. Donated blood can now be screened for the presence of the virus. Restrictions on blood donors are being proposed, but it is a very difficult area to control.

Other sexually transmitted conditions

Chancroid or soft sore is caused by a gram-negative bacillus *Haemophilus ducreyi* and is extremely contagious. Within a week of contact with the disease, small papules appear on the vestibule and labia minora. They quickly progress to become painful shallow ulcers. Further lesions may develop on the upper thighs and perineum. Inguinal lymph gland involvement usually occurs; abscesses may form and break down to form a single sinus. The diagnosis is usually made on recognition of the ulcer and by seeing its response to sulphonamide drugs. Culture of the discharge from the ulcers is done but this takes time and most doctors prefer to start treatment immediately. In severe cases, bed rest, with isolation if in hospital, relief of pain and frequent vulval wash-downs are required.

Non-specific urethritis causes symptoms in the male but very rarely in the female. Treatment is by the use of tetracyclines.

Vulval warts, pediculosis pubis, trichomonal and *monilial conditions* may all be transmitted sexually. They are discussed elsewhere under the appropriate headings.

Prevention of sexually transmitted diseases

Public campaigns educating the community about the symptoms, effects and dangers of these diseases are improving all the time. The minimising of promiscuous sexual activity is urged while an awareness of the pressures put upon people these days to be 'liberated' is shown. Where it is suspected that sexual restraint might not be practised, advice is given about the wearing of condoms, washing of the genitalia before and after intercourse, urinating immediately after intercourse and the immediate reporting of any suspicious symptoms.

Routine screening is carried out during pregnancy, at most family planning clinics, on all blood taken for donation, and, in some countries, as a prerequisite before the issue of a marriage licence.

Special clinics conduct contact-tracing as well as having diagnosis and treatment facilities. The staff of these clinics are chosen for their tact and patience, and are very aware of the reticence and difficulties involved in naming contacts.

Nursing aspects

The nursing approach to patients with sexually transmitted diseases is, of course, completely non-judgmental in word, gesture and expression. Barrier precautions must be observed for the protection of staff and other patients but these are done as discreetly as possible. If a lesion or discharge is suspicious of, or confirmed to be positive in, one of these diseases, they are not touched with bare hands. Disposable gloves are worn for all procedures involving the genital region, and all equipment, dressings and linen are disposed of carefully. Often patients should not know that they are being screened for these diseases; it depends greatly on the circumstances. Care should be taken to see that charts and record books are not left in places accessible to people who might misinterpret written information.

After diagnosis of, or recovery from, an acute attack of one of these diseases, referral is usually made to one of the special clinics. Nurses should be aware of the locations of these clinics and should be able to explain how they operate. The fact that the identity of the attenders is never disclosed and that the vital contact tracing is done using a file-number-slip system should be stressed.

Finally, nurses should consider the effects that these diseases might have on family and social life. In hospital, visiting hours may pass without company, or if there are visitors, their relationships may be strained. Guilt and worry may lead to depression or to a fear of going home and facing people. Social conditions may need to be looked into and so the services of a social worker may be of great benefit. In all cases the nurse must be ready and available to listen and explain and to help her patient through this difficult time. There is still a great stigma associated with these diseases. We should never make light of them but, by our attitude, we should help to lessen the rejection and censure that is so often felt.

14 Pruritus vulvae

Pruritus vulvae is an irritative condition of the vulva that brings about an intense desire to scratch. At least 10 per cent of women who attend a gynaecologist have this problem, although it may not be the overt reason for their visits.

There are many possible causes of pruritus and the management of this condition is dependent upon the cause. Every episode of scratching produces damage to the tissues, and this damage in turn leaves the tissues in a state of irritation that gives rise to further itching.

Three factors which seem to make any itching seem worse are warmth, weariness and attention to the symptom. So it is at night, in bed, that the woman with pruritus vulvae suffers most, and it is then that she will most likely scratch without inhibition or even without realising what she is doing.

Complaints of pruritus vulvae may not be clearly worded. Phrases like 'I'm nearly going mad with the irritation' may be used. Questioning about the nature of the irritation is necessary. Does it actually itch? Does it make you want to scratch? Is it worse at night? If it is indeed pruritus vulvae, these questions will be answered quickly and eagerly because the fact that somebody understands what it is like points to a possible hope for relief.

Causes

- *vaginal discharge:* not all vaginal discharges cause pruritus. The two that really do are those that occur with *Trichomonas vaginalis* and *Candida albicans*. The increased discharge and glycosuria associated with both pregnancy and the contraceptive pill can also cause itching
- *poor vulval hygiene:* encouraging the growth of micro-organisms
- *allergies* to chemicals, as in douching solutions, contraceptive creams, vaginal deodorants, perfumed soaps and even toilet papers. Pants and tights made of nylon or other synthetic materials are also sometimes responsible for pruritus
- *carcinoma of the vulva:* pruritus may sometimes be the only symptom of malignant change in the vulval tissues
- *chronic epithelial dystrophies:* epithelial changes may be atrophic as

in senile vulvitis; kraurosis, where the vulva is shrunken and thin; or hypertrophic—leukoplakia—where there are thickened white patches on the vulva. The term 'leukoplakia' is now regarded as descriptive only, as the types of hypertrophic changes vary

- *skin disorders* involving other areas of the body can also affect the vulva, eg psoriasis, seborrhoeic dermatitis, scabies, drug reaction dermatitis
- *as part of generalised pruritus:* as occurs with diabetes, jaundice, lymphadenoma and uraemia
- *post-menopause:* devitalisation of vulval tissues following oestrogen withdrawal. The vulva is thin and easily damaged, and the sensory nerve endings are exposed
- *deficiency states:* iron deficiency anaemia, gastric achlorhydria, avitaminosis A and B
- *psychological factors:* the itching sensation is determined and interpreted by the cerebral cortex. Cortical arousal may be the sole factor. Many people get itchy feelings when they see another person scratching. Even just talking about itching and itchiness can start them off. Sexual anxieties and frustrations have been blamed as the cause of pruritus vulvae in certain cases. But psychological factors appear most often in combination with one of the physical causes, making the effects of that cause far more obvious. If the nervous system is strained by anxiety, worry and fatigue, the sensation of itching is likely to be magnified.

Response to itching

The immediate and natural response is to scratch the itching area. This will, for a short time, bring relief from the itch. It will, however, bring about a sharp burning pain (which to many people is a preferable sensation).

The scratching will damage the surface epidermal tissue and, with it, the tiny superficial nerve fibres. Itching is absent until these tiny nerve fibres recover, when it returns. It will keep on returning because the damaged epithelial tissue will send irritative stimuli to the brain and so the cycle will continue. Prolonged scratching and epithelial damage can produce cellular changes that may ultimately lead to malignancy.

Management of pruritus vulvae

Local treatment is of little use unless it is aimed at removing the cause of the condition. Sometimes the cause is obvious from the history and examination. When it is not obvious, a wide range of investigations are carried out over a period of time, the simpler and more likely causes being eliminated first. While these investigations are in progress, a number of things can be done to minimise the itch, control the urge to scratch and prevent further damage to the vulva.

Investigations

- a careful history is taken of when the pruritus occurs, whether any specific factor starts it off, its intensity, frequency and duration. The woman is asked how long she has had the condition and what she does to relieve it. Details of her usual bathing and personal hygiene practices are discussed
- a general medical examination is carried out; it may reveal a general medical or skin condition
- rectal and vaginal examinations are performed, and the presence of any discharge is noted. A swab is taken for examination
- possible causes of allergic reaction are eliminated. This may involve mentioning the most simple and seemingly innocent agents and will include questions about laundry soaps and toilet papers. It will involve reviewing any medication, especially the contraceptive pill and antibiotics, that the woman may have been taking recently

Subsequent investigations

These include:

- repeated examinations of vaginal and vulval areas and tests for *Candida albicans* and trichomonas
- glucose tolerance test. A simple test for gylcosuria is not sufficient. More than a few diabetics have been diagnosed and so controlled because of investigation of pruritus. Figure 14.1 shows diabetic vulvitis

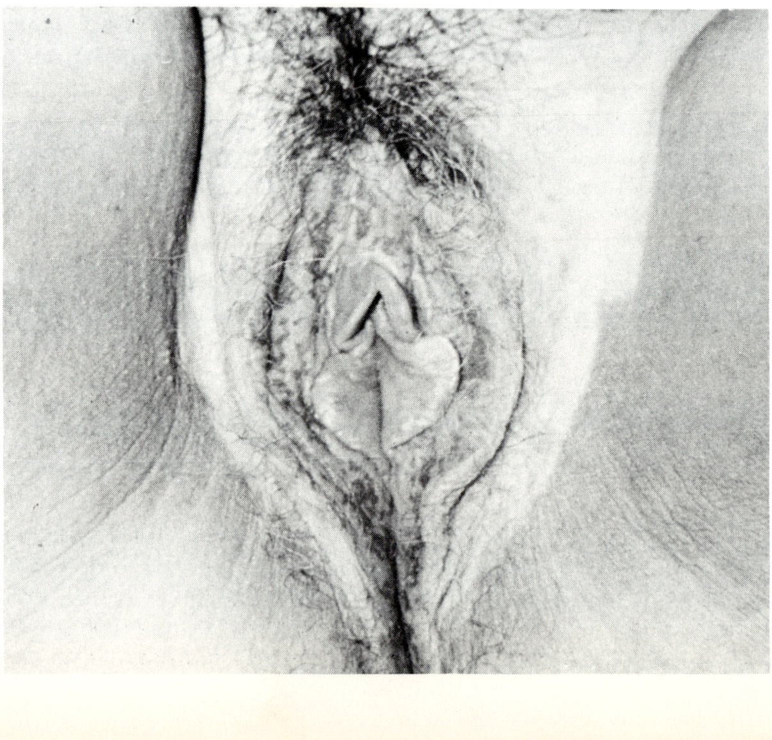

Figure 14.1
Diabetic vulvitis: pruritus may be one of the first symptoms of diabetes

- full blood examination
- fractional test meal for gastric acidity
- skin sensitivity tests
- biopsy of any suspicious lesion. In the absence of any obvious lesion and in the case of long-standing pruritus, especially where there is chronic epithelial dystrophy, the radioactive phosphorus (P^{32}) uptake test is performed. It indicates the sites for biopsy and so avoids missing any malignant area.

Psychological factors causing or contributing to pruritus are not always obvious. Time spent with the woman, discussing the effects of the symptom and learning about her home life, is well spent.

Treatment

When one or more definite causes are found, the specific treatment is commenced as soon as possible. In about 15–20 per cent of patients, however, no reason for the pruritus is discovered. If it persists, despite every effort to control it, it becomes known as *intractable* pruritus. In such a case, the woman may have no relief until the skin of the area is removed. This operation, simple vulvectomy, is done less frequently nowadays, but is still indicated for those older women who are very distressed by the symptom.

Measures to minimise itching, control scratching, prevent damage and aid healing

The woman is asked about what she has already tried in her effort to break the itch cycle. This is important because she is likely to be somewhat sensitive about her symptom and will not appreciate a dogmatic lecture on what she should be doing, when she has already tried every measure mentioned. If we are condescending in our approach, if we give her no credit for general knowledge or intelligence, her mental state is not going to contribute greatly to her recovery. Being admonished—'Don't scratch!'—rarely has a beneficial effect. It will only produce guilt, then anxiety about the persistence of the itch, or antagonism, a state that resists strongly most advice or help offered.

Minimising the itch

Consideration and discussion of all the points mentioned here is necessary. It takes time but is well worth it. Does the woman feel that she is able to keep the area properly clean? Does she use soap? What sort? Possibly it would be better to avoid soap, using just plain water or baby oil. Does she wipe from front to back after using the toilet? Does she find that it is difficult to clean herself properly following a bowel action? Could she try using baby oil then? Does she use non-coloured, good quality, soft toilet paper? Might cotton-wool or old soft cloth be better? Patting, rather than rubbing, the vulva to dry it can help. Does she use vaginal deodorants? Can she manage without for a while, and carry extra pants around instead? Does she wear firm, but not tight, cotton underwear? Cotton pants are more expensive than synthetic ones but they can make a big difference in this situation. Does she always wear pants under pantyhose, or tight jeans, or girdles? If she wears pads inside her pants for any reason, is she able to change them often enough? Are they lined with plastic? Are they securely attached or do they get too tight or too loose and chafe? What does she wash her underwear with? Is it a strong detergent or bleach? (It could well be, if discharge or urine has caused them to become stained.) Does she rinse them well, more than once? Do warm baths or showers start the itching off again? (Lower temperatures will help, and baths are better than showers because they stimulate the skin less.) Is it worse in bed at night? Is the bed too warm? Does she use an electric blanket? Can she manage without? Are her nightgowns made of synthetic material? Does she feel weary at night but not properly ('healthy') tired? Can she plan her day differently? If she has worries and anxieties, could she try to plan a time of mental relaxation, for example listening to music or reading before she goes to bed? (She won't itch if she sleeps soundly.) Might some suitable sedative be used at night just until this difficult period is over?

Controlling the urge to scratch

When itching does register, something other than scratching ought to be done. Local application of soothing substances such as weak bicarbonate of soda solution, calamine lotion, or a light dusting with zinc and starch powders are traditional but still effective measures. Patent 'cures' may not be suitable so are best avoided. If medications or creams, such as hydrocortisone cream, have been prescribed by the doctor, they should be used regularly. If they are to be applied whenever itching occurs, they should be kept close at hand.

Pressure applied over the itching area with the hand will stop the stimuli from reaching the brain. When the pressure can be maintained for a minute or two, the wave of itching will pass, but it might be difficult to do this in public. Cold dry applications are very useful. Large clean combine pads can be stored in any refrigerator and, when needed, worn inside firm cotton pants.

Admission to hospital for persistent pruritus can provide a welcome and often necessary change from the home environment while allowing supervision of, and assistance with, the treatment.

Preventing damage to the tissues

When the itching area is scratched, epithelial tissues are damaged. This damage can, to some degree, be prevented by making sure that the finger nails are short and the hands kept very clean. Cotton gloves can be worn, especially at night; they should not interfere with the woman's getting to sleep. Boxing gloves, which certainly keep the nails away from the itching area, are sometimes advised, but they are heavy and probably very uncomfortable.

Restraining the hands with 'shackles' or bandages should be the last resort. As an alternative to restrainers for hospital patients, the nurse can offer to do twice as many 'rounds' during the night to make sure that the woman is sleeping soundly, or to provide preventive measures if she is restless and likely to start scratching. During the day her visitors could effectively distract her; allowing them more flexible visiting times may enable this.

Healing of the damaged tissues

Most of the measures used to control the itching and scratching will contribute as well to the healing of tissues damaged by scratching. Apart from these, attention to the diet, the addition of vitamins, especially vitamin A, salt bathing, and exposure of the area to light and air (but not heat) are all useful. Systemic antibiotics may have some effect in aiding the healing process by preventing secondary infection.

Summary

Most women suffering from pruritus vulvae have tried to control it by themselves, for a while at least. Few go to the doctor on the first day of its appearance. But the longer it has been present, the longer it usually takes to clear up; so any woman with this problem should not continue indefinitely with self-medication. Pruritus by itself can have a number of undesirable effects, as well as being a possible symptom of several apparently unrelated and often serious medical conditions.

15 Dyspareunia

Dyspareunia is defined as pain or difficulty with intercourse. It differs from frigidity, where there is no interest in, or arousal for, intercourse. Dyspareunia may, however, have been the preceding factor in frigidity. Dyspareunia affects both partners in a relationship and they may both become disturbed. It is often a difficult matter to discuss with other people and many women with this symptom go to the doctor hoping that the doctor will introduce the subject (see Chapter 3).

Superficial dyspareunia

This is pain at the vulva or vagina felt during penile penetration of the introitus.

Causes

The causes of superficial dyspareunia include:

- inflammation of the vulva and vagina due to trichomonal, monilial or other infections; vulvitis caused by allergic response to sprays or soaps; vulval cracks and fissures; haemorrhoids
- urethral conditions—urethritis, urethral prolapse and urethral caruncle
- dryness, caused by postmenopausal atrophy, excessive vaginal douching, or disease or blockage of the Bartholin's glands and their ducts
- inelasticity of the introitus, caused by local adhesions, rigidity of the hymenal ring and scarring from episiotomy, perineal repairs or burns
- psychological factors (see below).

Deep dyspareunia

This is pain felt on, or after, deep penetration during intercourse. Causes of deep dyspareunia include:

- tender lesions in the pelvis, such as endometriosis, pelvic inflammatory disease or pelvic tumours

- uterine displacement such as retroversion where the ovaries have prolapsed into the pouch of Douglas, and prolapse of the uterus
- scar tissue in the upper vagina caused by repair operations or radiation therapy
- psychological factors which may be many and varied but which are affected by the woman's mental outlook on sex; unfortunate past experiences; physical, mental or emotional tiredness; bad home situations; lack of privacy; guilt; fear of pregnancy and labour; and lack of explanation and instruction following gynaecological operations or childbirth. Proven infertility, natural or induced, may occasionally be the problem.

Management of dyspareunia

Because of the psychological implications, dyspareunia is a difficult symptom to manage. It requires a doctor who is willing to spend time with the woman to discover the causes, if they are not obviously organic.

A careful and gentle pelvic examination is performed. The woman may need extra help in achieving relaxation during the procedure. If some organic cause is discovered, treatment is directed at that cause. Advice is given on the use of bland lubricants if necessary, and a warning given against using local anaesthetic ointments as these may cause reflex impotence in the male. Local lesions, adhesions or infections are treated. A rigid hymen may be incised; in some cases, gentle stretching may be all that is required. Hormone deficiency states are corrected by the administration of small doses of oral oestrogens or by the local application of oestrogen creams or pessaries.

Dilatation of a tight vagina may be achieved by the use of graduated vaginal dilators (Figure 15.1). Nurses are often asked to explain the procedure and to help the woman to insert the first sizes by herself. The lubricated dilators are worn twice daily for a period of ten to fifteen minutes. There are said to be significant psychological as well as physical benefits from successfully carrying out this procedure.

Surgical repair is sometimes necessary in the case of a poorly healed episiotomy or an extremely tight introitus.

Vaginismus

Because of the pain (actual or anticipated) during intercourse, vaginismus or reflex spasm of the levator ani muscles can develop. (Vaginismus has been likened to the 'shooting' rectal pains of proctalgia which most people experience occasionally.) The spasm is usually involuntary and causes the vagina to close tightly at the level of the levators. The adductor muscles of the thigh may also go

Figure 15.1
Vaginal dilator in position

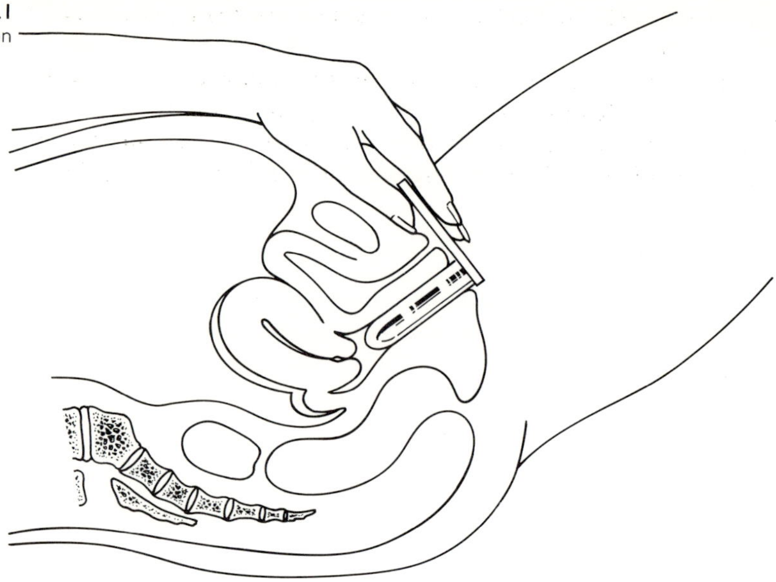

into spasm making it impossible for the woman to even open her legs. The sharp shooting pains of vaginismus are extremely distressing and each experience of this must profoundly affect the woman's attitude and response at subsequent attempts at intercourse.

Investigation of psychological factors

Investigation of the psychological factors involved in dyspareunia is often more difficult. It is not unknown for doctors to simply write a prescription for a tranquiliser or a referral to a psychiatrist as an easy way out as soon as difficulties with intercourse are mentioned. This approach is rather sad because these forms of treatment, when not absolutely necessary, may seriously undermine the woman's self-confidence and enlarge the problem out of all proportion. They are certainly necessary at times but not, one would hope, before a real attempt to uncover the causes has been made, and education to dispel any ignorance or fear has been given.

If at all possible the doctor should see the husband and wife together and should help them to discuss their sexual practices and attitudes. In many cases, this will be the first time that they have ever spoken seriously to each other about sex. Problems of which the other partner is entirely unaware may come to light, and the airing of these problems may result in resolutions to correct any bad situations or to bring about changes in their style of living.

The investigation of psychological aspects involved in dyspareunia is often accompanied by education in the positive benefits of achieving physical relaxation. Referral to a physiotherapist to learn how to relax the pelvic floor muscles may be of great value to the woman.

Abstinence from sexual intercourse is recommended during the period of investigation and treatment of dyspareunia. If intercourse is attempted before the causative problems have been resolved, the dyspareunia will probably return and be even worse than before.

16 New growths

New growths of the reproductive system may be benign or malignant. They can grow slowly or rapidly and may cause slight or severe symptoms. Benign growths may occasionally become malignant if untreated. One general observation, however, is certain—an early diagnosis results in early treatment, with a high percentage of successful cures. When one considers how much easier it is to discover abnormal conditions within the reproductive system in comparison with almost any other of the internal organs, it is hard to understand why certain growths, particularly the malignant ones, do become established and cause serious illness, even death. Ignorance of the importance of regular gynaecological examination and the fact that most of the warning symptoms are slight or do not have any real effect on the woman's daily life are the major reasons for delay in having these conditions discovered. Nurses, because they know of the effects of malignant growths and because they also understand the widespread reluctance to have gynaecological examinations have a tremendously important role to play in the community. As discussed in Chapter 7, what we are here for is, in this case, to know the reasons for delay and to be able to answer every one of them. We are also almost obliged to have these check-ups regularly ourselves, for our own benefit and for the very positive reason of setting an example to others.

Vulva

Benign tumours

Benign tumours of the vulva include:

- sebacious, epidermal and inclusion cysts
- Bartholin's gland cyst
- fibroma and lipoma
- vulval warts
- papilloma
- urethral caruncle.

Treatment

Simple cysts are excised. Bartholin's gland cysts are either marsupialised or, if the condition becomes chronic, excised. Vulval warts are treated with podophyllin paint or by cautery or cryosurgery. Papillomata may be cauterised although sometimes a simple vulvectomy may be necessary.

Malignant tumours

Vulval carcinoma is more common in women over the age of sixty-five. Pain is usually absent and, as a woman does not usually examine her own vulva, early changes are not noticed unless she has regular gynaecological check-ups or presents complaining of pruritus. Many women with carcinoma of the vulva do have a long history of pruritus and scratching, and many cases follow degenerative changes due to this. Sometimes a painless lump is present and this may ulcerate, or a cauliflower-like growth may be seen. (Figure 16.1.) Direct spread may occur to involve the vaginal introitus and

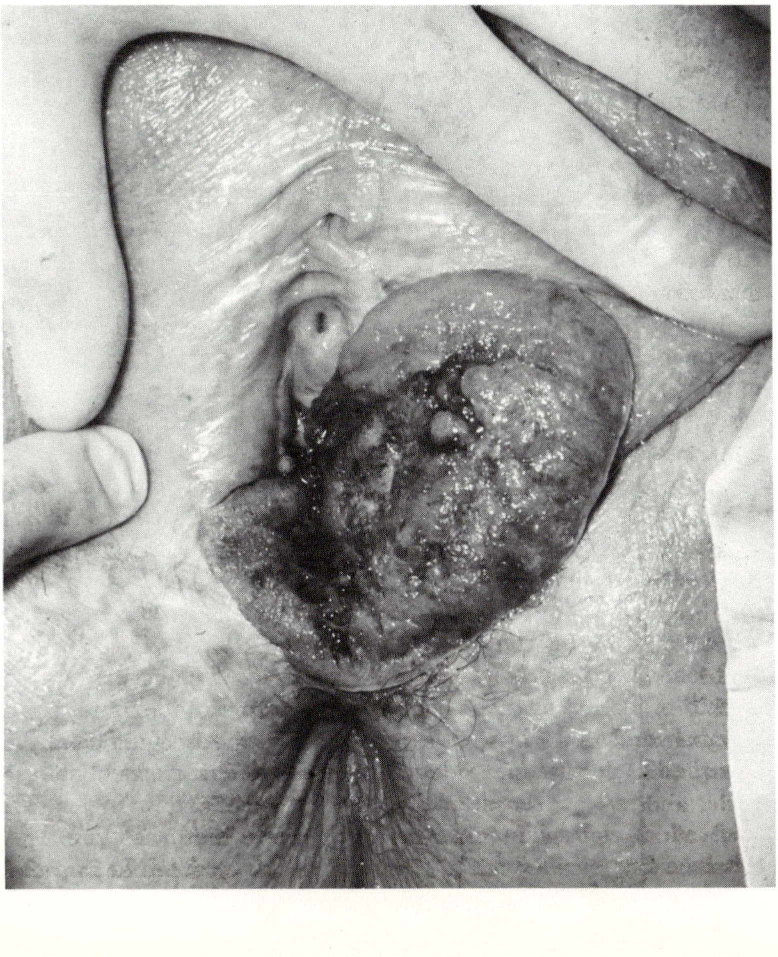

Figure 16.1
Carcinoma of the vulva

urethral orifice. Lymphatic spread occurs from the lesion to the groin, the external iliac chain and the lateral pelvic wall on the same or the opposite side.

Management

Skin biopsies are taken from any obvious lesions and from several areas on the vulva. If these prove to be malignant, a *radical* vulvectomy is performed (Figure 16.2 and 16.3). This involves wide excision of the vulva and removal of as much of the pelvic lymphatic network as possible. The operation is often long and recovery may be slow, especially in the older patient. Wound breakdown is common and is due to tension on the skin edges and to the relative ischaemia of the area following the ligation of its blood vessels. A skin graft may be applied to the raw area two or three days post-operatively.

Radiotherapy is not commonly used for carcinoma of the vulva except in those cases where the woman is too old or frail to undergo the radical operation, or where growths have recurred after surgery.

Vagina

Benign growths

Dermoid cysts, endometrial deposits, inclusion cysts, and cysts arising from wolffian duct remnants may occasionally be seen. If symptoms occur relating to these growths, the growths are excised.

Malignant growths

Primary carcinoma of the vagina is rare. Secondary carcinoma may come by direct spread from cervical growths or by metastases especially from endometrial carcinoma or choriocarcinoma. Vaginal and cervical adenocarcinoma has recently been discovered in a significant number of young women whose mothers received large doses of diethyl stilboestrol (DES) to treat threatened abortion, from 1945 onwards but especially in the middle and late 1950s. Many doctors and medical centres have traced girls whose mothers did receive this treatment and now keep them under regular observation with annual pelvic examinations, cervical smears and, if indicated, colposcopies. The girl's pregnancies would be supervised by an obstetrician who knows her history.

The treatment of vaginal carcinoma is by irradiation, radical surgery or cytotoxic drugs but, because of the usual lymphatic involvement, few patients with vaginal carcinoma survive longer than five years.

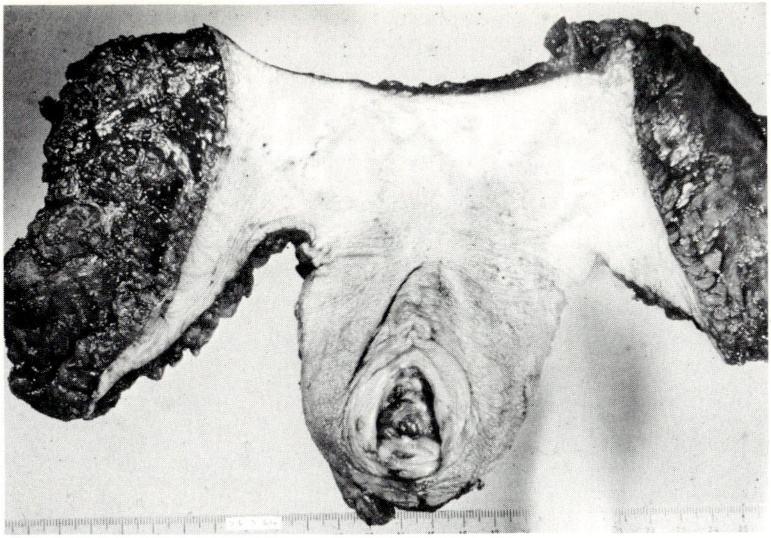

Figure 16.2
Radical vulvectomy specimen. The operation was performed for carcinoma of the vulva, involving the urethra

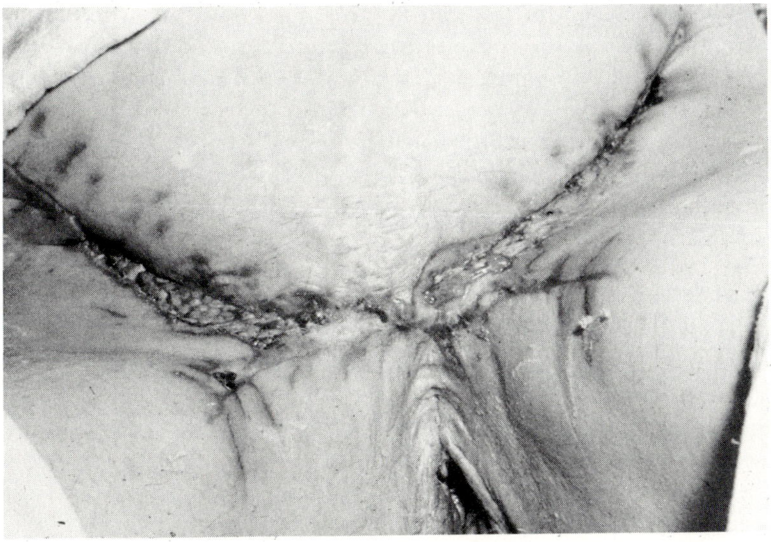

Figure 16.3
Wound healing five weeks after radical vulvectomy

Cervix

Benign growths

Cervical polyps are quite common, are mostly small, and may cause a slight discharge or bleeding. As they usually protrude through the cervix on a stalk, they can generally be 'twisted off' quite easily. A dilatation and curettage is done as an extra investigation and all tissue obtained is sent for histological examination to exclude malignancy.

Papillomata of the cervix, epithelial tags following childbirth, *small uterine fibroids* extruding from the cervix on pedicles and *Nabothian follicles* may also be seen. They are usually excised or treated by cautery or cryosurgery.

Malignant growths

Carcinoma of the cervix is the second most common malignant disease in women and occurs in the forty to fifty-five years age group. It can be diagnosed while still in the premalignant stage and so has a potentially high cure rate, especially as this premalignant stage may be evident for up to ten years before spreading.

Cervical carcinoma occurs more frequently in those women who have had intercourse early and who have children. It is more prevalent where conditions of hygiene are poor. It is seen less in nulliparous women and in those who lead a celibate type of life—it is almost unknown in nuns. It is very rare in orthodox Jewesses and this is most likely due to the strict prohibition of sexual intercourse before marriage, during (and for the seven days following) menstruation, during the entire term of pregnancy, and of any promiscuity at all. The immunity in Jewesses was once claimed to be due to circumcision of the males and the consequent absence of irritant smegma, but other groups such as the Muslims and Australian Aboriginals have practised circumcision since their history began and the incidence of cervical carcinoma is comparatively high in these groups.

Causes

The cause of cervical cancer is unknown but it is almost inevitably related to intercourse, especially when intercourse has occurred at certain times, such as adolescence and pregnancy, when increased hormonal output has caused high cellular activity in the area of the squamo-columnar junction (transformation zone). It is believed that certain irritants, viruses (especially the Herpes virus type II) or chromatin from the spermatozoa, may penetrate or irritate the cells of this area, leading to autonomous cell division which may in turn lead to dysplasia and then to carcinoma in situ. If not detected and treated at this stage it usually progresses to become invasive, although occasionally it may regress and become normal epithelium again.

Stages

Cervical carcinoma is allocated into stages (as shown in Figure 16.4) depending on the extent of its spread. The line of treatment varies according to each stage.

Figure 16.4
Staging of cervical carcinoma

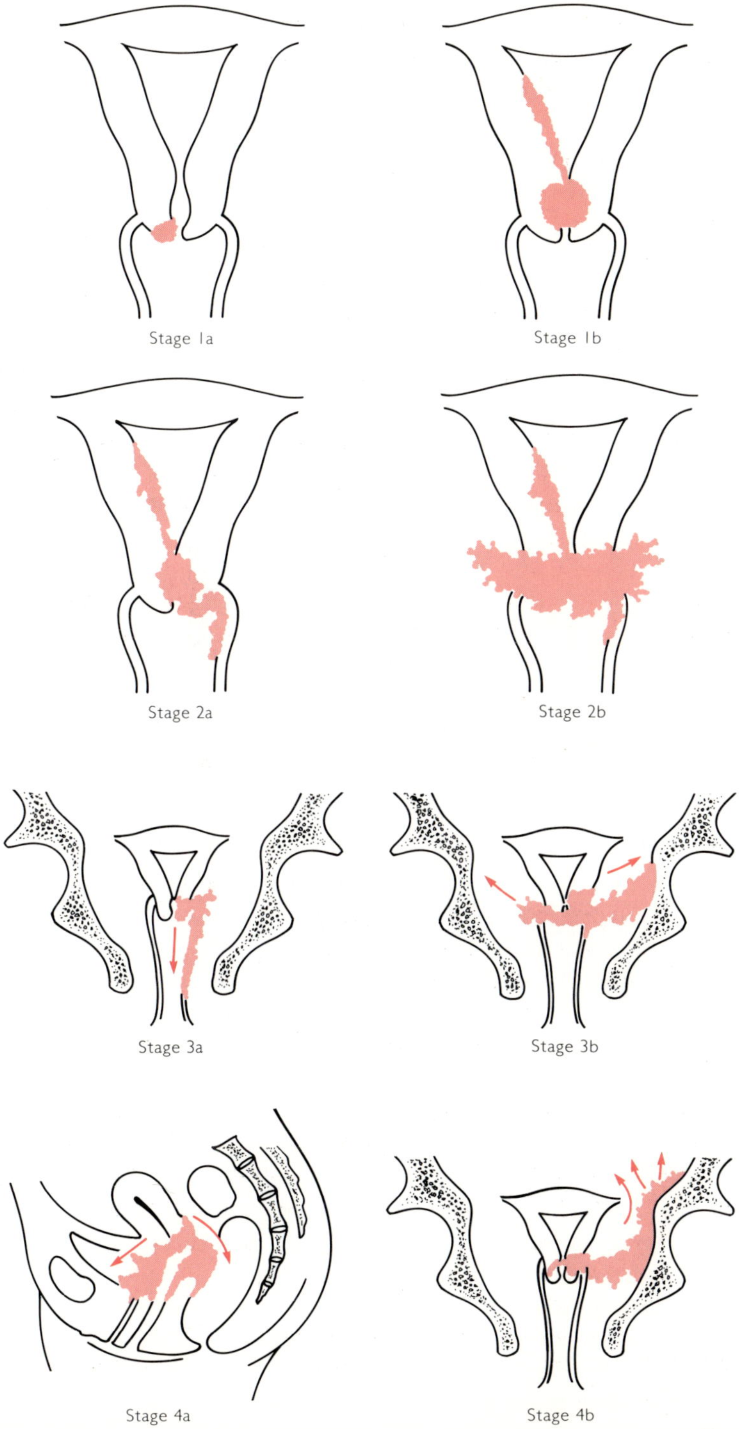

Stage 1: the growth is confined to the cervix. It has spread no further than the uterus

Stage 2: the cancer has spread from the cervix to the upper vagina. It does not extend to the lateral pelvic walls nor to the lower third of the vagina

Stage 3: the cancer has extended to the lateral pelvic wall or to the lower third of the vagina

Stage 4: there is involvement in the neighbouring organs, the bladder or the rectum, and in tissues outside the pelvis

Symptoms

The following symptoms may be present:

- abnormal or unusual bleeding, particularly following intercourse or vaginal examination and possibly a watery vaginal discharge are usually the only symptoms noticed by the woman, and these do not occur until the disease is well established.
- pain is a late sign and suggests invasion of the pelvic tissues and nerves
- urinary or faecal incontinence due to fistulae
- renal failure and uraemia due to constriction of the ureters.

Diagnosis

Cervical cytology: cells exfoliated from the cervix are examined. They are taken from the entire transformation zone (Figure 16.5) and from the posterior vaginal fornix. After staining, abnormal cells can be recognised under the microscope. If the smear is 'suspicious' or unclear, another smear is taken and the test repeated.

Figure 16.5
Papanicolaou smear, removing cells from the transformation zone of the cervix

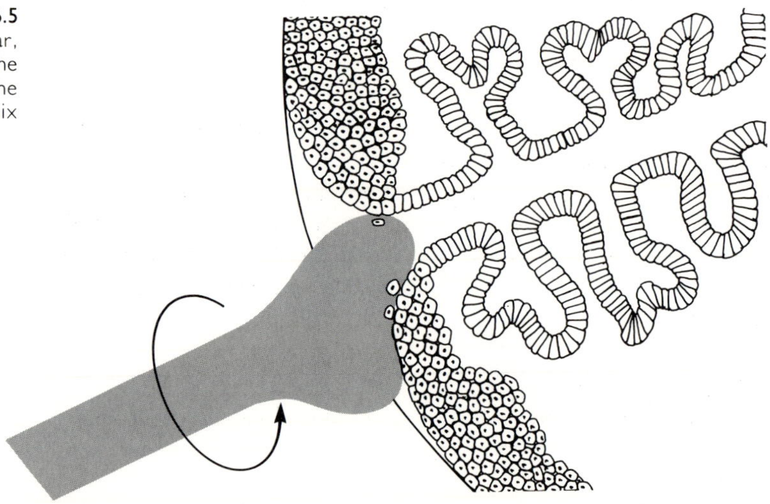

Schiller's test: this test involves painting the cervix and vagina with Lugol's iodine. Normal cells (containing glycogen) stain brown but the abnormal cells do not stain, and so indicate the sites from which biopsies should be taken.

Colposcopy is visualisation of the vagina and cervix using an illuminated magnifying instrument. It helps to differentiate between cervical erosions and atypical cells.

Biopsy of the cervix: either a punch biopsy, where small sections of suspicious area are removed, (see Figure 16.6), or a cone biopsy, which involves a circular tapering excision from the ectocervix to include the endocervical canal, is performed (see Figure 16.7). The

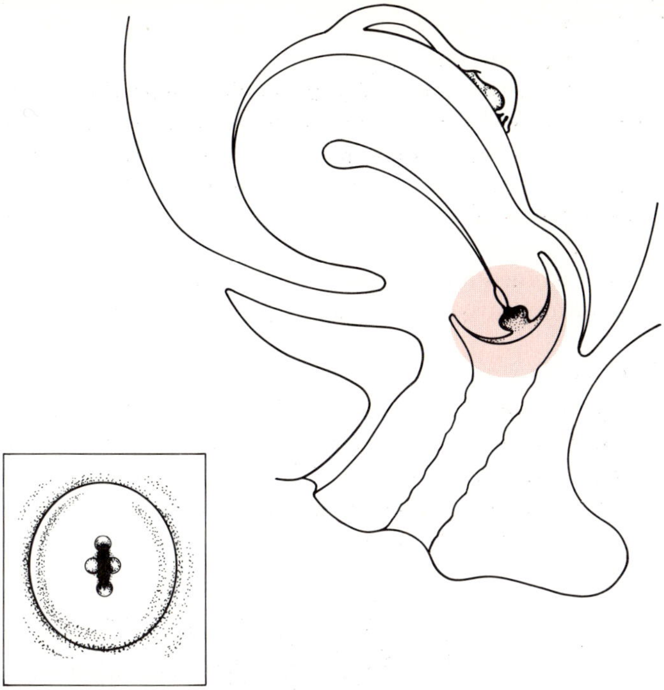

Figure 16.6
Sites for punch biopsy of the cervix

punch biopsy is done as an outpatient procedure and is relatively simple and without complications. A cone biopsy, on the other hand, involves admission to hospital and a general anaesthetic, and, although it is a more reliable biopsy, it can cause bleeding, lead to infection or result in cervical stricture. The tissues obtained at the biopsy are examined for malignant changes and, if positive, the degree of invasion or stage is assessed.

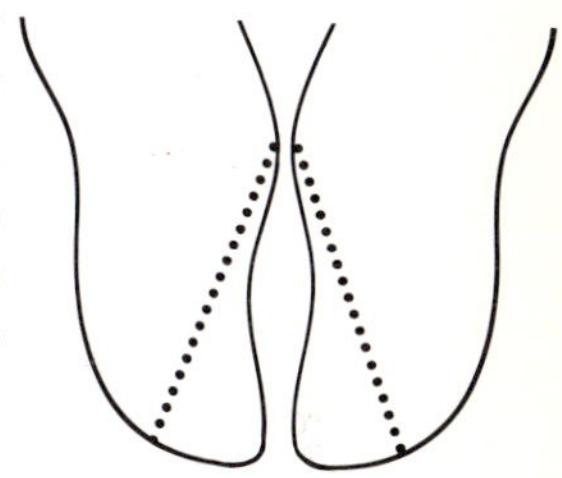

Figure 16.7
Cone biopsy specimen (shaded)

Treatment of cervical carcinoma

Treatment will depend on the stage of the disease.

Stage 0

If the woman is young and wants to have more children, a cone biopsy excision with follow-up cervical smear tests (every three months for the first year) may be all that is required. Any pregnancy which followed cone excision would need to be supervised by an experienced obstetrician and the delivery conducted in a well-equipped hospital. If the woman does not desire any further children, a total hysterectomy with removal of the upper vaginal cuff is performed. In some cases cautery or cryosurgery to the cervix is sufficient.

Stages I and II

Stage 1a may be treated by total hysterectomy. For Stages 1b and 2, intracavity irradiation, usually in the form of an insertion may be given, followed six weeks later by radical (Wertheim's) hysterectomy. The irradiation aims to destroy the primary growth and seal off the lymphatics, thus stopping the spread.

The operation of Wertheim's hysterectomy involves the removal of the uterus, tubes and ovaries, the pelvic connective tissue, the upper third of the vagina, and the regional (iliac) lymph nodes. The delay of six weeks before surgery is to allow the effects of irradiation to settle; increased vascularity and oedema will be present for three to five weeks and then fibrosis starts at about six to eight weeks following intracavity irradiation.

Stages III and IV

External irradiation is given, and is sometimes followed by intracavity irradiation. Where the bladder or rectum is involved, a pelvic exenteration operation (with diversion of the ureters and colon) is performed.

Intracavity irradiation

Preliminary admission: one week before insertion of the radioactive substance, the woman is admitted to hospital for a short (24-hr) stay during which she will undergo the following investigations:

- examination under anaesthesia, to assess the space available for the insertion
- intravenous pyelogram
- haemoglobin and blood urea investigation
- the taking of smears from the vagina and cervix to exclude infection
- chest X-ray.

The woman is given dietary instructions to follow so that a low-residue diet can be commenced two days before she is readmitted. Anaemia is corrected, by blood transfusion if necessary, and any infection is treated. At this stage it is extremely important to make sure that the woman and her family have been given a clear explanation about the coming procedure and what it will entail. If they are able to take a very positive approach to the aims of the treatment, the difficulties and discomforts involved will be made more bearable. Because the irradiation almost always causes the ovaries to cease functioning, the woman should be told that following the treatment she cannot expect to have any more children of her own, and in the light of this knowledge her consent to the treatment is obtained.

The woman is discharged, to be readmitted one week later.

Second admission (for insertion of the radioactive substance): on admission, the woman goes through a series of pre-operative preparation procedures including the usual pre-anaesthetic urinalysis, fasting and sedation.

Specific preparation will involve:

- shaving of the pubis, vulva and perineum
- a vaginal douche, if necessary, to clear the vagina of discharge
- an enema—by emptying the lower part of the bowel, the bowel itself is further from the radioactive substance and fistula formation is less likely. As well, the woman is less likely to need to use bed-pans with the associated danger of dislodging the insertion as she moves to get on and off the pans.

Insertion of the radioactive substance

The types of radioactive substance used, the dosage and the position and duration of the applicator(s) will vary according to the policies of different doctors or treatment centres. For example, caesium is most often used in Melbourne; cobalt and iodine are alternatives. The substance contained in special applicators is inserted in to the lateral vaginal fornices and the uterine cavity for a single period of five or six days or for two periods of three days each with a three-day interval between treatments. Figure 16.8 shows one method of intracavity irradiation. After-loading may be used for caesium insertions: the empty applicators are inserted in theatre as described, and the caesium loaded by machine into the applicators when the woman is back in the ward.

Figure 16.8
Intracavity irradiation

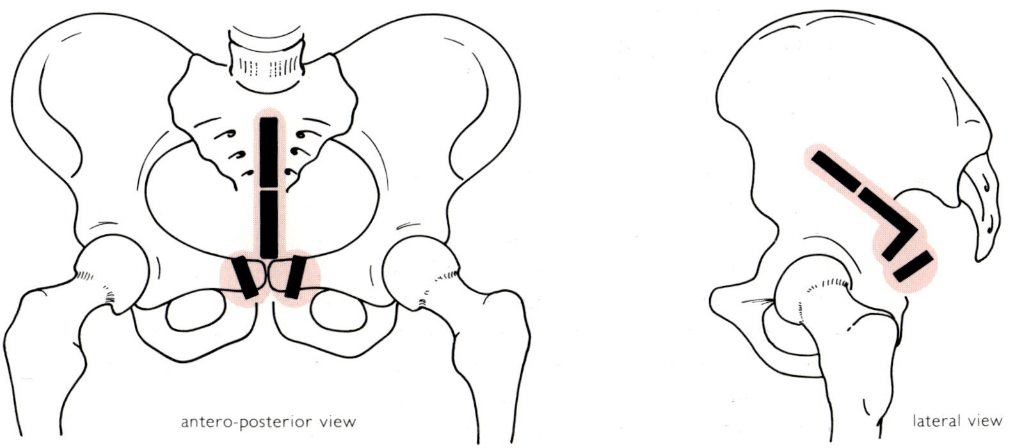

The applicators are inserted with the woman under general anaesthesia. The vagina is packed with gauze to help to keep the insertion in place and to protect the bladder and rectum from overdosage. Sometimes a perspex holding-device is used instead, or as well. Strings may be attached to the applicators; these are taped to the inner aspect of the thigh. An X-ray is taken at this point to check that the applicators have been correctly positioned.

Specific care after insertion

A bed will be prepared in a single room if possible. If the woman is to be nursed in a ward with other patients, the bed chosen should be one near to an outside wall and the bed next to it left unoccupied. If there are women of childbearing age in the ward, their beds may need to be moved, but without making a fuss. A radiation sign is placed on the door or bed. Long-handled sterile forceps are kept in the room to handle the radioactive insertion, should it fall out. A lead box is kept close by.

The woman is nursed on her back, with a maximum of three pillows. To avoid dislodging the applicator, her movement is restricted; she is allowed to turn on to her side for pressure care only. Careful attention is given to deep breathing and leg exercises.

Observations

Observations will include:

- four-hourly recording of temperature, pulse and respiration; temperature elevated over 37·8°C must be reported
- four-hourly check that the applicators are still in position and that there is no bleeding per vagina
- a fluid intake and output record is kept; oliguria should be watched for
- *severe* pain should be reported. Discomfort can be kept to a minimum by the regular use of effective oral analgesics; intramuscular analgesics should not be required after the first twenty-four hours
- nausea and vomiting are common but should always be reported.

Hygiene and comfort

A full sponge is given daily and pressure-area care is given at least four-hourly. The perineal area is swabbed down twice daily, and the perineal pad is changed at these times or more frequently if necessary. Only ointment that has been specifically prescribed should be used for vulval irritation. The woman will probably be concerned about odour from this area so attention to room ventilation and the provision of room deodorants is thoughtful. Vaginal deodorant sprays and talcum powder are *not* used during this period.

Diet

A low-residue diet is given. Small meals with high-protein and high-vitamin content are given. The meals should be attractive yet easy for the woman to manage from her semi-recumbent position. A variety of fluids is offered so that the fluid intake reaches three litres per day.

Bladder

Continuous urinary drainage via an indwelling urethral catheter is maintained for the duration of the treatment. Daily instillation of a suitable antiseptic solution may be ordered.

Bowels

The low-residue diet and the pre-insertion enema should confine the bowels until the treatment is completed. Loose stools, however, may occur and this could be an indication for early removal of the insertion. (If a bed-pan is used, a check should be made to ensure that the applicators have not been dislodged.) Antidiarrhoea medications may be ordered. Flatus causing discomfort may be relieved by insertion of a flatus tube.

Visitors

The comfort and support brought by her visitors are very important to the woman. She is often isolated, has the minimum number of staff involved in her care and can find it difficult to occupy her thoughts; her position and movements in bed are so restricted that she cannot even occupy her hands by knitting or writing. Visitors are asked to come—but not to stay for extended periods, nor to get closer to the insertion than two metres. They are advised not to come if they are pregnant, and should not bring young children.

Removal of the radioactive insertion

The date for removal will have been written in the patient's records. An explanation of the procedure should be given, so that the woman is not frightened. She is warned that the odour may be offensive, but that this is to be expected, and she will soon be able to shower. Sedation is usually given in time to take effect beforehand. The appropriate papers are gathered so that the number of applicators can be checked as they are removed. The urethral catheter is removed after instillation of antiseptic into the bladder. The vulva is swabbed and covered with a clean pad until the doctor is ready to remove the insertion.

The techniques for removal, cleaning and storage of the radioactive insertions and their applicators vary from place to place. The nurse should ensure that she is familiar with the local procedures before she is involved in these tasks. In every centre, however, the records of these materials are most important and must be accurate.

After care

Aftercare of the patient who has had a radioactive insertion involves douching with a weak solution of sodium bicarbonate, one hour after removal of the insertion. The return should be observed and any bleeding noticed. A bath or shower with assistance will be given a few hours later. The patient will be able to go home the next day if she is voiding well and has no bowel problems. She should continue her low-residue diet for a further three weeks.

After she has been discharged from hospital, she will continue to need daily douches for the first week, then every second day for the second week, then every third day for the third week. These will be given by a visiting nurse.

New growths of the body of the uterus

Benign growths

The two kinds of benign growths that can be found in the body of the uterus are endometrial polyps and fibromyomata.

Endometrial polyps

Endometrial polyps are small overgrowths of normal endometrium. They are frequently multiple, usually no larger than a pea and they are often associated with endometrial hyperplasia. They may protrude through the cervix.

Symptoms

- menorrhagia
- mild cramping pains
- bleeding between periods or postmenopausal bleeding

Treatment

When endometrial polyps are suspected, a dilatation and currettage is always performed. The polyps are removed by the curette or by avulsion—twisting the polyp on its pedicle.

As endometrial polyps can undergo degenerative and malignant changes, all of the currettings obtained, including polyps, are examined to exclude malignancy.

Fibromyomata

Fibromyomata (fibroids) are benign growths of fibrous and muscular tissue within the wall of the uterus. They are usually multiple and may vary in size from that of a very small seed to that of a large grapefruit. They are firm, usually round or oval in shape, and have a pseudocapsule. When cut across, the fibroids are pearly white, with the fibres arranged in a whorled pattern (Figures 16.9 and 16.10).

Fibroids are very common, occurring, it is believed, to some degree in almost all women. About 15 to 20 per cent of women show symptoms, usually in their mid-thirties. Fibroids very rarely arise after the menopause.

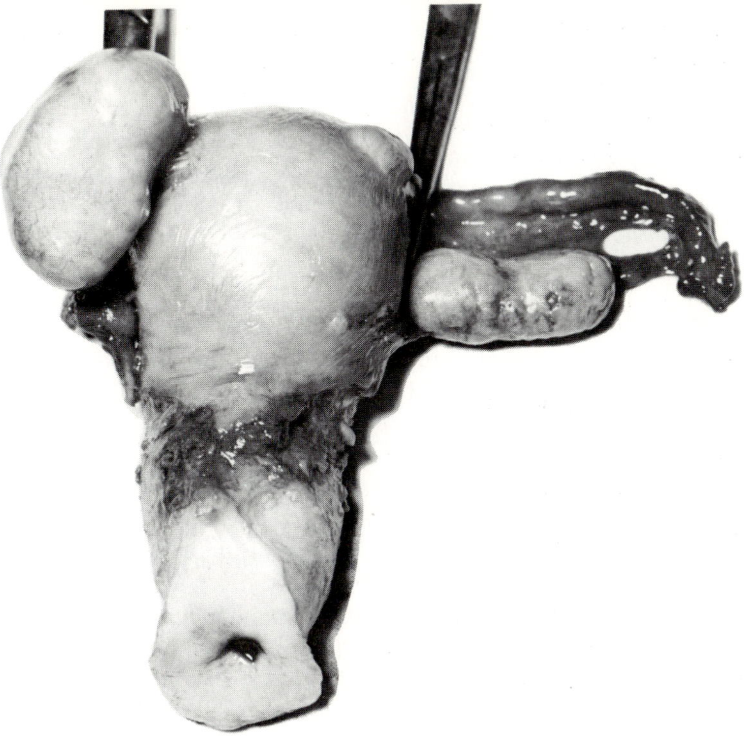

Figure 16.9
Hysterectomy specimen showing fibromyomata

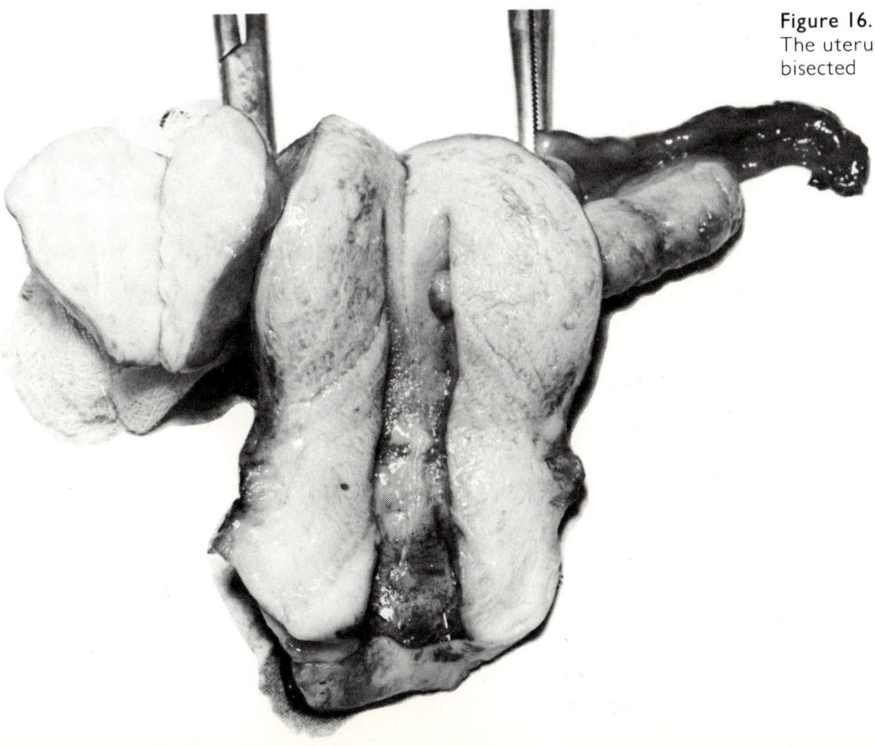

Figure 16.10
The uterus in Figure 16.9 bisected

Cause

The exact cause of fibroid growths is unknown, but there is a definite association with hormonal imbalance—an elevated production of oestrogen, or a lack of progesterone opposition. That fibroid growth is related to oestrogen levels is shown by their marked growth during pregnancy and also by their usual atrophy after the menopause.

Sites

Uterine fibroids arise in three main sites (Figure 16.11):

- just under the endometrium, ie *submucous* fibroids, which bulge into the uterine cavity and enlarge its surface area. Sometimes they pedunculate to become fibrous polyps
- within the myometrium, ie *interstitial* fibroids, where they can enlarge without really affecting the endometrial cavity, but where they are likely to interfere with the contractions of the uterus
- just below the outer (peritoneal) layer of the uterus, ie *subserous* fibroids, which will project away from the uterus and may press upon adjacent organs. Subserous fibroids may become pedunculated and grow out into the abdominal or pelvic cavity.

Fibroids may also develop in the pelvic ligaments and within the cervix.

Figure 16.11
Sites of uterine fibroids

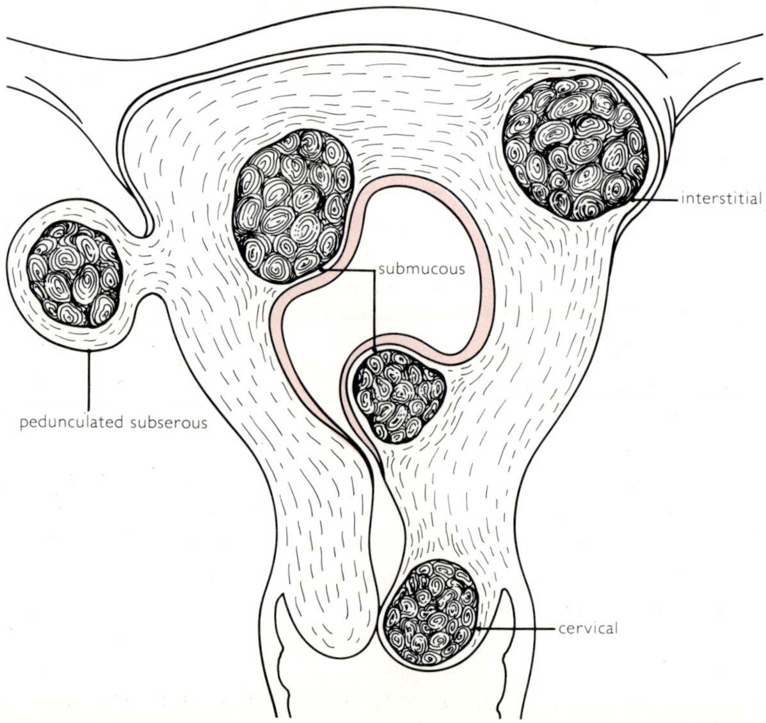

Complications

Degeneration may occur and is usually due to interference with the fibroids' blood supply, eg torsion of a pedicle, pressure upon the blood vessels, or excessive enlargement of the fibroid (during pregnancy).

Hyaline degeneration can occur, with the muscle fibres being replaced by hyaline connective tissue and, if extensive, with liquid forming in the centre of the hyalinised area leading to cystic degeneration. This can in turn lead to calcification—'womb stones'.

Red degeneration is usually seen only in pregnancy. The fibroid is large, dark red (from haemorrhage into the substance of the fibroid) and causes considerable pain.

Malignancy: a uterine fibroid may undergo sarcomatous changes, but this is quite rare.

Signs and symptoms

Signs and symptoms depend upon the number, location and size of the fibroid growths. Many fibroids cause no symptoms and are discovered incidentally on routine pelvic examination. The following symptoms may be present:

Swelling: the woman may see or feel a swelling in the lower abdomen.

Menorrhagia may occur and is due to:

- an increased endometrial (bleeding) surface
- interference with uterine contractions
- the associated elevated or unopposed oestrogen levels, which encourage endometrial hyperplasia.

The menorrhagia is often accompanied by clots; it may lead to anaemia.

Pressure symptoms: fibroids causing pressure on the bladder can limit its capacity and thus cause frequency of micturition. Pressure against the rectal wall may result in difficulty in bowel evacuation. Backache can be troublesome when there is pressure from a fibroid upon pelvic nerve plexuses.

Infertility: fibroids are more common in nulliparous women or women with only one child. The lowered fertility is probably associated with distortion of the uterine cavity by submucous fibroids or to the state of hormonal imbalance.

Pregnancy complications: when pregnancy does occur, the presence of large fibroids may be the cause of habitual abortion, premature labour, or obstruction to the birth canal. As mentioned before, red degeneration of fibroids can occur during pregnancy and can cause considerable pain.

Treatment

Treatment is usually given only when the fibroids are large or causing symptoms. Iron replacement is given if there is a lowered haemoglobin level as a result of menorrhagia. Hormone therapy may be ordered to suppress or balance excessive oestrogen levels.

Surgical treatment may be necessary. Choice of operation depends largely on the age of the woman, her desire (or otherwise) for more children and the size, number, and accessibility of the fibroids. The operation may be:

Myomectomy: the fibroids are shelled out of their pseudocapsules, and the uterus is thus retained for childbearing purposes. (In the treatment of infertility, a myomectomy would be done only when all the other factors necessary for conception are proved to be present.) Myomectomy removes the symptom-causing fibroids, but adhesions may result and small fibroids can be missed with the possibility of recurrence of growth, as happens in about 10 per cent of cases.

Hysterectomy: removal of the uterus is performed when the woman is over forty years of age, when the uterus is no longer required for childbearing, and for inaccessible fibroids, eg in the broad ligament and cervix. As the uterus is usually enlarged, the operation is done via the abdominal route.

Malignant growths

Carcinoma of the endometrium (adenocarcinoma)

Malignant changes originating in the glandular epithelium of the endometrium are referred to as carcinoma of the body of the uterus. This is the second most common cancer in the female genital tract, the incidence being nearly one-half of that of cervical cancer.

Carcinoma of the endometrium is more often found in woman aged fifty-five to sixty-five years, although it is seen occasionally in younger women. It is far more common in women who have few if any children—in about 30 per cent of cases, the patient is nulliparous.

Causes

No definite cause is known. There is a familial tendency towards the disease. Carcinoma of the endometrium is often associated with a higher than average production of oestrogen. It may be preceded by endometrial hyperplasia, especially if this occurs at the time of the climacteric and afterwards. The menopause has usually occurred comparatively late.

Obesity, hypertension and diabetes are also associated factors. These conditions (plus the fact that the woman is usually not young) increase the risks of surgery and make post-operative complications such as infection, chest complications and venous thromboses more likely.

Spread

Invasive carcinoma of the endometrium is believed to be preceded by a carcinoma in situ which, unlike that of the cervix, sometimes remains dormant and may even be reversible.

Direct spread occurs by extension of the growth along the endometrial surface and, as well, into the myometrium. Further spread can then involve the cervix and vagina. Cells may also spread along the fallopian tubes and thus involve the ovaries and peritoneum.

Indirect spread occurs late, via the myometrial lymph channels to the pelvic and para-aortic lymph glands.

Blood-born spread is rare, but sometimes metastases occur in the lungs. liver and lower vagina.

Signs and symptoms

Irregular spotting or bleeding, especially postmenopausal bleeding, is the first and major sign and must never be ignored. Even though bleeding occurs comparatively early in this condition widespread education is needed if women are to appreciate the importance of seeking advice promptly.

A clear brown watery discharge with an offensive odour may appear.

Pain is rare, but may occur when the cervix is stenosed and the uterus becomes filled with pus or blood.

Very occasionally, suspicious endometrial cells are discovered on a routine Papanicolaou smear.

Investigations

All postmenopausal women who suffer from hypertension, obesity, or diabetes or who have a family history of carcinoma should be regularly 'screened' by endometrial aspiration or lavage which can be performed as a simple outpatient procedure.

When there has been bleeding, a 'fractional' curettage of the cervix and uterus is done. The curetting is done systematically, starting with the endocervical canal and progressing upwards to the fundus, and the specimens placed separately into carefully labelled containers. This system aims to show both the location of the growth and whether or not the cervix is involved.

A complete physical examination is carried out, to exclude other medical conditions, eg diabetes.

Treatment

If the carcinoma has spread to the cervical canal, the treatment is the same as that for carcinoma of the cervix because of the probable pelvic lymph gland involvement.

Surgical treatment: where the growth is confined to the body of the uterus, a total hysterectomy with bilateral salpingo-oophorectomy is performed. The upper third of the vagina is removed to prevent vaginal vault recurrences.

Irradiation is often used in conjunction with surgery, either as insertions into the uterine cavity and vaginal vault six weeks before surgery, or post-operatively (after healing) as implants into the vaginal vault. Irradiation without surgery is used in those cases where the woman is a very poor operative risk, where the carcinoma has been discovered incidentally after a simple hysterectomy, or where vaginal vault recurrence has occurred.

Hormone therapy: progestogens, because of their effect of opposing oestrogenic activity, are used to inhibit cell division and so control the growth. They are given in large doses initially, for advanced growths, and must be continued for the rest of the woman's life. Some doctors prescribe smaller doses of progestogens routinely for the full twelve months following hysterectomy for carcinoma of the body of the uterus.

Fallopian tubes

Benign tumours and primary carcinoma of the fallopian tubes are very rare. When primary carcinoma does occur, it spreads early in the course of the disease to the peritoneal cavity and into the lymphatic system. Secondary carcinoma is more common and results from the direct extension of an endometrial or ovarian growth.

Broad ligaments

Cysts may arise from the remnants of the mesonephric duct or from the epoophoron (mesovarium). The cysts can grow extremely large, filling the abdominal cavity and causing pressure symptoms. They do not become malignant, and are treated by simple excision.

Ovaries

Ovarian tumours may be cystic or solid, and either type may be benign or malignant. About 20 per cent of the ovarian tumours discovered are malignant. Many of the new growths arising within the ovaries are symptom-free for a long time. They may enlarge considerably but because the ovary is insensitive to stretch, pain is usually absent. Abdominal enlargement can be attributed to 'middle-age spread' or to overeating.

Pain does occur at times, but this is usually associated with complications such as infection, adhesions, rupture of a cyst, torsion of a pedicle or haemorrhage into the cyst. Symptomless ovarian cysts are often discovered during a routine gynaecological check-up, providing further proof of the importance of these examinations for women of *all* ages. (Any ovary that is easily felt on pelvic examination is probably abnormal.) If discovered and removed early the cysts cannot progress to malignancy.

Types of ovarian tumours

Retention cysts

Follicular cysts occur when the graffian follicle fails to rupture. They are associated with excessive FSH stimulation. Menstrual irregularities and menorrhagia may result.

Corpus luteum cysts

These arise when the corpus luteum fails to degenerate; it continues to produce progesterone and so causes amenorrhoea.

Teratomata

These may be benign or malignant. The commonest benign teratomata are *dermoid cysts*, which are derived mainly from embryonic ectoderm and may contain sebaceous fluid, hair and teeth. The cysts are usually unilateral and are seen mostly in women between the ages of twenty and thirty-five years. (Figure 16.12.)

Malignant teratomata are solid tumours occurring mainly in young girls. The cells divide very rapidly and the malignancy spreads quickly via the bloodstream to the lungs.

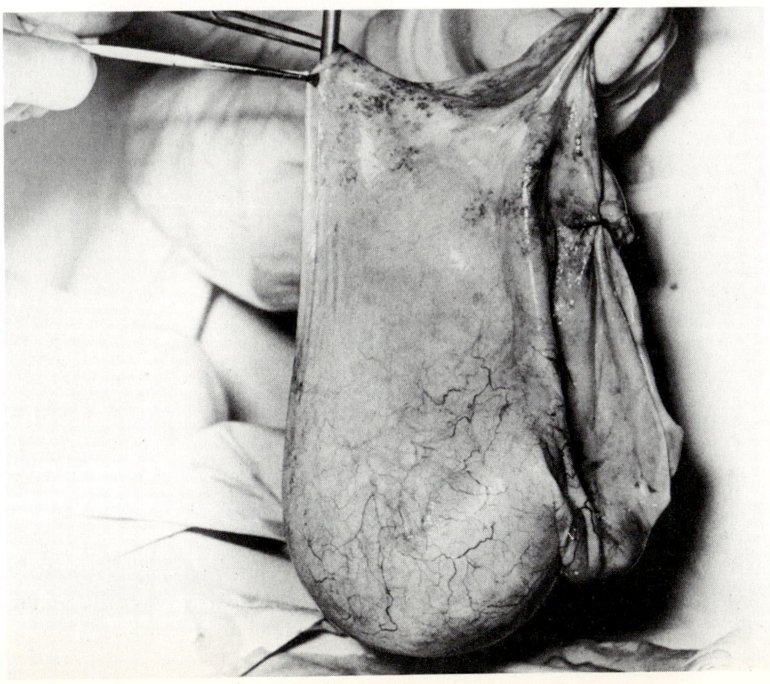

Figure 16.12
A dermoid cyst (teratoma) of the ovary, which had contained 4.5 litres of fluid. It was removed from a young woman aged 24 years

Polycystic ovaries

Both ovaries are enlarged and the cortex contains multiple small follicular cysts, which are not true tumours but are due to an endocrine disturbance. Associated amenorrhoea, anovulation and hirsutism make up the Stein-Leventhal syndrome (see page 99).

Endometrial cysts

These are deposits of endometrium filled with old blood, and appearing as 'chocolate cysts'. They are common on the ovaries as part of endometriosis.

Serous cystadenomata

These are common single-cavity ovarian cysts, filled with a watery serous fluid. They are often bilateral and occur in the thirty to forty age group. Serous cystadenomata occasionally develop papillary processes on their walls. These cysts, although classed as benign, are considered to be potentially malignant.

Mucinous cystadenomata

These are large, usually multicavity ovarian cysts, filled with a thick fluid resembling mucin. They continue to grow and may become

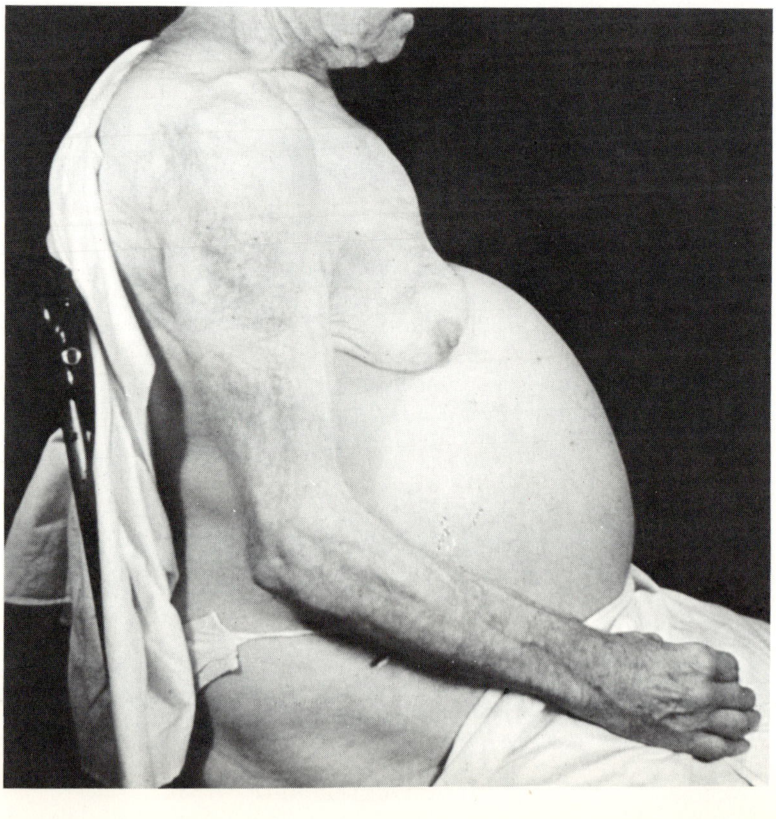

Figure 16.13
Pre-operative photograph of a woman with a large abdominal mass which had been present for several years

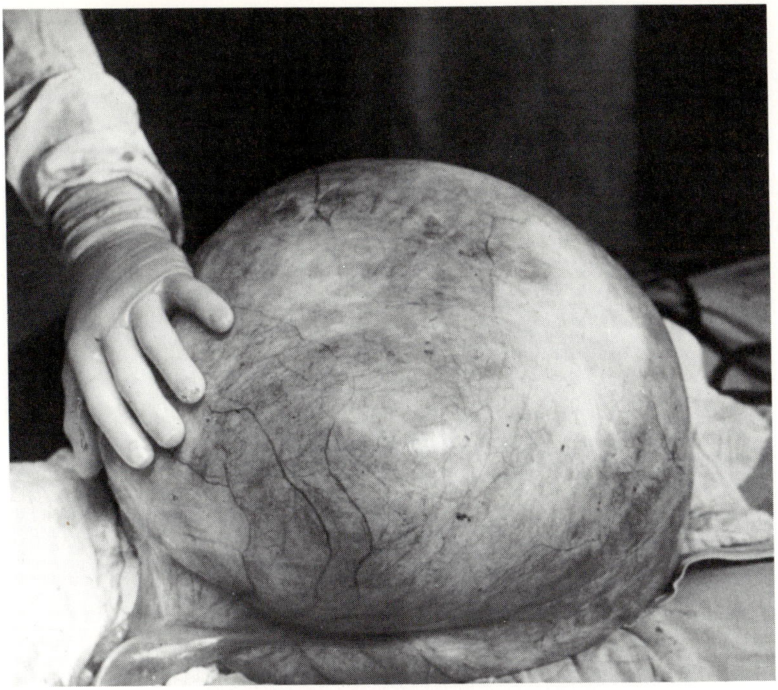

Figure 16.14
Laparotomy on the patient shown in Figure 16.13 revealed an enormous benign fluid-filled ovarian tumour

immense (see Figures 16.13 and 16.14), to occupy the whole peritoneal cavity, and even cause difficulty with walking and breathing. The cysts tend to be unilateral and generally occur later in life, around sixty years of age. They are also potentially malignant if there has been papillary development.

Ovarian fibromata

These are small, solid and hard, white benign tumours. They occur in women aged around forty years, and are usually unilateral. Ascites and pleural effusion may be associated with ovarian fibromata—Meigs' syndrome. Removal of the fibroma results in the spontaneous cure of the condition.

Hormone-producing tumours

Feminising tumours, affecting the granulosa and theca cells, cause excessive oestrogen production. They may occur at any age, causing precocious puberty in children, cyclic disturbance and menorrhagia during the reproductive years, and postmenopausal bleeding in older women. Malignancy occurs in about 25 per cent of these tumours.

Virilising tumours of the ovary, of which arrhenoblastoma is the most common, cause virilising changes due to the production of significant amounts of androgens by the tumour cells. Atrophy occurs in the genital organs and the breasts. Scanty periods occur and are followed by amenorrhoea. The clitoris may enlarge and there may be hirsutes, skin problems and deepening of the voice. These tumours become malignant in about 20 per cent of cases.

Carcinoma of the ovary

Primary carcinoma may occur at any age but is more likely to arise in women around fifty to sixty years old. It spreads rapidly, mainly by seeding directly into the peritoneal cavity.
Secondary carcinoma is due to metastases from other organs, especially the uterus, stomach, intestines and breasts.

Treatment of ovarian tumours

Treatment depends upon the extent of ovarian enlargement when it is first discovered, upon associated symptoms (if any) and upon the woman's age.

Surgery

Some doctors will perform a diagnostic laparoscopy and may remove tissue for biopsy or aspirate cystic fluid for cytological examination. In most cases, however the doctor will operate to excise the tumour. The cyst may be able to be removed from the ovary, leaving ovarian tissue to function. Polycystic ovaries are treated by Wedge resection. If there is any suspicion of malignancy, both ovaries are completely removed and the uterus and the omentum are removed as well. Very large fluid-filled cysts are sometimes tapped first to drain off most of the fluid. This relieves the pressure symptoms and enables the operation to be performed through a relatively small incision.

Radiotherapy and chemotherapy

Radiotherapy is sometimes used to inhibit malignant tumour growth.

In some cases of carcinoma of the ovary, there has been good response to certain cytotoxic drugs, some of which can be applied locally through a tube into the peritoneal cavity, or can be given by injection or orally. Chlorambucil is frequently the drug chosen as its side effects are less toxic than many of the other drugs available.

Early detection

Malignant growths of the genital tract have been known to regress spontaneously, possibly because of some immunological resistance to the tumour cells. These cases are, however, very much the exception to the rule. The most sure way of preventing death or suffering from pelvic malignancies is by their early detection.

Annual pelvic examination, cervical cytology smears, and immediate attention to abnormal bleeding or discharge must be encouraged by every person involved in health care. Cervical and endometrial carcinoma need never become invasive, and ovarian tumours could, in many cases, be found and removed *before* malignant changes occur in benign growths.

17 Endometriosis

Endometriosis is *ectopic endometrium*, that is, functioning endometrium which is in a site other than the lining of the uterus. The deposits of ectopic endometrial tissue (covered by stroma) follow the same pattern of proliferation, becoming secretory, and breaking down and bleeding as the normally situated endometrium does in response to ovarian hormone stimulation during the menstrual cycle. In most cases of endometriosis, however, there is no escape route for the blood flow, so it becomes trapped and small dark blood-filled cysts are formed. Some of the blood serum is absorbed between menstruations, leaving a thick tarry fluid which resembles chocolate—'chocolate cysts'. Endometriosis may occur within the uterine muscle wall, *adenomyosis*, or it may be scattered throughout the pelvic cavity and occasionally beyond it, *extra-uterine endometriosis*. Endometriosis only rarely undergoes malignant changes.

Adenomyosis

This condition usually affects the thirty to forty years age group and is more commonly seen in parous women. The endometrial deposits are spread throughout the myometrium, and lie between the muscle fibres. Cells from the basal layer of the endometrium extend downwards to infiltrate the muscle tissue; the uterus enlarges and its muscular contractions are interfered with. Menorrhagia, dysmenorrhoea and pelvic pain may result.

The management of adenomyosis follows the same lines as that for extra-uterine endometriosis, but with one exception—conservative surgery is not attempted because it is almost impossible to successfully remove individual deposits from the myometrium.

Extra-uterine endometriosis

This occurs more commonly in nulliparae or in women who have only one or two children. The predisposing factor for the establishment of extra-uterine endometrial deposits seems to be a history of long spells of uninterrupted menstrual cycles. Where pregnancies have occurred, they have usually been at a relatively late age.

Sites

The commonest sites are the ovaries, the pelvic peritoneum, the uterosacral ligaments, the pouch of Douglas, the lower bowel, vagina and the rectovaginal septum (see Figure 17.1).

Less common sites include the appendix, umbilicus, abdominal wounds, bladder and extra-pelvic sites such as lymph nodes, the lungs and the breasts.

Dense adhesions may occur around the endometrial deposits, causing distortion of the pelvic organs and disturbances of function.

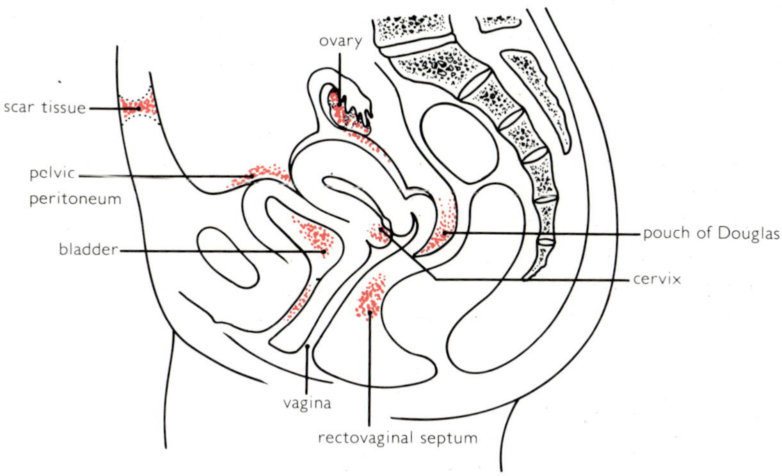

Figure 17.1
Sites of extra-uterine endometriosis

Symptoms

Dysmenorrhoea: secondary congestive dysmenorrhoea with pain felt both during the one or two weeks preceding menstruation (as the deposits enlarge) and for the whole duration of the flow.

Dyspareunia: deep dyspareunia occurs when the deposits are in the pouch of Douglas, and the rectovaginal septum.

Menorrhagia and irregular periods are due to disturbances of hormone production by affected ovaries. There is also pelvic congestion from an increased blood supply.

Bowel disorders may arise where there is colonic involvement, either by deposits or adhesions.

Infertility is common and could be due to disturbed ovarian function, or to adhesions causing displacement and immobility of the tubes, or fixed retroversion of the uterus. Thirty to 40 per cent of infertile women are found to have some degree of endometriosis.

Diagnosis

Diagnosis is based on the clinical history and from pelvic examination preferably done in the premenstrual week. Examination under anaesthetic and ultrasound may be used. Laparoscopy will confirm the diagnosis but may be difficult to perform because of adhesions.

Causes

Although the exact cause is unknown, endometriosis is most likely to be primarily due to retrograde menstruation, where uterine contractions or reverse tubal peristalsis may force endometrial tissue through the fallopian tubes and out into the peritoneal cavity. The tissue would fall first on to the ovaries, then on to the peritoneum, especially that portion which covers the uterosacral ligaments and the pouch of Douglas. Endometriosis may be spread during pelvic or abdominal surgery and deposits are sometimes seen in scar tissue. Endometrial fragments may be carried through the lymphatic or vascular systems as emboli.

Treatment

General

Suitable non-habit-forming analgesics and local warmth are recommended for dysmenorrhoea. Iron replacement may be required where menorrhagia has been a problem.

Hormonal treatment

As it is known that endometriosis regresses and often disappears during pregnancy, progestogens or oral contraceptives are given to create a pseudopregnancy. The treatment is given continuously for at least six months, producing a decidual reaction in the endometrial tissue and atrophy in the cysts. In this way the endometriosis may die down, but adhesions may continue to cause symptoms. Another hormonal drug, danocrine, which acts in a similar way is reserved mainly for those trying to achieve a pregnancy as it is very expensive.

Sometimes there may be unacceptable side effects from the hormonal treatment (eg marked depression from progestogen; masculinising changes from danocrine); in such cases surgical treatment may be preferable.

Conservative surgery

Endometrial deposits from the ovaries, uterus and any other accessible area are excised, while conserving the reproductive organs. Adhesions are divided and the round ligaments shortened to keep the uterus anteverted (ventrosuspension). A presacral neurectomy may be performed when deep and painful deposits cannot be removed.

Radical surgery

When other methods have proved unsuitable, and particularly towards the end of the childbearing years, total hysterectomy with bilateral salpingo-oophorectomy may prove to be the best way of relieving the symptoms of endometriosis. Following ovarian removal the condition will disappear and hormonal replacement therapy can be given without fear of reactivating the endometriosis.

Irradiation

Irradiation to cause the cessation of ovarian function may be indicated when excision is too difficult or when there is a danger of damaging important nearby structures.

18 Displacements of the pelvic organs

Retroversion of the uterus

The uterus in maturity is normally anteverted and slightly anteflexed, and it can be made to move in all directions. The cervix of the anteverted uterus projects into the posterior vaginal fornix and is thus immediately accessible to spermatozoa deposited there. The anteversion also permits the growth of the pregnant uterus upwards and out of the pelvic cavity without the danger of becoming caught (incarcerated) under the sacral promontory. In about 20 per cent of women, the uterus is retroverted or turned backwards (Figure 18.1). Because retroflexion (of the uterine body from the cervix) very often accompanies retroversion, the term 'retroversion' is commonly used to include both backward turning and backward flexion of the uterus. The fundus of the retroverted uterus will lie in the pouch of Douglas and can be felt through the posterior fornix, on vaginal examination.

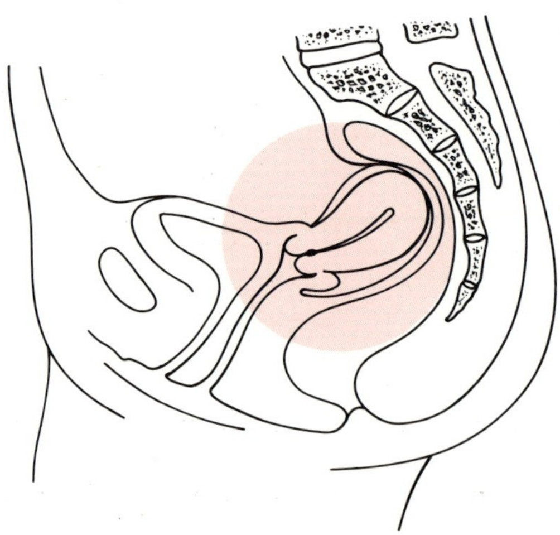

Figure 18.1
Uterine retroversion

Causes

Retroversion may be *developmental* and be due to the failure of the uterus to turn forward when the fundus grows rapidly to its adult size at the time of puberty. Sometimes there is an inherent laxity of the pelvic supports. In these cases the uterus is not fixed; it remains mobile and can be manipulated forward, although it will probably retrovert again if not supported in the anteverted position.

Acquired retroversion may occur following childbirth, when the pelvic supports, having been stretched and weakened, are ineffective in holding the uterus forwards. In most cases this will spontaneously correct itself within two or three months unless the uterus was retroverted before the pregnancy began.

Fixed retroversion is caused by the presence of some other condition in the pelvis. Tumours such as fibroids or cysts may push the uterus backwards; adhesions or endometriosis (in the pouch of Douglas) may pull the uterus backwards.

Symptoms

Retroversion in itself causes few symptoms. The underlying causes of the fixed retroversion are responsible for any symptoms that do arise. Many doctors do not tell a woman when she has a simple mobile retroversion because of a tendency, in the past at least, of many women to discover all sorts of symptoms once they found out that they had 'something wrong inside'.

Dyspareunia may occur when the ovaries have prolapsed and lie in the pouch of Douglas. The dyspareunia is deep and may be severe, and aching in the pelvis may continue for several hours after intercourse.

Backache may occur because of the increased tension upon the uterosacral ligaments as the cervix pulls them forward.

Infertility is probably never directly caused by retroversion itself, but the retroverted uterus, with its cervical os pointing towards (and sometimes almost occluded by) the anterior vaginal wall is less accessible to spermatozoa deposited in the posterior fornix. Surgical correction of the condition to improve fertility is usually only done after all other possible causes for the infertility have been excluded.

Abortion and incarceration of the pregnant uterus with acute retention of urine are very rare complications of retroversion. In the majority of cases, the pregnant uterus will grow out of the pelvis without mishap.

Figure 18.2
Hodge pessary in position

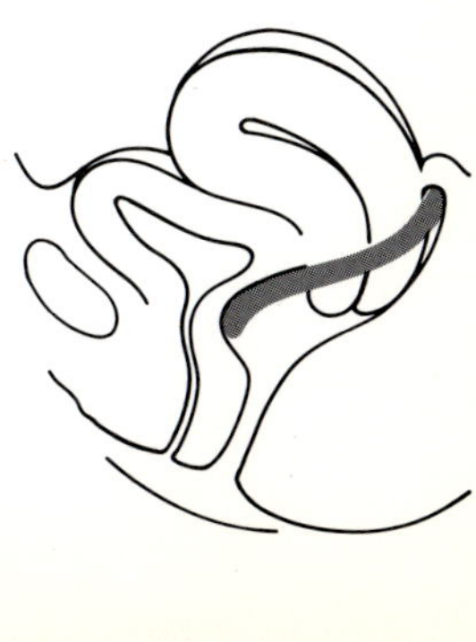

Treatment

Treatment for retroversion of the uterus will depend on whether the uterus is fixed or mobile. The doctor determines the mobility or otherwise by attempting to move the cervix backwards and push the fundus forwards.

'Pessary test' treatment

Successful manipulation of a mobile uterus is usually followed by the insertion of a special oblong-shaped device, the Hodge pessary (Figure 18.2). This maintains the anteverted position but does not cure the basic retroversion; when the pessary is removed the uterus usually becomes retroverted again. The pessary should not be felt while in position. It is worn for about six weeks. If it has not relieved the woman's symptoms, they are unlikely to be due to the retroversion and so further investigations are made. If the pessary has given relief from the symptoms and these symptoms return again after the pessary is removed, surgical correction of the retroversion is indicated.

Operative treatment

The uterus is brought forward and the round ligaments are shortened. There are several techniques to achieve this, but they all come under the heading 'ventrosuspension' (holding forward) operations.

Inversion of the uterus

Acute inversion (turning inside out) of the uterus is a rare and dangerous immediate postpartum complication, usually caused by the excessive use of fundal pressure or cord traction to deliver the placenta. Severe shock usually arises; it is an obstetrical emergency.

Chronic inversion of the uterus may arise gradually from an unnoticed partial inversion following childbirth. It may also result from the uterus itself attempting to expel a securely fixed tumour such as a pedunculated intracavity fibroid. Sometimes it arises spontaneously in old age as a result of laxity of the uterine supports, especially following cervical amputation operations.

The symptoms of chronic inversion are irregular or unusual vaginal bleeding and a feeling of something coming down in the vagina. After diagnosis, the treatment is surgical, either repositioning (if a partial inversion) or removal of the uterus. Because infection is almost always present, the surgery may be preceded by several days bed rest and antiseptic vaginal packing to minimise post-operative complications.

Uterovaginal prolapse

Prolapse means 'a falling or slipping downwards'. In gynaecology it refers to either the descent of the uterus into, or through, the vagina or to the herniation or 'bulging' of the structures adjacent to the vagina, into the vagina. The vaginal walls may prolapse without associated descent of the uterus, but a uterine prolapse is always accompanied by the prolapse of at least the upper part of the vagina. Prolapse occurs most often in parous women who have reached the age of the menopause.

Causes

Prolapse occurs when there is weakness of the structures that support the pelvic organs in their normal positions. It is made worse by any prolonged or constant increase in intra-abdominal pressure.

Weakening of the pelvic supports may be due to:

Congenital laxity of the fibromuscular tissues. This might not become evident until after the woman has borne children or until after the climacteric with its attendant atrophy of the pelvic tissues.

The effects of pregnancy and labour, after which the stretched muscular and fibrous tissues of the pelvis and vagina never completely regain their former tone. Repeated pregnancies, close together, give these tissues little chance to recover. Unnoticed or poorly repaired vaginal tears and the failure to do an episiotomy for a prolonged second stage can both lead to loss of support from the perineal body (Figure 18.3).

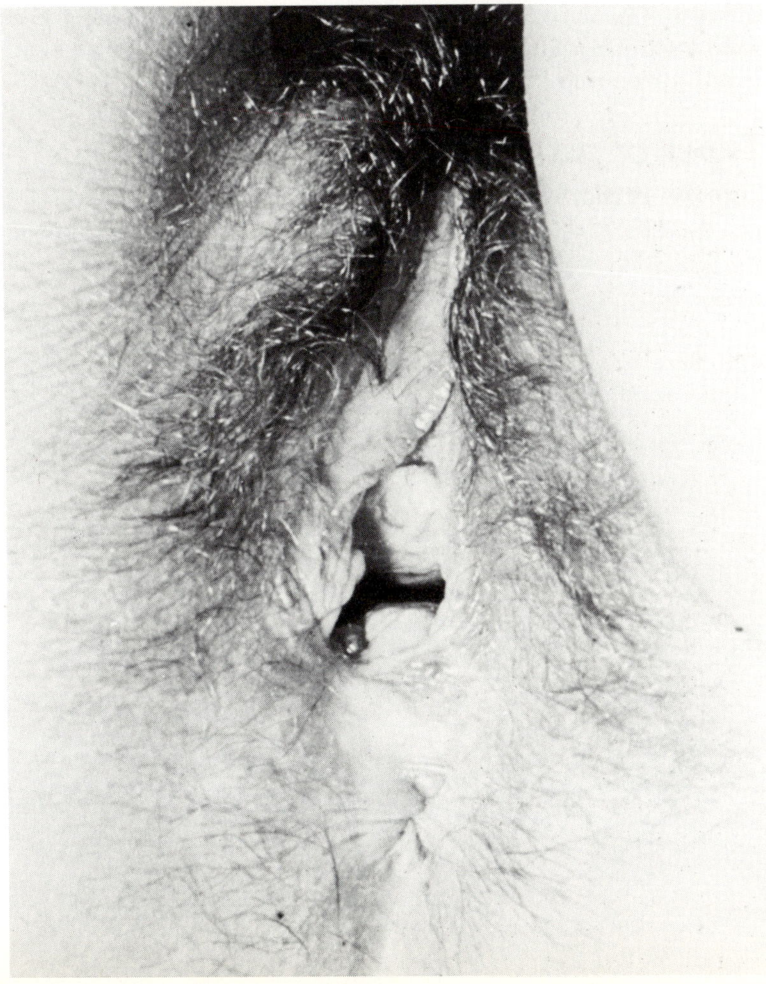

Figure 18.3
Badly-healed episiotomy

Age: the pelvic tissues are dependent upon oestrogen for their health and vitality. When the tisses become slack postmenopausally, there is less support for the uterus and vagina. Increased intra-abdominal pressure due, for example, to chronic coughing, obesity, a large abdominal tumour or 'straining' because of chronic constipation, causes pressure upon, and eventual weakening of, the pelvic floor. It also, of course, worsens any existing weakness.

Prevention of uterovaginal prolapse

The attention now given to providing good antenatal, labour and postnatal care will almost certainly result in a great reduction in the incidence of prolapse in the years to come. The use of well-timed episiotomies in the case of prolonged second stage, especially if the baby is expected to be large, education and supervision of postnatal exercises, and impressing the need for sufficient rest and recovery from each childbirth experience are all important points in which nurses are involved. In addition, we can be alert for evidence of those conditions that cause increased intra-abdominal pressure and direct attention to these conditions so that they may be relieved.

Types of prolapse

Uterine prolapse

The uterus descends into the vagina because of weakness of the uterosacral and cardinal ligaments. There are three degrees of uterine prolapse:

First degree: the uterus has descended slightly, is often retroverted, and there is usually some elongation of the cervix. The cervix remains inside the vagina.

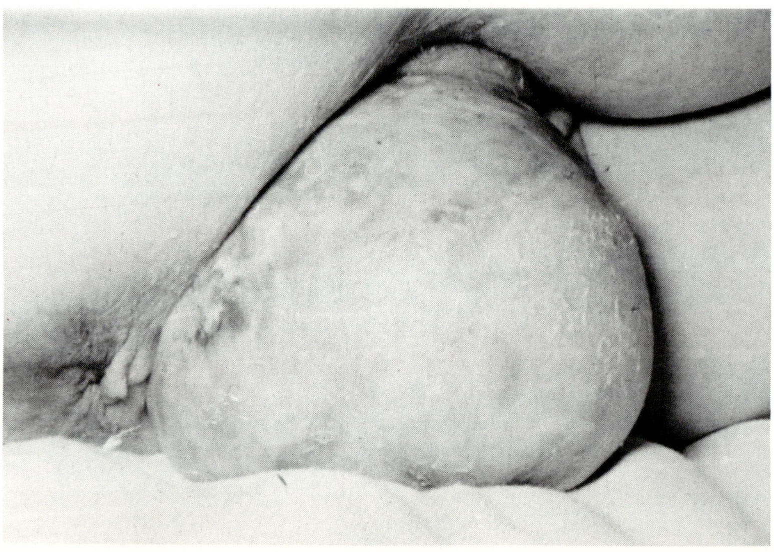

Figure 18.4
Complete (third degree) prolapse of the uterus—procidentia. The exposed epithelium is dry and cracked, and prone to ulceration

Second degree: the cervix protrudes from the vulva. It may become ulcerated due to its exposure to air, friction and to interference with its normal circulation.
Third degree: (procidentia): the uterus is completely outside the vulva, and the vagina is completely inverted (Figure 18.4).

Vaginal prolapse

Because of their closely connecting fascia, any weakening and descent of the vaginal walls will cause the adjacent organs to descend with them (see Figure 18.5). The type of prolapse is thus named according to the organ lying behind it. Herniation is seen when the woman pushes down.

Figure 18.5
Displacements of the pelvic organs (genital tract prolapse)

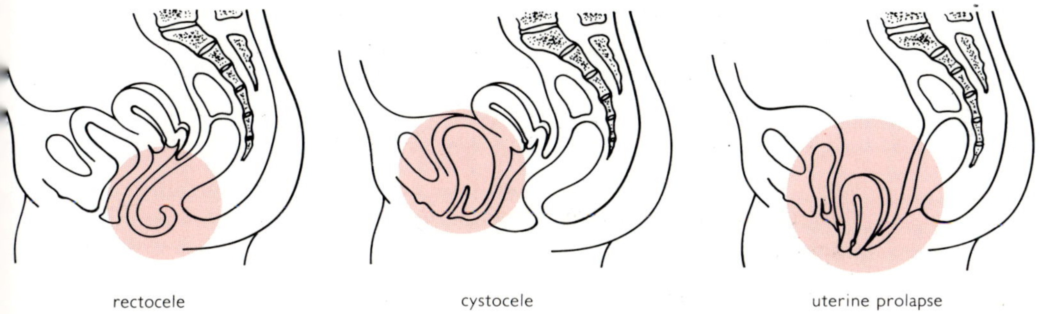

Urethrocele: herniation of the urethra through the anterior vaginal wall, with displacement of the bladder neck.
Cystocele: herniation and descent of the bladder through the anterior vaginal wall.
Rectocele: herniation of the rectum through the posterior vaginal wall.
Enterocele: herniation of the pouch of Douglas and intestines through the posterior vaginal wall.

Symptoms

- discomfort, dragging pains and low backache occur, but vary in relation to the type and degree of prolapse. Large prolapses are often less uncomfortable than lesser ones, as resistance and tension offered by the ligaments have by then completely disappeared
- the woman feels 'something coming down' in the vagina. There may be difficulty in walking in the case of procidentia
- vaginal discharge, sometimes bloodstained
- urinary symptoms, especially frequency and inability to empty the bladder completely. With a large cystocele, much of the urine is below the level of the urethral sphincter, and so cannot be voided unless the cystocele is lifted up via the vagina. Many women learn to do this instinctively but are shy to mention it to the doctor. Where there is a chronic state of residual urine, cystitis

is more likely to occur. Stress incontinence may also appear, especially where there is distortion or displacement of the bladder neck and urethra (urethrocele)
- bowel symptoms appear with rectocele. There is often constipation and difficulty in complete evacuation of the rectum without resorting to digital support via the vagina

Treatment

A prolapse that is discovered incidentally and is causing no symptoms is not treated.

Supporting pessary

This treatment is used when the woman is too frail or ill or if she refuses to undergo surgery. It is also used in the younger woman who wishes to have more children in the near future, and in cases of prolapse during early pregnancy. The most commonly used pessary is ring-shaped (Figure 18.6) and is made of a non-irritative polythene or vinyl material. Use of the pessary will not cure the prolapse, nor will it relieve any stress incontinence, but in some cases, because it lessens the continual strain on, and stretching of, the uterosacral and cardinal ligaments, the ligaments may regain some of their former tone.

Figure 18.6
Supporting (ring) pessary

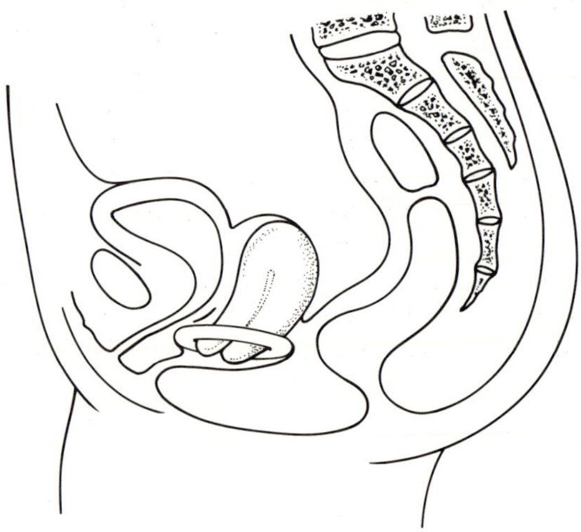

Operations for prolapse

Vaginal repair (colporrhaphy) operations aim to restore strength and support to the vaginal walls. The wall is opened, the fascia tightened and reinforced by suturing, and redundant tissue from the vaginal wall is excised.

A cystocele is repaired by anterior colporrhaphy.

A urethrocele is treated by anterior colporrhaphy with special attention to elevation of the bladder neck or by one of the urethral sling operations.

A rectocele is repaired by a posterior colpoperineorrhaphy which includes repair of the perineum by bringing together the levator muscles adjacent to the perineal body.

An enterocele is usually repaired as part of a Manchester repair operation or during an extended posterior colpoperineorrhaphy.

A uterine prolapse may be treated by:

- Manchester repair (Fothergill's operation) which is done when there is prolapse of the vaginal walls and some descent of the uterus. The cervix is dilated (to prevent later stricture and allow drainage), its vaginal portion is amputated and the cardinal ligaments are shortened. The uterus is thus elevated and the vaginal vault strengthened. This procedure is followed by anterior and posterior repair operations
- vaginal hysterectomy and repair is performed for procidentia. As well, it is done when the uterine prolapse is less marked but where there is some other indication to remove the uterus. (The uterus cannot be removed by the vaginal route if it is large or fixed by adhesions.) The uterus is removed after incising through the vaginal walls, the uterine ligaments are shortened and joined together at the midline, and the operation is completed by repairs of the anterior and posterior vaginal walls.

Nursing management during the pre- and post-operative periods of these operations is discussed in Chapter 21.

Repair operations are generally effective in relieving the symptoms of uterovaginal prolapse. As in all operations for herniation, much depends on the patient's understanding of the need to prevent strain or pressure on the newly repaired area. If this is not understood, the prolapse may recur.

Other complications of vaginal repair are stress incontinence and dyspareunia. If either of these occur, the woman should seek advice early so that they do not cause her misery and make her feel that her 'cure' is worse than her original complaint.

19 Urinary problems in gynaecology

Urinary problems are unpleasant. They can interrupt daily life to an enormous degree yet they are not really acceptable topics of conversation. So the sufferer, young or old, has to be silent.

Urinary problems in women are, in many cases, related to gynaecological conditions because of the close anatomical relationships between the urinary and the genital tracts. The effects of the reproductive functions—intercourse, pregnancy and labour—can all cause urinary symptoms, the common ones being the various types of incontinence, and frequency. The student nurse will find it helpful to revise the anatomy of the urinary tract and the physiology of micturition as a basis of understanding the urinary problems of gynaecology.

True incontinence

True incontinence occurs when there is a fistulous communication between the urinary and genital tracts. The most common site of fistulae is between the bladder and the vagina, through the anterior vaginal wall—vesicovaginal fistula. The other sites illustrated are less common (Figure 19.1). The urine drains through the vagina and the woman is wet all the time.

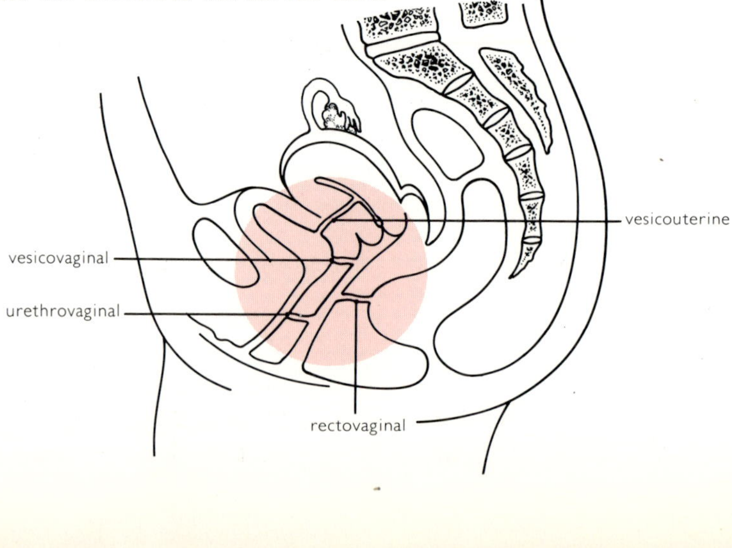

Figure 19.1
Sites of fistula formation

These fistulae are less common now that obstetric care is so much improved. Their main cause used to be delay in the late first or early second stage of labour, when the pressure of the presenting part was constant and prolonged. This pressure caused ischaemia, necrosis and ultimately fistula formation. It is still an obstetric complication in some underdeveloped countries.

Fistulae may also occur from the spread of carcinoma, following irradiation, or as a result of damage during pelvic operations. Very occasionally the fistula is congenital; in such cases it would be treated early in childhood.

Management

Where there is only one fistula, and that one is small and where infection can be controlled, an indwelling urethral urinary catheter may be passed. This will drain the bladder and so may allow natural healing to occur over a period of several weeks.

Surgical repair of the fistula will be attempted when spontaneous closure and natural healing seem unlikely. The operation is followed by continuous catheter drainage for at least a week, and antibiotic coverage to prevent wound breakdown due to infection. The other problem that may arise is that of bladder tone; the bladder may have 'forgotten' the stimulus of being full or, alternatively, it may not be able to cope with any significant quantity of urine before it registers full. Carefully timed clamping and release techniques are part of the important post-operative care.

Overflow incontinence

Overflow incontinence occurs when the bladder is filled to its limit but is unable to empty itself either because stimuli are not registered (as in certain disorders of the nervous system, eg spinal cord injury, multiple sclerosis, or following damage to pelvic nerves during surgery) or because there is an obstruction to the proper exit of the urine. A common cause of overflow incontinence is bladder atony due to advanced old age. Urine is retained in the bladder, and what comes in from the ureters subsequently results in urine 'overflowing' from time to time, via the urethra.

In the first case, where stimuli are not registered, the condition is chronic and usually not painful. Acute retention due to some obstruction is extremely painful. In both cases, ascending infection is a problem.

Management

The bladder is gradually drained and any infection treated; any obstruction is relieved. Bladder tone is aided by drugs such as bethanechol chloride which stimulates bladder muscle contraction.

In chronic cases, bladder drainage may need to be continued for a month or more until bladder tone returns. Then the woman must be asked to void at no greater than two-hourly intervals to avoid further distension.

Urge incontinence

Urge incontinence is the term used to describe the situation where the woman has the desire to void but this desire is followed almost immediately by voiding—she cannot get to the toilet in time. Urge incontinence comes without warning and is, by itself, not related to specific events such as coughing or laughing as happens with stress incontinence. It may, however, occur as well as stress incontinence, and so may be the cause of continuing problems after treatment for stress incontinence has seemed to be unsucessful.

Urge incontinence is due to irritability of the bladder; the bladder is hypertonic and contracts strongly even when it contains only a relatively small amount of urine. The sphincter muscles are normal but they cannot cope with such increased force from the bladder contractions.

Management

The causes of bladder irritability are investigated and treated. Infection is controlled by antibiotics. In cases where the bladder is hypersensitive to volume because of years of deliberate frequent emptying—to prevent accidents or having to go to the toilet when out of the house—the bladder will have to be re-educated so that it will not respond so often or so violently to stimuli. Antispasmodic drugs, eg propantheline bromide, are used to reduce the tone of the bladder and its contractions. The bladder is re-educated as well by deliberate voiding at regular intervals, starting one- to two-hourly and gradually increasing over a period of weeks until the woman can comfortably manage intervals of up to four hours between voiding.

Stress incontinence

Stress incontinence is incontinence which occurs as the result of a sudden increase in intra-abdominal pressure as may occur when laughing, coughing, sneezing, jumping or running. The extra force from the diaphragm pushes down the abdominal contents, and they, in turn, exert pressure on the bladder. The bladder is normally able to withstand this pressure, but when the bladder neck is weak or not well supported, the sphincter will be forced open and some urine will escape (Figure 19.2).

Stress incontinence occurs most often in parous women following the menopause, though it can happen before this and in women who have not had babies. It is entirely due to the inefficient action of the internal urethral sphincter and this inefficiency can be the result of weakness, stretching and loss of tone of the urethral suspensory ligaments. The weakness may be congenital; there may be a congenital weakness which does not cause symptoms until the extra weight and pressure caused by pregnancy is too much for it; or it may not be evident until the effects of labour, or oestrogen withdrawal, or both, appear later in life. Surgical interference with, or near, the urethrovesicular junction (eg an anterior colporrhaphy) may cause damage to the urethral sphincter.

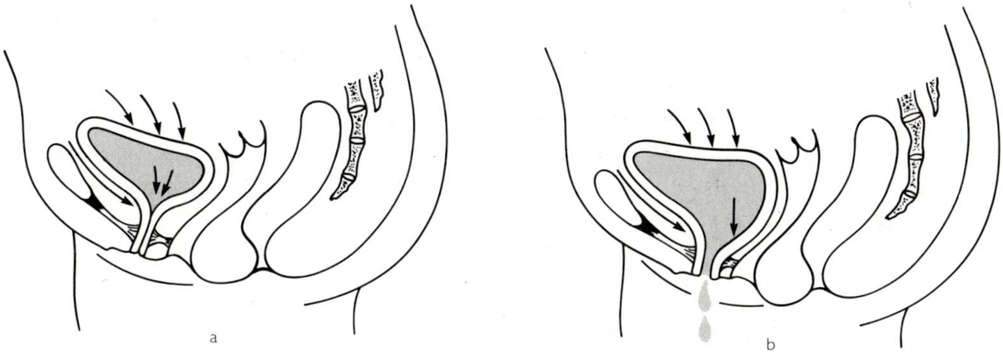

Figure 19.2
Effects of increased intra-abdominal pressure upon bladder and (a) normal proximal urethra (continent) (b) displaced proximal urethra (stress incontinence)

Demonstration of stress incontinence

The woman who complains of stress incontinence undergoes a careful vaginal and pelvic examination. She is asked to cough and any escape of urine is noted. When urine does escape, she is asked to cough again, but this time the urethra is supported by direct pressure. If urine does not escape, it is presumed that the bladder neck support is deficient, and surgery is aimed at improving that support. Sometimes it will be necessary for the woman to stand upright to demonstrate stress incontinence, as gravity may change the situation; the urine may not escape when the woman is lying down.

Management

Any contributing factors are discovered and treated. Frequent laughing probably should not be suppressed, but frequent or chronic coughing should certainly be investigated. Obesity may require a weight reduction programme. Both of these factors need attention in any case, for the sake of the woman's general health as well as to lessen post-operative risk. Their elimination may, on its own, reduce the stress incontinence to the degree that the woman can cope with it.

Physiotherapy: pelvic floor exercises may be used to improve the line of secondary defence and so prevent incontinence. Pelvic floor exercises are simple and in many cases effective. The woman is asked to 'squeeze up inside and hold', with her legs crossed, as if she were trying to stop urine from coming away. If she does this ten times every two hours (with about ten seconds rest between each contraction) and holds each squeeze for at least four seconds, she will be exercising and strengthening the pelvic floor, including that part which compresses the urethra. Additional exercises include deliberately stopping the flow two or three times whenever she voids normally, and placing one or two fingers into the vagina when she practises squeezing so that she can feel the muscles tightening (Figure 19.3).

Figure 19.3
Squeezing exercise to re-educate the pelvic floor muscles

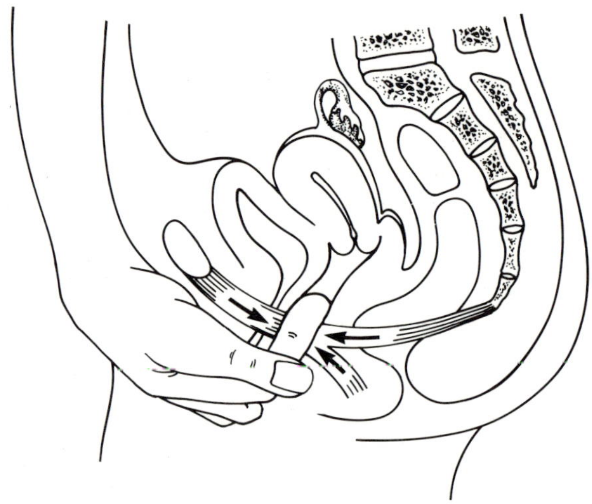

Surgery: many women with stress incontinence will require surgical correction of the pelvic problem that has led to the symptom. The operation chosen (usually anterior colporrhaphy) will depend on whether or not a cystocele is present and whether or not a previous anterior colporrhaphy has been performed. The Marhsall-Marchetti operation is an abdominal procedure that fixes the urethra (with sutures) to the back of the symphysis pubis. Other operations involve the tightening and reinforcement of the paraurethral tissues (vaginal urethroplasty) or the use of muscle 'slings' to elevate and support the urethra.

Nursing aspects of incontinence

Nurses must, at all times, be sensitive to the widespread effects that even the slightest degree of urinary incontinence can have on a person's daily activity. When in our care in hospital, she may be what is sometimes described as 'unco-operative' in her attempts to keep this personal shame to herself: wanting to keep her pants on in bed, refusing to do post-operative coughing (just as the woman described in the first chapter of this book must have seemed unco-operative to her nurses). When people do know about her incontinence, she still has to cope with the embarrassing and uncomfortable investigations that must precede diagnosis and treatment. If we are there, she needs our support.

Local skin care is of great importance. The constant presence of dampness and the ammoniacal substances from the urine will soon cause soreness and excoriation of the skin of the vulva and inner thighs. The wearing of pads that may chafe and particularly the wearing of plastic pants will make the situation much worse. Skin care involves washing the area at least twice daily with plain water, the application of a waterproofing agent, eg silicone cream, or when necessary a healing agent, eg zinc cream with cod liver oil. Thick disposable incontinence pads that can hold urine while staying dry on the surface can be obtained from chemist shops. They are better suited and probably cause less chafing than do menstrual pads. Alternatively, the one-way fabric that is now popular for use inside infants' napkins can be most useful in these conditions, and can be worn with a simple thick combine pad and knitted or flannel pants.

It is acceptable for babies to be incontinent; good mothers don't mind and they make every effort to care for the delicate skin. With older people, and nurses, the same must apply.

Frequency of micturition

Frequent passage of urine is the other major urinary problem in gynaecology. Urine is passed because the bladder is stimulated to contract. It is stimulated to contract frequently because it (or the urethra with which it is intimately associated) is irritated. The woman is not incontinent; she is able to use the voluntary powers to help to contract the urethra until it is convenient to void, but it happens often. When the irritation is severe and accompanied by infection, dysuria with pain, and sometimes bleeding, will occur.

Causes

Polyuria may be caused by a number of medical and renal conditions. It is also the result of a very large fluid intake.

Pressure on the bladder occurs in the early and then the last months of pregnancy, or from a large pelvic tumour.

Vulvourethral causes: acute vulvitis, gonoccocal urethritis, chronic urethrotrigonitis ('the urethral syndrome', see below) postmenopausal urethritis, and urethral prolapse or caruncle can all cause frequency and burning on micturition.

Cystitis: acute or chronic inflammation of the bladder. A symptomless low-grade infection is present in the bladder of most adult women especially once they have been sexually active. Cystitis may result from the introduction of further organisms, for example at catheterisation, or from incomplete emptying of the bladder (as in cystocele) resulting in residual urine in which organisms can multiply quickly. Post-operative cystitis is a special problem following gynaecological surgery.

The 'psychogenic' bladder: a number of nervous and emotional factors may lead to a woman or girl adopting the habit of going to the toilet whenever possible. This can lead eventually to the bladder being unable to fill to any degree before the stretch receptors are stimulated.

Management

Frequency, especially when accompanied by dysuria, is a distressing problem; the cause has to be found and treated. A mid-stream specimen of urine (for culture and sensitivity) will be the first investigation after the history-taking and local and pelvic examinations have been completed. Swabs from the vulva and vagina are examined. Urinary antiseptics, alkalinisers, and, when indicated, antibiotics may be prescribed. Further investigations may include cystoscopy, bladder capacity tests, and intravenous pyelogram.

Chronic urethrotrigonitis—'The urethral syndrome'

This syndrome is also known as 'honeymoon cystitis'. Its symptoms are acute, but it is essentially a chronic condition which may take months or years to clear up or even just to keep under control. The effects of the syndrome, and the enormous number of women who suffer because of it, are very well described by Angela Kilmartin in her book *Understanding cystitis* (Pan Books, London, 1973).

The syndrome affects susceptible women; some women, but not others. It is said to be due in most cases to damage to the short, sensitive urethra by the movements of the penis during intercourse. Added to this, bacteria from the outside may be pushed into the urethra and may colonise there. The symptoms are frequency, pain and burning on micturition, and lower abdominal discomfort. In some cases the pain may be so bad that its anticipation results in the inability to void, or only being able to void in a bath of warm water. And, as one girl said, 'I can't keep having baths *all* day; I have to go to work. But at work I can't pass urine. It's *terrible*.' The symptoms usually do not appear until about thirty-six hours after intercourse, and so the connection may not be realised. But unless the condition is recognised and managed well, it can have serious effects. Intercourse will not be welcome when the symptoms are present because the area hurts so much, and it will be unwelcome later if it is going to start the whole business off again.

Management

A mid-stream specimen of urine is routinely collected, for culture and sensitivity testing. Often this test is negative or shows only a very mild infection, to which the symptoms are disproportionate.
Surgical: some doctors have treated this condition successfully by dividing the hymenal ring anteriorly on each side of the urethra.
Medical: antibacterial therapy may be prescribed and also prophylactic urinary antiseptics. Advice is given on various methods of preventing attacks.
Self-help: this involves diluting the urine by doubling, at least for a while, the daily fluid intake. The use of urinary alkalinisers may be advised as well, and potassium supplements may be necessary.

The woman should void just before intercourse, and immediately afterwards. This will help to flush out any organisms that may have been introduced, before they colonise in the urethra. In addition, she should drink at least two glasses of water straight away. Using a lubricant during intercourse and altering the position used may help some.

These measures have made a considerable difference to the lives of those women and their partners—they suffer jointly—who have been afflicted by the urethral syndrome.

Part IV Gynaecological surgery

20 Common operations, their indications and implications

This chapter is meant as a summary of facts relating to the more common gynaecological operations, which are discussed in greater detail as they appear throughout the text. The implications (in other words, what will happen to the woman and how it will affect her) are also very briefly covered here.

Surgeons, nurses, and hospitals differ in their practices. Patients differ in their responses. Even so, it is a definite responsibility of every nurse to ensure that no patient in her care suffers because of fear, anxiety or ignorance about her operation or its effects. There are many examples illustrating how the use of medical terminology has confused, bewildered and made fools of the most intelligent of women. Or showing how the lack of a few words of advice about the resumption of intercourse has resulted in the readmission to hospital of women who have undergone recent repair operations and now are bleeding or infected, or now suffering from dyspareunia. One woman told of her hospital experiences to a nurse friend who could only feel, in response, rather ashamed of her profession.

> In April I went in for a curette operation. That was simple; I was home two days later. But it didn't do much good so I went back to the doctor. He decided that my problems (heavy periods and a prolapse) weren't going to get much better without an operation; so he told me that he would book me in for a vaginal hysterectomy and repair, and that I wouldn't have any more periods. Then I read a few articles about hysterectomy and talked to some people who had had it done, and decided that there really wasn't much to be worried about. The scar

> mightn't be right for bikinis but wouldn't be *too* ugly. So in July I went back in there and was on the same floor and was glad to see some of the same staff. Everything went well until I woke up properly after the operation—I had an intravenous drip in! I though that something must have gone wrong because don't you only have those when you're really sick? Then a bit later I thought about the operation and bandages and things. There weren't any. Then I thought that they hadn't done the operation at all because I must have got sick. I did feel rather awful. The next day they came and took out a pack of something from the vagina and I saw that there was a catheter draining the urine. The doctor didn't seem worried; he said everything was going very well. I didn't say anything then, but I wanted my husband to phone the doctor but he said not to be silly. After a few days they took out the catheter but they kept on putting it in again because apparently I wasn't passing enough. Once I asked a nurse if the doctor would still do the hysterectomy on me after all this. She told me not to worry, of course I had had it done: didn't I know? And she said the bladder business was quite routine after these operations; I was progressing really well. But I *did* feel a fool.

Eventually this woman found out the meaning of 'vaginal hysterectomy and repair' and understood why she did not have an abdominal wound. She had, however, experienced a week of anxiety and misunderstanding because nobody had properly prepared her for her experience.

Whose responsibility was it to tell the woman what we take for granted and yet what she, despite her reading and discussions, did not know? Intravenous therapy, residual urines, operation routes, vaginal packs—all accepted and understood by the initiated. But all frightening to the person whose interests and talents are in other fields.

The first task is to find out how much the pre-operative patient does know about her operation. It is not sufficient to ask if her doctor has told her anything about her operation. The doctor in the example just quoted had indeed told his patient something about her operation. So in response she would probably have assured the nurse that, yes, she did know about it and so the conversation would close. Yet although gynaecological topics in general fascinate a lot of people, talking specifically on a one-to-one basis is different. Shyness and embarrassment have to be overcome to start with. Then the gaps in knowledge have to be filled, in a manner that shows sensitivity and takes into account such things as the woman's age, marital status, diagnosis, prognosis and previous experience of hospitals, medical personnel and surgery.

The following points are useful as guidelines where appropriate:

- what will be done (or taken out) at the operation?
- what will be left (specific)?
- would a diagram help?
- what effect will this operation have on the general functioning of her body?
- will it have any effect on her normal sexual activity?

- will it affect her ability to have children?
- will there be a scar?
- should she be warned about any special post-operative problems or procedures?
- will there be a vaginal blood loss?
- how long will she be in hospital after the operation (if there are no complications)?

Table 20.1 lists some of the answers to the above list of questions for the more common gynaecological operations, and also gives indications for these operations.

Figures 20.1 and 20.2 illustrate some of the features associated with some of the gynaecological operations.

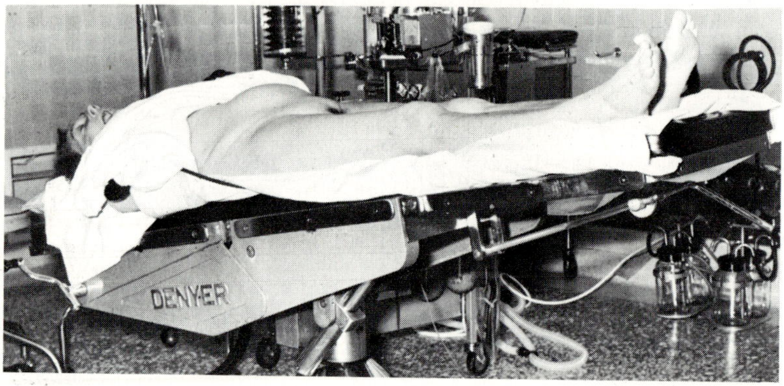

Figure 20.1
Trendelenburg position is used for abdominal gynaecological operations. Gravity moves the bowel out of the pelvis

Figure 20.2 (opposite)
Lithotomy position is used for vaginal operations

Table 20.1
Common gynaecological operations—useful guidelines

Operation	Description	Indications	What remains after operation (specific)	Effect on body functioning
Total hysterectomy (abdominal)	uterus (including cervix) removed via the abdominal route	dysfunctional uterine haemorrhage; fibroids causing symptoms; endometrial carcinoma confined to the uterine cavity	ovaries; vagina	no more periods; if premenopausal will not have a sudden climacteric
Pan-hysterectomy (bilateral salpingo-oophorectomy)	uterus, tubes, ovaries removed	endometriosis; chronic pelvic infection; malignancy	vagina	climacteric will result, possibly with symptoms; no more periods; oestrogen replacement may be ordered

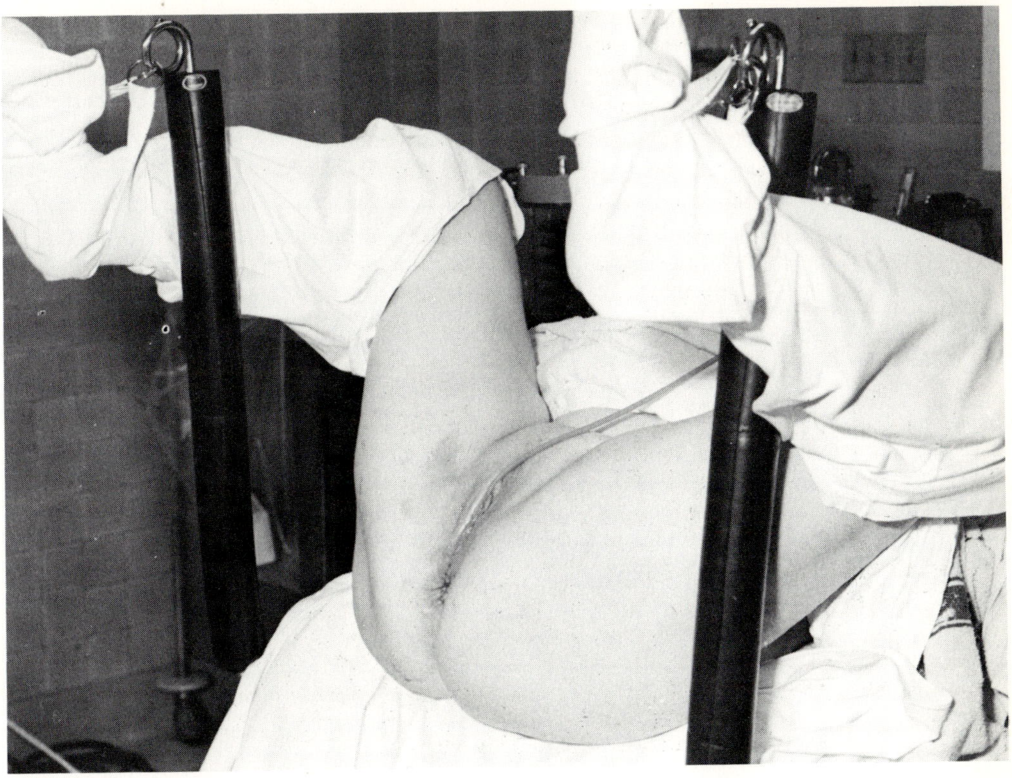

Physical effect on sexual activity (once healed)	Effect on reproductive ability	Will there be a scar?	Specific post-operative points	Vaginal blood loss	Days in hospital after operation (approx)
nil	ceased	yes—lower abdominal	IV; possible wound drain tubes; possible urinary catheter for 3–5 days	yes	8–10
oestrogen withdrawal; dryness etc, otherwise nil	ceased	yes—lower abdominal	IV; possible wound drains; possible urinary catheter for 3–5 days	yes	8–10

Figure 20.1 continued

Operation	Description	Indications	What remains after operation (specific)	Effect on body functioning
Wertheim's hysterectomy	uterus, tubes, ovaries, upper third of vagina, pelvic lymph nodes all removed	stages one and two of carcinoma of the cervix	lower vagina	will have climacteric, menopause; no oestrogen replacement given
Myomectomy	fibroids shelled out from their pseudo-capsules	fibroids causing symptoms when the uterus is to be conserved for pregnancy purposes	uterus and all other reproductive organs	nil
Salpingectomy	fallopian tube(s) removed	ectopic tubal pregnancy; chronic pelvic infection; malignancy	uterus; ovaries; vagina	nil
Abdominal tubal ligation	fallopian tubes cut; 2·5 cm removed from each; ends tied separately	sterilisation (contraception)	uterus; ovaries; vagina	nil
Ovarian cystectomy	cyst tissue removed from ovary but remaining ovarian tissue conserved	benign ovarian cysts	uterus; tubes; vagina; some ovarian tissue	nil
Oophorectomy	ovary(ies) removed	ovarian cysts; malignancy; bad endometriosis; chronic pelvic inflammation; carcinoma of breast	uterus; vagina	if unilateral—nil; if bilateral—climacteric will occur; no more periods
Ventrosuspension	round ligaments shortened to hold uterus forward	retroverted uterus causing symptoms	everything	nil

Physical effect on sexual activity (once healed)	Effect on reproductive ability	Will there be a scar?	Specific post-operative points	Vaginal blood loss	Days in hospital after operation (approx)
shortness of vagina is not main problem; if operation preceded by radiation treatment, there could be contraction; lack of secretions (oestrogen withdrawal)	ceased	yes—lower abdominal	IV; possible wound drains—closed suction; urinary catheter for 3–5 days; oedema of vulva may occur 7–10 days after operation	yes	10–14
nil	retained; often improved; labour closely supervised	yes—lower abdominal	possible wound drains	probable	6–8
nil	if both removed—ceased	yes—small lower abdominal	depends on indication for operation; in itself, none	possible	5–7
nil	ceased	yes—small lower abdominal	nil	possible	5–7
nil	retained	yes—lower abdominal	nil	possible	5–7
nil, if unilateral; oestrogen withdrawal effects if bilateral	if bilateral—ceased	yes—lower abdominal	depends on indication for operation; in itself, possibly only wound drainage	possible	5–7
nil	nil	yes—small lower abdominal	nil	possible	5–7

Figure 20.1 continued

Operation	Description	Indications	What remains after operation (specific)	Effect on body functioning
Examination under anaesthesia (EUA)	vaginal (pelvic) examination under anaesthetic	obesity; prior to radioactive insertion; inability to relax—pain, fear; vaginismus	everything	nil
Dilatation and curettage (D&C)	cervix gradually dilated; lining of uterus scraped	*diagnostic*: abnormal uterine bleeding; postmenopausal bleeding; to establish if ovulation is occurring *therapeutic*: abortion, missed abortion, incomplete abortion: hydatidiform mole; removal of polyps; postpartum haemorrhage; menorrhagia; dysmenorrhoea	everything	nil
Vulvectomy 1 simple	labia majora, minora and clitoris removed	intractable pruritus; leukoplakia carcinoma of the vulva	urethral orifice; vagina	nil
2 radical	whole vulva, skin and fat of femoral triangle, pelvic lymph nodes removed		urethral orifice; vagina	chronic oedema of legs is common
Vaginal repairs: Colporrhaphy	nothing removed; cutting into vaginal wall and sewing the underlying fascia more firmly to strengthen it	anterior repair—cystocele, cystourethrocele; posterior repair—rectocele, enterocele; perineal—weakness of perineal body	everything	nil

Physical effect on sexual activity (once healed)	Effect on reproductive ability	Will there be a scar?	Specific post-operative points	Vaginal blood loss	Days in hospital after operation (approx)
nil	nil	no	nil	no	1–2
nil	retained	no	nil	yes	1–2
still capable of intercourse but different because clitoris absent	retained	yes—vulval	urinary catheter for 3–5 days	possible wound drainage	3–5
younger women should be capable of intercourse; vaginal delivery has been reported after this operation	retained	yes—vulval and lower abdominal	IV; urinary catheter; closed suction wound drainage; raw wound—skin grafting possible	wound drainage	3–12 weeks
still possible; may improve or worsen difficulties	retained; second stage of labour closely observed	not obvious (inside vagina)	possible IV; urinary catheter for 3–5 days; may have voiding problems; residual urine estimates; pack in vagina; stitches will dissolve 9–10 days—yellowish discharge	yes	7–10

Figure 20.1 continued

Operation	Description	Indications	What remains after operation (specific)	Effect on body functioning
Manchester repair	uterus lifted up by shortening its supporting ligaments; vaginal part of cervix removed; anterior and posterior vaginal walls repaired	descent of the uterus and laxity of the the vaginal walls	everything but vaginal portion of cervix	nil
Vaginal hysterectomy and repair	vaginal wall opened; uterus removed via vagina; vaginal walls repaired	prolapse plus an indication to remove the uterus (uterus not large or with adhesions)	ovaries; vagina	no more periods; will not have artificial climacteric
Laparoscopy	direct inspection of pelvic contents; forceps fitted to cervix to help move uterus around, using cold light illumination through hollow; CO_2 insufflated into peritoneal cavity to displace intestines	acute or chronic pain; removal of tissue for biopsy; diagnosis of ectopic pregnancy; infertility; tubal interruption, eg by diathermy; removal of ovum for fertilisation outside the uterus	everything	nil
Vaginal urethroplasty	paraurethral tissues tightened, urethra raised and supported by stitching	stress incontinence	everything	nil
Sling operations	elevation and support of bladder neck by stitching it to the back of the symphysis pubis	stress incontinence	everything	nil
Bartholin's marsupialisation	Bartholin's gland opened and edges sewn to vaginal wall thus creating a pouch or channel for drainage	blocked Bartholin's duct	everything	nil

Physical effect on sexual activity (once healed)	Effect on reproductive ability	Will there be a scar?	Specific post-operative points	Vaginal blood loss	Days in hospital after operation (approx)
as for vaginal repair	fertility may be lowered because less cervical mucus will be produced; possible cervical imcompetence; otherwise as for vaginal repair	not obvious (inside vagina)	as for vaginal repair	yes	7–10
as for vaginal repair	ceased	not obvious (inside vagina)	as for vaginal repair	yes	7–10
nil	retained unless diathermy used specifically to occlude tubes	one or two tiny incisions near umbilicus	nursed flat for 8 hours	possible	1–2
as for vaginal repair	retained as for vaginal repair	not obvious (inside vagina)	possible IV; possible vaginal pack; catheter 3–5 days; usually no voiding problems afterwards	possible wound drainage	7–10
nil	retained	yes—small lower abdominal	as above	no	7–10
improvement of lubrication	retained	small pouch opening into vagina; not obvious	pack in 48 hours	some drainage after pack out	3–5

21 Gynaecological surgical care

All people who undergo operations and surgical procedures have basic physical and psychological needs in common. The assessment of those needs and the planning of actions to meet them, the implementation and ongoing evaluation of the planning and actions are all part of the nursing process that the nurse will have been following since she began her nursing career.

As these principles are, in one form or another, well and thoroughly covered by nursing educators and the authors of many excellent textbooks written about the care of the surgical patient, it is necessary here to add only those specific points that apply to the woman undergoing surgery for gynaecological conditions. It should not be forgotten, however, that any patient could be suffering from one or more other conditions, totally unrelated to her gynaecological condition or operation, with which she is far more concerned. Apart from this, there are some important considerations to remember as we approach the nursing care of our gynaecological patients.

A gynaecological operation, whether it be large or small, involves organs of a system that is, or has been, of special significance in a woman's concept of herself as a female. Some women go through life without ever having 'used' their reproductive system in any way. Such a woman may never have had intercourse; she may never have borne children. Even so, the system is still an integral part of her person and any threat to that integrity will not be without some conscious or unconscious effect. Where her reproductive system has been an active influence in the woman's life, she will regard it in a different way again, but she *will* regard it as important to her bodily integrity.

Certain other parts of the body—the tonsils, the appendix, the gall bladder—are rarely invested with any emotional significance; their loss is rarely mourned. This does not mean that the gynaecological patient coming into hospital is going to be 'another neurotic hysterectomy' or that she is going to feel 'only half a woman' or 'a shell of a woman'. It means nothing of the kind; such generalisations are foolish and dangerous. In most cases, the pre-operative patient will be seeing the very positive aspects of her operation; the anticipated relief from whatever symptoms she has had, the prevention of more serious consequences of an existing condition, the control of a life-threatening condition. We should not be over-excessive in our enthusiasm to discover a psychological reason for our patient's every word and deed. But we must give our attention and special help to the highly strung, the over- or under-emotional, and the embarrassed patient. This special help given from the time she comes into our care may make a great deal of difference in the post-operative period and beyond.

Every person who comes into hospital has to make several adjustments. The woman who is used to making decisions has to submit to, and agree with, the decisions of other people, made for her. She has to behave in an acceptable manner, obeying rules that may seem unfair or ridiculous to her. She has to be a 'good patient'. She must establish a relationship with strangers who not only know a lot more about her than she does about them, but who are comfortable in their surroundings and to whom the procedures and operations like hers are probably everyday events. She may have to adjust from being the one upon whom a husband and family depend for the stability of their daily lives—the giver—to being dependent herself—the receiver. Any initiative that she takes for herself may be unacceptable because it interferes with ward routine or the ideas of the staff or her own safety and recovery.

For the woman's stay in hospital to prove a positive and therapeutic experience, the development of an honest, open and considerate relationship between the nursing staff and the patient and her family is the first important task of those who have the responsibility of her care.

Pre-operative period

Admission to hospital

The woman is usually admitted two days prior to major elective surgery, in order to undergo essential pre-operative investigations and physical preparations. This period will also be used to help her adjust to the hospital environment, to prepare her for post-operative experiences, and to ensure that she is physically rested and in the best possible state of health to undergo surgery.

Ceasing of the contraceptive pill. The admission procedure should always include questions about any medications the woman has taken recently. Where appropriate (and not forgetting the younger or unmarried woman), the contraceptive pill is specifically mentioned. This is important because many women take the pill so routinely that they do not regard it as a medication or a drug. Most doctors will have ensured that the pill is ceased at least six weeks prior to admission, but we should still ask about it and if she has been taking it within that time, we must inform the doctor. A recent Health Commission survey in New South Wales has reported that venous thrombosis is four times as likely to occur when synthetic oestrogens have been given in the period shortly before a major operation.

The date of the woman's last menstrual period is always checked, and any possibility of pregnancy excluded; a pregnancy test may be done if there is doubt. Many surgeons try to arrange to do the operations between periods, when there is less likelihood of pelvic congestion, but this is not always possible. The presence of menstruation seems to be more embarrassing to people than the presence of a post-operative or postnatal blood loss.

Consent forms may require the signature of the patient (and her husband if she is married) if infertility will be a result of any operation. The policies of each hospital may differ on this, so it is wise to check and make sure that it is done when necessary. The necessity of giving a clear explanation of the possible effects of the operation has been mentioned. It is repeated here to emphasise its importance.

Specific investigations

Micro-urine

As well as urine being tested routinely in the ward, a mid-stream specimen is collected and examined microscopically to exclude urinary tract infection which could cause discomfort and difficulties with post-operative voiding.

Chest X-ray

This is performed if there is any indication of possible chest problems.

Blood tests

Blood is taken for assessment of haemoglobin, serum urea and electrolytes. Typing and cross-matching is also done if it is thought that a transfusion may be necessary.

Vaginal examination

A vaginal examination may be carried out to exclude the possibility of local infection. If infection is suspected, a high vaginal swab is sent for culture and sensitivity testing. A cervical (Papanicolaou) smear is taken if this has not been done already.

Specific preparations

Skin preparation

For abdominal operations, the abdominal and pubic areas are shaved. For vaginal and perineal procedures, a full (pubis to anus) vulval shave is done, extending to the mid-thighs. Some doctors do not require this shaving before a D and C operation; it is wise to check first.

Bowel preparation

A 1200 mL tap-water enema is usually given on the evening before surgery. A disposable enema or suppository may be ordered instead, for the less extensive operations.

Vaginal preparation

Pre-operative cleansing douches are no longer a routine practice in most hospitals because the healthy vagina is self-cleansing and douching can upset the natural defence mechanisms and so defeat the purpose. It is, however, done to remove excessive or infective discharge in certain cases.

Ulceration of the vagina or cervix (as may occur with procidentia) is treated by admission to hospital several days prior to operation. Bed rest (sometimes with the foot of the bed elevated to reduce oedema) and twice-daily packing of the vagina with gauze soaked in a suitable antiseptic solution, eg acriflavine and glycerine are carried out. Oestrogen cream is sometimes applied locally as an aid to healing.

Post-operative care

General early care

Unless there is a specific contraindication (eg after laparoscopy or after spinal anaesthesia) the woman, when she has fully recovered consciousness, is nursed supported by three to five pillows and sitting on a softly inflated air-cushion.

Deep breathing and coughing (with wound support) is supervised at least two-hourly when she is not asleep. Limb movements and exercises are done at the same time.

Early ambulation is encouraged, depending, of course, on the patient's condition and on the type of tubings that she has attached to her. Even with intravenous and urinary catheter tubes she should be able to be helped out of bed and to walk a few steps some time within the first twenty-four hours after her operation.

Sips of fluid are offered hourly and increased as tolerated; a good fluid intake should be encouraged.

Observation of the patient's post-operative condition is carried out according to the accepted routine of the hospital. Specific observation for evidence of haemorrhage includes frequent (half-hourly for the first four hours, then hourly for at least the next four hours) recording of the pulse rate, respiratory rate, blood pressure and the vaginal loss. If a blood transfusion has been, or is being, given, the temperature should be recorded as frequently. After eight hours, if there are no indications to do so more frequently, the recording of vital signs and assessment of loss is usually done four-hourly. Vaginal loss should not fill more than two perineal pads each hour.

Voiding, in those operations not followed by catheter drainage, must be observed. Distention of the bladder could cause pressure on newly sutured pelvic structures as well as discomfort or pain. It is difficult to palpate a distended bladder if lower abdominal dressings are present. The woman should be allowed out of bed to sit on a proper commode (not a pan balancing on a chair!) to facilitate complete emptying of the bladder. The provision of adequate pain relief will often prevent reflex retention of urine. Catheterisation is done only after nursing measures fail.

Pain relief must be attended to promptly and before the need for analgesia is too desperate. Any unusual or prolonged pain must be reported. Intramuscular analgesia, eg pethidine, is given as ordered (perhaps four-hourly for the first twenty-four hours; twice only within the following twenty-four hours). It is then replaced by adequate oral analgesia given whenever necessary.

Specific gynaecological care

Vaginal packs

The vagina is packed with gauze after some vaginal operations to provide firm pressure to stop bleeding and to prevent adhesions across the vagina. There should be almost no loss draining through the pack. Voiding may be difficult while the pack is in, because of pressure on the urethra and bladder neck. The pack is removed after twenty-four hours or as instructed. This must be done gently as sometimes the packing is very tight; giving an analgesic before-hand will help. (The removal of the pack is recorded in the patient's notes.) Following this, some vaginal loss will occur and should be carefully observed.

Bladder management

Urinary tract infection and retention of urine are the commonest problems encountered after pelvic surgery, especially after vaginal repair operations. Fluid intake is encouraged; it must be kept up to at least three litres per day. Accurate and detailed recording of intake and output is essential. The voiding of frequent small amounts of urine should be reported promptly as it may be an indication of urinary retention with overflow. Frequency accompanied by pain or burning can mean cystitis, which, without good management, can lead to infection of the ureters and kidneys.

Following most of the major gynaecological operations and especially following repair of the anterior vaginal wall, the bladder is drained through a catheter to prevent pain, distension and dysuria. The procedures followed will vary according to different surgeons' wishes. Most surgeons, however, prefer continuous urinary drainage for three to five days, followed by a four-hourly clip and release programme for twenty-four to forty-eight hours before the catheter is removed.

Urinary antiseptics are often prescribed as ascending infection is common. A specimen of urine is obtained prior to the removal of the catheter, and this is sent for culture. The catheter is removed early in the morning to allow observation of the woman's voiding ability during the day. There may be difficulties in attempting to void, most especially after repair of the anterior vaginal wall; the woman will have been warned of this but usually needs extra reassurance at this point. If she tries too hard to void, she may cause strain on the muscles and suture line and possibly ruin the intended benefit of the operation. If she senses any impatience from the staff or imagines that she is 'on trial', she *will* try too hard. She should be recatheterised if she is unable to void, and this catheter should be left in overnight, to be removed the next morning.

Once she has voided naturally, residual urine estimations are made by recatheterising the bladder immediately after voiding, twice-daily, morning and evening, until the residual urine is less than 100 mL on two consecutive occasions, after which they may be discontinued. If the evening residual urine is over 300 mL, the catheter is usually left in overnight. The whole process of regaining the ability to empty the bladder properly may take up to a week, sometimes even longer, to achieve. Repeated catheterisations with their associated exposure and discomfort, no matter how gently they are performed, can be extremely wearing to the patient. Anxiety can inhibit the ability to pass urine, making matters worse. She must never get the impression that she is causing the staff a lot of work or that she is taking a long time to get over the problem—even if she is.

A lot of the difficulty associated with bladder management is prevented when a *suprapubic catheter* is used instead of the traditional urethral catheter. The suprapubic catheter is inserted by the surgeon at the time of operation and is not removed until the woman is voiding normally. The catheter is a fine-bored plastic tube with a two-way tap, which can be connected to regular urinary drainage equipment. Urinary tract infection seems to occur less frequently when these catheters are used. After the usual four to six days of continuous or intermittent drainage (often, in fact, earlier than this) the woman is asked to void naturally. It does not matter if she cannot, because the bladder can be emptied simply by releasing the tap. Residual urine can be measured in a matter of minutes. The woman consequently has less interest invested in her voiding ability and so has less anxiety about it.

The suprapubic catheter is held in place with a square of adhesive or one or two silk sutures; this tiny wound must not be ignored. It requires, like any other lower abdominal wound, twice-daily application of antiseptic and redressing until the catheter is removed. Time will tell whether or not the suprapubic catheter will replace the urethral catheter after vaginal surgery. Some surgeons do not use it because they feel that it could not possibly drain the bladder completely unless the woman lies flat on her front; others do not think that this is a significant factor. But the method is certainly appreciated by both nurses and patients.

Bowel management

It is important to avoid constipation, as this and its associated straining can place undue stress on a new suture line; it also worries and upsets the patient. Because, however, the lower bowel has in most cases been cleared by pre-operative enema, medications to assist bowel movement are not usually given before the third night after surgery. Milk of magnesia and plain coloxyl are suitable agents to give at this stage, as they will soften the faeces without causing peristaltic stimulation. If spontaneous bowel action has not occurred by the fifth post-operative day, two glycerine suppositories are used; if these fail, an olive oil enema is given. Where perineorrhaphy has been performed, any enema must be given with great care to avoid damage and pain at the repair site.

The first bowel action after surgery may be feared because of the general tightness and discomfort which the patient feels in this area, but, if the faeces have been softened with the above-mentioned or other suitable agents, the fears are likely to be worse than the action. The patient should be told this. Proper dietary management and encouragement of ambulation are, of course, very necessary factors in the restoration of full and normal bowel functioning.

Vulval care

Any operation which is followed by vaginal drainage requires attention to vulval hygiene and comfort. Warm water, sometimes with a mild antiseptic, is poured over the vulva and the vulva swabbed from front to back. This vulval toilet procedure is repeated twice-daily until the woman is allowed to bath or shower daily, and continued after this if indicated; it makes a great deal of difference to her comfort. Vaginal douches are sometimes, but not often, indicated as well.

A clean vulval pad, held in place by a T-binder or stockingette, is worn at all times, and is changed before it becomes necessary to change it. The presence of blood in the area will only encourage the growth of micro-organisms. When the woman is able to change her pad by herself, she should be reminded of the necessity of careful handwashing before and afterwards, and of the reasons for front to back pad application and wiping after using the toilet.

Perineal care

After a perineorrhaphy, it is necessary to keep the perineum clean and dry. Perineal dressings are done three times a day using a weak antiseptic solution such as chlorhexidine 1 in 5000. Catgut sutures are usually used; these dissolve and fall out by themselves after about ten days. The woman may well be worried when she finds these on her pad if she has not been warned. Sometimes if the sutures are cutting into the perineum and causing pain, they will be removed before this.

A ray lamp is used after the fifth day to aid healing, applied for ten minutes twice-daily, followed by the application of a drying paint, eg Tinc Benz Simplex. The ray lamp is of no use unless the rays have access to the perineum, so the patient is best placed in the left lateral position and asked to lift her right buttock to expose the area. The lamp itself must be safely placed away from where the patient could knock or kick it over. Hand-held hairdryers, on low heat, are sometimes used instead of ray lamps.

When the perineum or vulva is bruised or oedematous, ice packs are applied and heat treatment withheld. (Oedema does, however, occur more often in the early post-operative period.) Sitz baths (with salt added) relieve pain and aid healing and are used as soon as the woman is allowed to bath or shower. Air cushions should be provided and adequate analgesia given, especially around the sixth and seventh day when the restoration of full blood supply to the area occurs and seems to bring with it a heightened sensitivity to pain and discomfort.

Wound care

Abdominal incision

Dressings are changed as necessary and according to the wishes of the surgeon. In some cases the wound is not dressed at all; in others, the dressing is left undisturbed until the sutures are due to be removed. It is important to note whether or not a wound drain has been inserted, and to follow carefully the instructions for its shortening and removal. After the more extensive operations, especially those involving pelvic lymph node removal, continuous slow suction may be applied through fine tubing to drain the operation site. Patency of the vacuum is checked four-hourly, and the drainage noted, then either emptied or its level marked for the appropriate time, whichever way the system allows.

Sutures are removed when healing has occurred; usually alternate sutures on the seventh day and the remaining sutures on the eighth day. Michel (or other) skin clips are usually removed by the seventh day. Special instructions will be given for the removal of tension sutures.

Vaginal incision

Internal vaginal sutures dissolve themselves and fall out around the ninth or tenth day. Healing of the vaginal wall, and especially the vaginal vault, is usually by second intention. The wound granulates and so gives rise to a yellowish discharge, which appears at the ninth or tenth day and may take three to six weeks to taper away completely. No treatment apart from daily warm baths is necessary.

Major complications following gynaecological surgery

Thrombosis

Deep vein thrombosis is the major risk in gynaecological surgery today. The site of surgery, with its interruption to venous return, and the positions used for operation are the specific contributing factors. Clot formation has been shown to start in the calves during the operation, and if it later extends into the popliteal and ileofemoral vein, there is a real danger of the clot being swept up to the pulmonary artery or its branches as a pulmonary embolus, the consequences of which can be fatal.

Prevention of thrombus formation begins in the pre-operative period by eliminating or treating contributory factors and discouraging pre-operative lying in bed 'because there is nothing else to do'. It continues during the operation itself with special attention to padding and support of the limbs, and by calf stimulation while the patient's muscles are affected by relaxant drugs. Post-operatively, the supervision of limb physiotherapy, standing the woman out of bed within twenty-four hours of surgery and the encouragement of her early ambulation (not just sitting in a chair beside her own bed) are vital points and are very much the responsibility of the nursing staff unless there are specific instructions to the contrary in individual cases.

Haemorrhage

Reactionary haemorrhage may occur in the first twelve to twenty-four hours after operation, when the blood pressure has risen sufficiently to dislodge an insecure or loose ligature. Bleeding can be severe, and swift action is necessary. Internal bleeding is recognised by the usual signs of shock; the first indication can be a rapid feeble pulse. External vaginal bleeding may be much in evidence. It is to be remembered that the saturation of more than two pads per hour is regarded as above the norm and should be reported.

On the other hand, a lot of blood can collect in the vaginal vault and so a vaginal loss that does not seem excessive is no indication that bleeding is not continuously occurring. In fact, it is an accepted practice in gynaecological nursing to refrain from post-operative elevation of the foot of the bed except in the most necessary circumstances, because of the problem of pooling of blood in the vagina. Any signs of reactionary haemorrhage must be reported immediately so that the patient can be taken back to theatre to have the bleeding vessels ligated before she loses an excessive amount of blood.

Secondary vaginal haemorrhage usually occurs on about the tenth post-operative day. It may be preceded by warning signs on the previous day—a minimal but *bright* vaginal loss and a slight elevation of temperature. The haemorrhage is due to low-grade infection in the suture line which becomes very friable (like a wet paper bag), starts to break down and ooze blood. If this oozing is not noticed and not treated immediately by rest, institution of antibiotic therapy and perhaps cautery of oozing capillaries, it can proceed to severe and alarming haemorrhage. Heavier bleeding is treated by tightly packing the vagina immediately in the ward; the procedure for this is described in Chapter 9.

The pack is left in place for twenty-four hours and, if bleeding starts again after its removal, another pack is inserted. Voiding may be difficult when a vaginal pack is in situ; this factor should be considered. A blood transfusion will frequently be necessary. Antibiotics are given to combat the infection that has caused the secondary haemorrhage.

Pelvic haematoma

Bleeding into the tissues may drain and form into a haematoma which might subsequently become infected. This is suspected if the patient has an otherwise unexplained high fever on about the seventh day, despite antibiotic therapy. Her haemoglobin estimation may be low if she has not already been transfused. She will have lower pelvic pain, and a purulent vaginal discharge may appear. The haematoma will eventually discharge itself through the vagina, but, once diagnosed, it is usually treated by artificial rupture to allow free drainage through the vagina. The drainage is cultured and specific antibiotics ordered. Nursing management involves extreme care with vulval hygiene and pad changing, observation of the drainage and relief of pain.

Injuries to urinary structures

Because of the close anatomical relationship between the urinary and reproductive organs, injury during gynaecological operations is possible. The ureters may be inadvertently cut or clamped, or they may be caught up in a position which results in their distortion and oedema. The bladder may be perforated, leading to an open communication between bladder and vagina. Other types of fistulous communication may develop (see Chapter 19).

In most cases, such injuries are discovered and dealt with immediately. Bilateral injury to the ureters is rare; undiscovered, it results in anuria, hence the need for careful observation of urinary output. Damage to one ureter may be less easy to recognise. If urine is escaping into the pelvis, it may collect and cause peritoneal irritation and inflammation, or it may drain out via the vagina and present itself as continuous dribbling of urine. This may go unnoticed in the early post-operative period, where there is a reasonable amount of vaginal blood loss.

Discharge from hospital

In the absence of complications, the woman is allowed to go home when both she and her doctor agree that she is well enough to manage without hospital care. The number of days spent in hospital depend on a variety of factors; the woman's age, general state of health, the particular operation, and the home conditions that she will be returning to. The average stay for each of the common operations is listed in Table 20.1.

We must make absolutely sure that the woman knows what should be done, in the interests of her health and recovery, when she returns home. Whether she needs to continue any treatment or medication. Whether or not she can bath or shower. Whether she can take aperients or analgesics. How to observe discharge and what might be abnormal. If she is likely to be sexually active, she should be reminded that it is usually wise to wait until she has had her post-operative check-up. Her doctor may have prepared her well for her discharge from hospital, but it is still wise to check that she has understood such things.

A vaginal examination is usually made just before discharge to ensure that there are no signs of infection and to separate any adhesions that may be starting to form. An appointment is made for the post-operative check-up at the doctor's rooms or the outpatients' department.

Her return to full strength and health will be considerably hastened if she allows her body to recover quickly by sufficient rest and avoidance of exertion.

Part V
Conditions related to pregnancy and conception

22 Family planning

There is probably no other area in which the familiar 'You're a nurse—you'll know!' is more likely to be said than in relation to the area of family planning. Until recently, there was almost no reason why the nursing profession should have been expected to have much knowledge in this field. Nurses in general hospitals rarely come across family planning as such in the course of their work and theoretical instruction was given little emphasis in most places. In some states, family planning is not yet included on the curriculum for general nursing education.

Nowadays, nurses are able to do postgraduate training to enable them to specialise in this work. But questions still come frequently to other nurses; for example those in general medical or surgical wards. Patients about to go home may want to know if their treatment will have made any difference to their usual method of contraception or sexual activity. Other questions may come from the nurse's own friends and relatives, seeking interpretation of their doctors' instructions or voicing worries about the effectiveness or side effects of various contraceptive methods.

The main reasons for the nurse being approached so often for advice about such matters are, once again, centred on the fact that many people do see that nurse as someone who is able to discuss intimate things without being embarrassed and whose knowledge of medical matters is likely to be reasonable and sensible. She is also seen as one who is likely to have time to listen.

If only for these reasons, we have an obligation to be fully informed of the facts and to be aware of the fallacies and anxieties that people have about the various methods of birth control. Any advice has to be quite impartial and must recognise the great number of factors that will influence people in their approach. As the decision on whether to achieve or avoid conception is made by the couple, what they do about it should be acceptable in all ways to both of them. Their ages, marital status, family and cultural backgrounds, religious commitment and their emotional and physical health will all combine to influence their motivation to practise family planning. Anyone who is asked for advice will also be affected by these factors and so the task of giving full and impartial advice is not an easy one.

Nurses should be capable of answering simply and factually many of the questions that are likely to be put to them. They should also be able to tell people where they can obtain expert advice, particularly when there is a reluctance to visit the local general practitioner. Many hospitals, community health centres and infant welfare centres conduct clinics or have staff trained in family planning counselling. If not, they are usually able to arrange referrals. Information on natural regulation of fertility can be obtained from natural family planning centres, where the ovulation method is taught.

Family planning is not solely concerned with the avoidance or spacing of pregnancies. It covers as well the problem of infertility, but because this is such a complex subject it is discussed separately, in Chapter 24.

There are three main ways by which contraception can be effected:

1 preventing (inhibition of) ovulation
2 allowing ovulation to occur, but preventing the ovum and sperm from meeting
3 allowing fertilisation but preventing successful implantation in the endometrium.

Inhibition of ovulation

Oral contraceptives—the pill

Oral contraceptives are tablets containing the hormones oestrogen and/or progestogen in various combinations. The oestrogen, given for three weeks out of every four, prevents the normal feedback stimulus to the hypothalamus and pituitary, thus preventing the release of FSH. Ovarian follicles are not stimulated to ripen and so ovulation does not occur. The progestogen is included to balance the oestrogen and to prevent undesirable side effects. The endometrium is built up to a much smaller degree than during a normal cycle, and the menstruation (withdrawal bleeding) is slight. The cervical mucus becomes thick and impenetrable by spermatozoa. (A low-dose progestogen pill—the mini pill—is sometimes given to achieve this cervical mucus state without suppressing ovulation.)

There are two main types of oral contraceptive; the 'combined pill' and the 'triphasic pill'. The combined pills contain both oestrogen and progestogen in the same tablet. Some companies include an extra seven pills, made of an inert substance, to complete the four week programme; the woman finishes one pack and immediately starts another. The pills are commenced on the 5th day of menstruation. In a 21-day course, bleeding will start two or three days after the last pill was taken. The woman should have exactly seven days without taking tablets before starting a new course. Because the oestrogen content in modern contraceptive tablets is as low as possible, breakthrough bleeding may occur. This usually only happens during the first one or two cycles; if it continues it should be reported, as the type of pill may not contain enough oestrogen to suppress ovulation in that particular woman.

The triphasic pills aim to mimic the ratio of oestrogen and progesterone in the natural cycle while keeping the levels as low as possible. The tablets must be taken in the proper sequence. If a tablet is missed, the woman should take it as soon as she realises, even if that means taking two pills in one day. If two or more tablets are missed, she should use another form of contraception for the rest of the cycle, and she should ask her doctor's advice about completing the course. The same precautions apply in the case of vomiting up the tablets.

Oral contraceptives may only be issued on prescription. This law, although challenged by some, means that the woman must return regularly for renewal of the prescription, and this provides an opportunity for any adverse effects to be discovered.

Advantages

Oral contraceptives are almost 100 per cent effective if taken according to instructions. While on these tablets, the woman will have regular 'periods' with reduced blood loss, with little pain or discomfort, and with a reduction of premenstrual problems. The habit of taking a pill each day is soon acquired, and intercourse can take place without the fuss and bother involved with some of the other methods.

Disadvantages

A number of side-effects have been attributed to oral contraceptives. Nausea, vomiting, skin changes, breast discomfort, and various mood changes including depression and loss of libido are among the less serious but nonetheless worrying symptoms sometimes reported. Many of these settle after one or two months. If they persist, the doctor may decide to discontinue the treatment or prescribe a pill with a different hormone ratio.

Monilial vaginitis occurs more frequently in women taking oral contraceptives. Post-pill amenorrhoea occurs in a small percentage of cases, especially where there has been a previous history of long or irregular menstrual cycles. The hypothalamic gonadatrophin releasing factors, suppressed by the pill, are sometimes not released again when the woman stops taking the pill.

Blood clotting factors are known to be altered by oestrogen. The incidence of thromboembolism is increased in women on the pill, especially women who smoke. Oral contraceptives are not prescribed when there is a history of thrombophlebitis or pulmonary embolism. Many doctors require that the pill be discontinued four to six weeks before elective operations, especially those involving the abdominal or pelvic regions.

Other contraindications include liver disease or damage, unstable diabetes mellitus, certain problems with sight, steroid therapy, and carcinoma of the breast.

The pill gives no protection against the venereal diseases; the rising incidence of these diseases is known to be related to the widespread use of the pill.

Long-term hormone therapy

Long-term hormone therapy is sometimes used for contraception in special cases or where motivation by the couple may be low. Depo Provera, which contains slow-release progestogens, is usually given at three-monthly intervals, by intramuscular injection.

Oestrogen implants, inserted subcutaneously as a pellet, usually in the forearm, contain oestrogens which are released over a six-month period. These are most suitable for women approaching the end of their reproductive years. The dose is reduced gradually. Oral progestogen is taken for seven days each month, to complement the oestrogen.

Slow-release progestogens are also sometimes incorporated into rings which are inserted into the vagina: these have the advantage of being able to be removed easily. As well, some of the intrauterine devices contain slow-release progestogens, which act locally and do not, therefore, interfere with the menstrual cycle.

Preventing the ovum and sperm from meeting

Limiting intercourse to the woman's infertile periods

There are three methods used to avoid contraception by restricting intercourse to those days of the cycle upon which the woman is naturally infertile.

The rhythm method

This is based upon the calculation of the day of ovulation by counting back fourteen days from the date upon which the next menstrual period is due to begin. Allowing for sperm survival (dependent on the type of cervical mucus present) of three to five days and ovum survival of thirty-six hours, intercourse is avoided from the eighteenth to the twelfth day *before* the next period is due. This method relies heavily upon the regularity of ovulation and constancy of the luteal phase. It is thus unsuitable for those women who have irregular cycles and those approaching the menopause. It cannot be applied during lactation. Unless the period of abstinence is greatly extended, this method has a fairly high failure rate; it is no longer taught in Australia.

Basal temperature charting

Because of the thermogenic action of the hormone progesterone, the basal body temperature rises approximately 0·5°C when progesterone levels are increased. Thus, with the formation of the corpus luteum following ovulation, the temperature is elevated and this elevation is maintained until the corpus luteum degenerates, one or two days before the onset of menstruation (see Figure 22.1). The woman is instructed to take her temperature, either orally, vaginally or rectally, but without changing the location, immediately after she wakes each morning before rising. She keeps a chart to record these daily temperature readings, and to note any obvious cause for temperature variations, such as respiratory infections. The woman cannot predict ovulation by this method; she can only realise it after it has occurred, because the temperature does not rise until after ovulation. Therefore, strict application of this method will involve abstinence from intercourse from the onset of menstruation until three days after recognised ovulation. Ovulation is presumed to occur when there has been a definite and sustained elevation—three higher recordings over the previous six lower

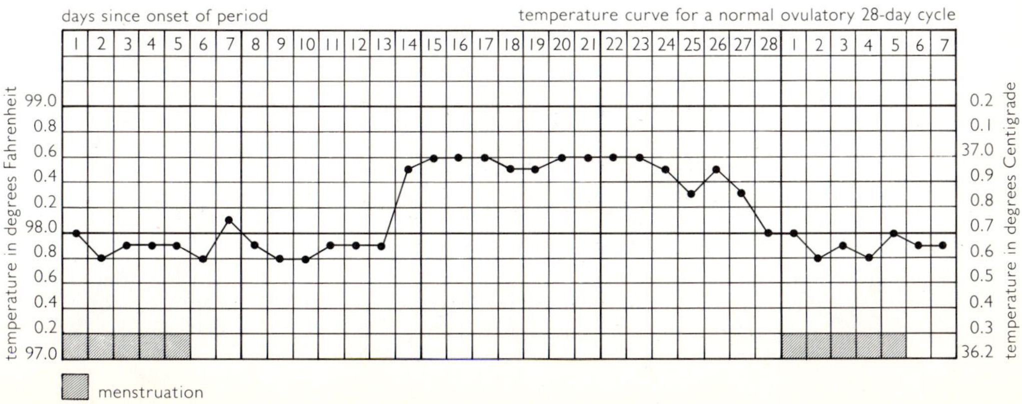

Figure 22.1
Basal temperature chart, showing temperature changes around the time of ovulation

recordings. Sometimes a step-ladder rise is noted in which case five higher recordings over the previous three lower recordings indicate ovulation in that particular cycle.

Basal temperature charting is an improvement on the simpler rhythm method but, as not all cycles are ovulatory, it can sometimes involve greatly extended periods of abstinence from intercourse and thus be unacceptable. Its application in the field of infertility and as a method of timing endometrial biopsy are its major uses today.

The ovulation method (Billings)

The ovulation method has superseded both the rhythm and basal temperature charting methods for those who wish to avoid or space their pregnancies without using artifical contraception. This method, properly applied by a well-motivated couple, has now been scientifically verified by research involving the measurement of ovarian hormone levels throughout the menstrual cycle.

The ovulation method is based upon the observation and interpretation, by the woman, of the symptoms which accompany the hormonal changes throughout the cycle, but particularly those changes which occur before and around the time of ovulation. It aims, by teaching the woman the significance of these symptoms, to make her aware of her own fertility so that, if she wishes to avoid pregnancy, she will avoid all genital contact from the time that she recognises the approach of ovulation until three days after ovulation has occurred.

The glands within the cervical canal respond to elevated levels of oestrogen by increased mucus secretion. When oestrogen levels rise towards the end of the proliferative phase of the cycle, the most fertile mucus will be secreted. This mucus, which is necessary for sperm survival, becomes obvious a few days before ovulation. At its 'peak' secretion, it is thin, clear, slippery and stretchy (Figure 22.2).

Figure 22.2
Cervical mucus

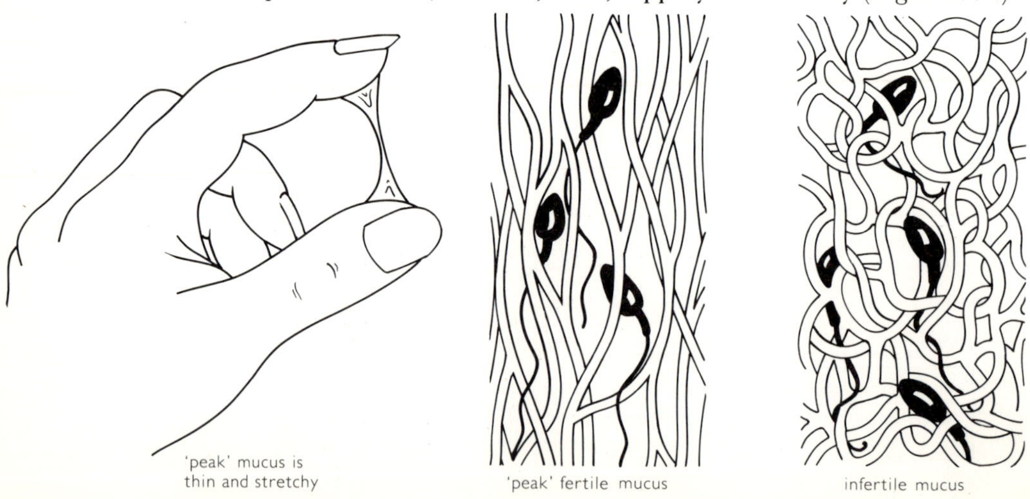

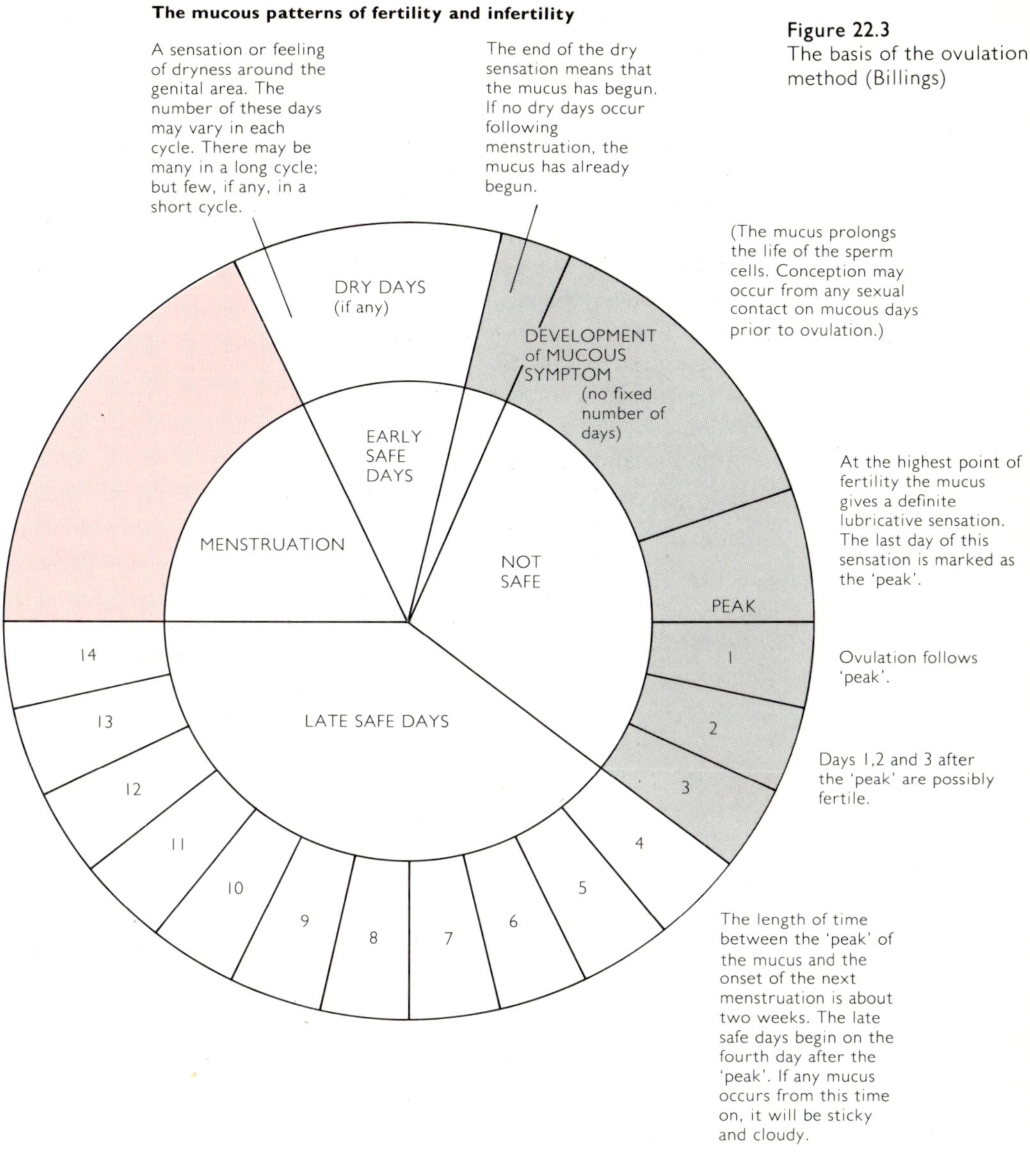

Figure 22.3
The basis of the ovulation method (Billings)

Also during this time wetness is felt and spotting may be noticed. The 'peak' is on the last day of any of these events. When ovulation occurs (and the corpus luteum is formed) the presence of increased levels of progesterone changes the character of the mucus; it becomes thick and opaque and is very much reduced in quantity.

These are the changes that the woman learns to observe and interpret as indications of her state of fertility (Figure 22.3). She does not have to explore her vagina and cervix to find the mucus. These practices are, in fact, discouraged. What she does have to learn is to be aware of the sensations of wetness (in contrast to the usual dryness) of the perineal area, and to be particularly observant when wiping this area with tissue paper.

The ovulation method is taught to couples by trained counsellors who are themselves experienced in its practice; these women, in turn, are advised by doctors. It involves an initial period of abstinence from intercourse for one full month, while the woman is learning to recognise the symptoms, because seminal fluid can be confused with mucus. Fill-in charts are provided with the instruction books; these are used until the woman is completely familiar with the symptoms.

The teachers of the method prefer to have the woman and her partner present at the first sessions, at least, so that the couple together understand the principles and application of the method and so that the teachers can anticipate and help to resolve early problems. Evening sessions are usually available to allow the couple to attend together.

Advantages

Once the method has been learnt, it can be used successfully whether the woman's cycles are regular or irregular. It can be used to predict and recognise the return of ovulation in the absence of an established menstrual cycle, for example during lactation, after coming off the pill and at the approach of the menopause, a time when some other methods may be contraindicated. The mucus secretion is not affected by any known medications other than oestrogen and progesterone.

The ovulation method is a safe, easy and effective method by which a couple can avoid conception and space their family.

Disadvantages

The method requires the full understanding by both partners of the need for abstinence during the woman's fertile period. It is difficult to imagine its success in very unstable or casual relationships. It may not be able to be used by those women who have disturbed or absent cervical secretions, as can occur following cauterisation of the cervix, cone excision or amputation of the cervix (as is done as part of the Manchester repair operation).

Douching

The practice of douching the vagina immediately after intercourse to wash out spermatozoa is no longer taught by health professionals. It is, however, traditional in some cultures, and douching appliances (the bulb syringe and the douche bag and tubing) continue to be available from chemists and medical-appliance shops. Douching solutions can also be bought, but these rarely have any advantage over plain water. Douching, when it works, probably does so by reducing the number of sperm available to reach the ovum. To achieve this, it must be done immediately after intercourse, thus detracting from the pleasure of the experience. Douching is the least effective method of contraception.

Coitus interruptus (withdrawal or 'being careful')

Coitus interruptus is the withdrawal of the penis from the vagina before ejaculation. It has probably been used since humans discovered the connection between intercourse and pregnancy. It has a fairly high failure rate because spermatozoa are often present in the lubricating fluid which precedes ejaculation. Also, pregnancy can result from sperm deposited even as far away as the vulva.

Advantages

This method has very few advantages. It does not cost money and requires practically no planning. Its only advantage would be in an 'emergency'.

Disadvantages

This method can cause considerable psychological strain and tension for the couple involved. There is always the fear that the man will not withdraw in time. The woman is less likely to experience orgasm and this factor has been blamed at times for several vague gynaecological complaints, where no organic cause can be found, such as menorrhagia, dysmenorrhoea and low backaches.

Physical barriers

Male barriers—the condom or sheath

The condom and sheath are rubber or skin coverings rolled on to the erect penis and worn during intercourse to prevent sperm from being deposited in the vagina. Although basically the same as the sheath, the condom is thinner and is usually regarded as disposable. The sheath is of a stronger but thicker rubber and so may be washed and reused. These devices are known by various names—'prophylactic', 'safe', 'rubber', French letter, or by their brand names, eg Durex.

Advantages

They are widely available and can be bought from dispensers or over the counter; and, if used correctly (especially in combination with a spermicidal agent), are an efficient form of contraception. They form a physical barrier against infective organisms as well as against pregnancy. There are no side effects.

Disadvantages

The condom or sheath cannot be put on until the penis is erect and thus can interrupt spontaneity. Unless it is put on carefully it could be damaged by rough handling, fingernails or rings. Some women find the condom uncomfortable, especially when there is insufficient lubrication, and both partners may find that it reduces sensation. The male partner must withdraw very soon after ejaculation to prevent the condom from slipping off as the erection subsides. The cost factor has to be considered; individual condoms are not expensive, but if they are used frequently or exclusively the cost can mount up.

Figure 22.4
Correctly-placed diaphragm

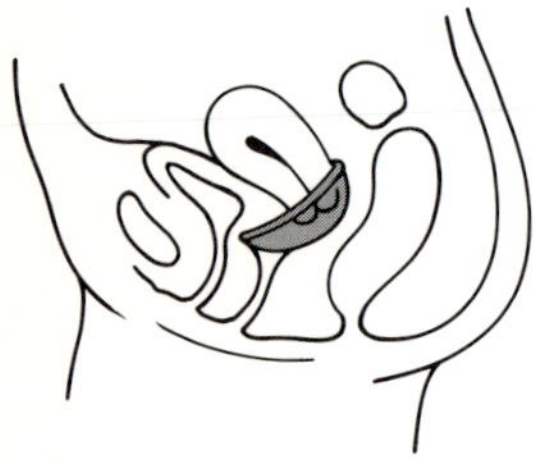

Female barriers

The diaphragm and the cervical cap are the two most commonly used of the female barriers. The diaphragm (Figure 22.4) is a saucer-shaped rubber cap with a spring inside the circular rim. When inserted, it lies in the fornices of the vagina, and so occludes the cervix. The cervical cap is thimble-shaped and fits directly on to the cervix (Figure 22.5).

Figure 22.5
The cervical cap in place

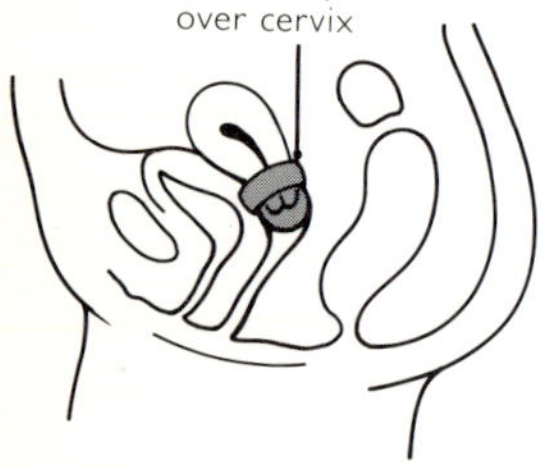

The diaphragm and cap both come in a variety of sizes and the decision as to which type and size is most suitable for a woman must be made by a doctor or specially trained nurse. The diaphragm is prescribed more frequently than the others because it is the easiest to learn to manage. A spermicidal agent is often recommended for use in conjunction with the female barriers—it should be spread over the inside and rim of the diaphram.

Advantages

They have no effect upon the body and may even afford protection to the cervix. They may be inserted up to two hours before intercourse and so need not interfere with spontaneity. They can be retained in place after intercourse and so do not interrupt post-coital contact. In fact, they *must* be retained for at least six hours after intercourse to allow the spermicidal agent to be fully effective. They are not felt by either partner when correctly in place and they do not reduce sensation.

Disadvantages

Not all women can be fitted, especially those with displacements of the uterus or laxity of the vaginal walls. Also, local conditions can change after miscarriage or childbirth, after significant weight loss or gain and especially after vaginal surgery, necessitating the refitting of the diaphragm or cap. All diaphragms need to be checked frequently in the first few months and at least every year after that. Some women may not like handling their genital organs. If a woman does not like using tampons, she is unlikely to be happy inserting a diaphragm or cap high into the vagina, especially when she is not in any state of sexual arousal. She will need to practise inserting the diaphragm and learn the correct ways of cleaning and storing it.

There are two other disadvantages: the diaphragm may dislodge during intercourse and, like the condom, it may become damaged during use or by handling.

Chemical barriers

Vaginal spermicidal agents are used to destroy or inactivate sperm cells. They are chemicals combined with a base agent that serves to form a blocking film across the cervix. They are in the form of creams, pastes, dissolving pessaries, aerosol foams (the most effective) or jellies. Instructions are provided with the products and must be followed carefully.

They are most effective when used with a cap or diaphragm, and the spermicide should be applied to both the outside and the inside of the barrier so that it comes into contact with the cervix. If used with a condom, they must be injected high into the vagina. A thin smear on the outside of the condom will give no more protection than a condom used on its own.

Advantages

Spermicidal agents can be purchased without prescription and are widely available. They help to lubricate the vagina.

Disadvantages

They are messy to use, and may increase lubrication to the extent of reducing sensation. Creams and jellies have to be applied just before intercourse, thus causing an annoying interruption. Pessaries and tablets must be inserted ten to fifteen minutes earlier to allow time to dissolve and spread. Either partner may be allergic to the chemicals and may suffer burning and itching. Used on its own, this form of contraception has a high failure rate.

Sterilisation operations

Tubal ligation or diathermy in the female, and ligation of the vas deferens in the male, are the most common of the operations performed solely for contraceptive purposes. These operations involve the severing or blocking of the tubes which carry the germ cells; they do not 'sterilise' in the sense of removing or inactivating the gonads, and so they do not affect hormone production.

Because most sterilising operations are regarded as permanent, any decision to undergo such surgery should only be made with a clear understanding of the operation's effects. The decision is best made when the couple concerned is not under any sort of stress. Most doctors insist on seeing the couple for a full discussion about the procedure and its effects, and very few will perform the operation without a written consent signed by both.

Tubal ligation

There are several methods used to interrupt the pathway of the fallopian tubes. A widely used method (Pomeroy) involves the removal of 2·5 cm or more of the central portion of the tube. The free ends shrink away from each other (Figure 22.6). This operation requires a fairly small lower abdominal incision and a hospital stay of four to five days.

Tubal diathermy, using the laparoscope, is becoming more popular as the stay in hospital is reduced to one or two days. It involves two tiny incisions, each 1–2 cm long, one for the passage of the laparoscope and one for the cannula through which the diathermy forceps are passed. A portion of each tube is coagulated by diathermy.

Temporary tubal ligation methods are now being tried using small clips applied under laparoscopy.

Figure 22.6
Tubal ligation (Pomeroy)

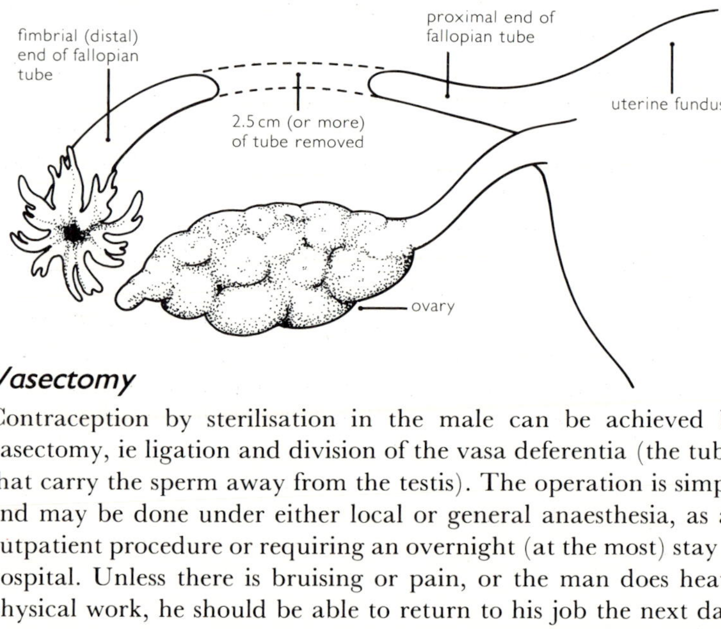

Vasectomy

Contraception by sterilisation in the male can be achieved by vasectomy, ie ligation and division of the vasa deferentia (the tubes that carry the sperm away from the testis). The operation is simple and may be done under either local or general anaesthesia, as an outpatient procedure or requiring an overnight (at the most) stay in hospital. Unless there is bruising or pain, or the man does heavy physical work, he should be able to return to his job the next day.

Vasectomy involves two small incisions into the scrotum. About 6 cm of each vas is removed and the ends are turned back and sutured or diathermied. The contraceptive effect of a vasectomy is not achieved until all remaining sperm above the excised portion of the vas have been removed from the body. This may take twenty to thirty ejaculations, for which alternative protection against pregnancy must be found. (Some clinics issue this number of condoms to the man routinely.) The man is asked to submit specimens of ejaculate for examination at monthly intervals until two consecutive specimens show no sperm. In most cases, sperm are absent by four months after the vasectomy.

Reversible sterilisation

Procedures involving the clamping (rather than crushing, cutting or coagulation) of the fallopian tubes or vasa deferentia to provide a temporary interruption to the passage of the ova or sperm are being tried, but without great success to date. Injection of a fluid plastic substance to create a plug (later surgically removable) is another advance in this field.

Reconstruction operations

When life situations change, for whatever reason, a person who has had a sterilising operation may want to be able to have children. He or she may ask the doctor to 'untie the tubes'. This may sound very easy to them, especially if their understanding of the original operation was incomplete. The more thorough the sterilising procedure, the more difficult reconstruction is likely to be. The operations are generally done by microsurgeons working with a gynaecologist.

In the female, the blocked portion of the fallopian tube is removed and an end-to-end anastomosis is performed. A plastic or polythene tube may be inserted to keep the lumen open until healing has occurred, after which it is removed via the uterus. Doctors rarely guarantee success following tubal reconstruction and most will warn that should conception occur, the incidence of ectopic pregnancy is high. Where there is insufficient length of the tube to attempt end-to-end anastomosis, the ovary may be sutured on to the outside of the uterus and a channel made through the uterine wall. This is rarely successful because the fertilised ovum has little time to develop sufficiently to embed upon reaching the endometrium.

In the male, reuniting of the ligated vasa deferentia may result in a patent pathway for the sperm, but the absorption of sperm into the man's system which may have occurred during the period of blockage, could have created an additional problem—that of formation of antibodies against his own spermatozoa—to render him 'sterile'.

Advantages of sterilisation

Sterilisation operations provide a permanent and (almost 100 per cent) effective form of contraception. In women they are effective immediately; no further contraception is required. The general functioning of the body is not affected; hormonal activity, menstrual cycles, sexual urge and intercourse should remain as they were before surgery.

Disadvantages

The permanency of the operation is not always an advantage. Life is unpredictable and situations may change, but once a permanent barrier to conception is established in one partner of a relationship, there is very little chance of that couple achieving pregnancy. Psychiatric and sexual problems may arise after, or at any rate, be blamed on the operation. The response to the loss of fertility may show itself in disorders such as depression, dyspareunia, frigidity or impotence. Finally, there is the risk of the operation itself, simple though it is. Abdominal operations and anaesthesia *are* still accompanied by a number of hazards.

Prevention of implantation of a fertilised ovum

Intrauterine devices (IUD)

These devices are small plastic and/or metal objects inserted into the endometrial cavity to prevent pregnancy. There are several different types of intrauterine devices to suit different women. Commonly used ones are: the Lippes loop, the Saf-T-Coil, and the Copper-7 (see Figure 22.7). Other IUDs are available, including some that contain a reservoir of progesterone, releasing a small quantity every day to create a 'hostile' cervical mucus. The devices are inserted (as a sterile procedure) after being drawn through a special applicator, and they spring back into their original shape after insertion. Most of them have a small attached thread which hangs down into the vagina so that the woman can check its presence; but it does not interfere with intercourse.

It is still not known precisely how the IUD prevents pregnancy. It may be due to an increased peristalsis of the fallopian tubes, which would bring the fertilised ovum to the uterus before it is ready to

Figure 22.7 Types of intrauterine devices

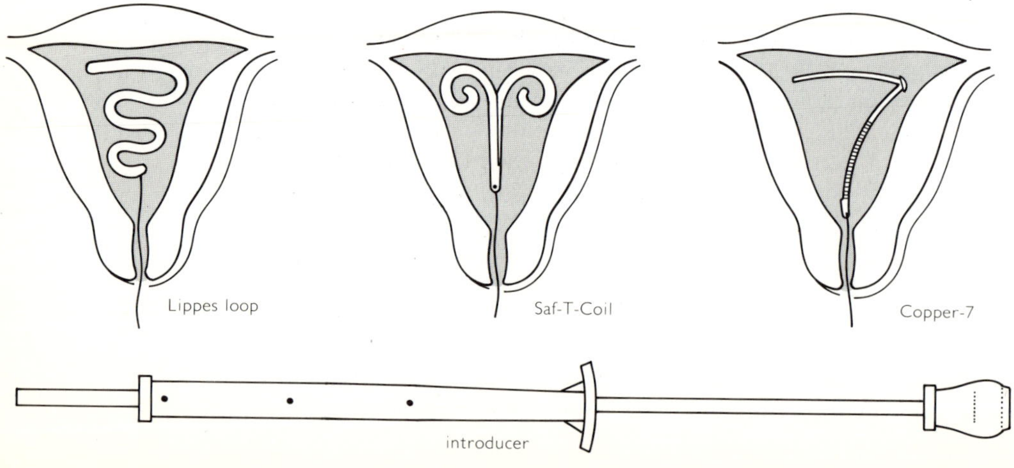

implant. As well, there is possibly a local endometrial reaction (to the presence of a foreign body or foreign chemicals) and this changed endometrium is unsuitable either for implantation or for the provision of nutrients should implantation occur.

Intrauterine devices are usually inserted on the second last or last day of a menstrual flow. The cervix is still open at that time, making the insertion easier, and also, there is little likelihood of a pregnancy being present then. Postnatally, the device is not inserted until at least six weeks have passed; before this, it is more likely to be expelled and, because the placental site is still raw, infection must be avoided. The wearing of tampons is discouraged for the first forty-eight hours after insertion of the device.

The woman is usually asked to return for a check-up following the first period after insertion of the IUD. She should also seek advice if she misses a period or if she cannot locate the thread in the vagina.

Advantages

After the initial expense of consultation and insertion, there is no further cost. There is a 97 per cent success rate, and no deliberate action at the time of intercourse is necessary. When pregnancy is desired, the device is simply removed (by the doctor) so there is no period of waiting for the body to adjust.

Disadvantages

Bleeding—heavy and prolonged menstruation and intermenstrual spotting—is a common problem. It may be due to the uterus receiving a larger blood supply (pelvic congestion) as a response to the endometrial reaction. The device may also cause a flare-up of a pre-existing or low-grade pelvic inflammation, especially salpingitis. Pregnancy does occur sometimes, and could be due to failure of the device to change local conditions, or to an unnoticed expulsion. Expulsion occurs in about 20 per cent of cases. Occasionally the device perforates the uterine wall and may even escape completely into the peritoneal cavity. Pain and cramping during menstruation is often increased, particularly for the first three months. The devices are rarely suitable for nulliparous patients as the cervix is usually too tightly closed for their easy insertion. They cannot be used when the endometrial cavity is distorted, eg by a septum or by fibroids. Some of the newer devices such as the Copper 7 have to be renewed every two years, as the extra effect of the metal gradually wears off. (NB Microwave treatment should not be given to the abdomen or back when a copper device is in place.)

23 Abortion, ectopic pregnancy and hydatidiform mole

Abortion, ectopic pregnancy and hydatidiform mole are pregnancies that have gone wrong. These three are conditions in which, after the conception and establishment of a new human being within the body of a woman, some factor arises to prevent that new being from developing into a baby capable of independent existence.

Before dealing with the details of the causes and management of these conditions, it is worth considering some of the aspects surrounding them, and how they may be affecting those people who come under our care. To start with the obvious—a pregnancy has occurred, as the result of sexual intercourse between a man and a woman. So there is more than one person involved. In the *ideal* situation, the couple are healthy, established in their relationship, have welcomed the pregnancy, and are able to support each other in a crisis. They are saddened by the loss of their future child, but are concerned for each other's suffering and the experience ultimately brings them even closer together.

The situation becomes less ideal when there is some complicating factor such as: the pregnancy was achieved only after years of waiting or trying; other pregnancies had ended in a similar manner; the pregnancy was unwelcome and the woman, or the man, or both, had considered abortion; the woman didn't even know that she was pregnant. The interruption to pregnancy has caused the woman pain, made her weak, put her into hospital, possibly threatened her life. Who is feeling the blame? The woman (because she played tennis, or kept working)? The man (because he 'got her pregnant, didn't he?')? Both of them (because their 'cuddle' progressed to an exciting, orgasmic intercourse and then the bleeding started)?

There are as many variations on the responses to pregnancy and its problems as there are babies conceived. It would be foolish to think otherwise and it would be very poor nursing practice to adopt the same approach to every person who has a similar diagnosis. Excessive sympathy can be exhausting to the people involved. The stiff upper lip treatment can, at times, be cruel. Disapproval of any aspect of a situation as it appears is intolerable.

The admission to hospital is, in these cases, usually without much warning. There is no time to gather a collection of best nightgowns and toiletries. She must simply leave her home even though emergency arrangements may be unsatisfactory. Total patient care involves concern for and appreciation of all such anxieties. It involves action in the form of contacting (with the patient's permission) the appropriate helper, be it a social worker, clergyman, relative or special friend.

To return to the 'ideal' situation of the couple who welcomed their pregnancy: they probably announced it with joy to their friends and family. When the man leaves his partner in our care and goes home, maybe to an empty house, he faces the task of letting people know what has happened. If we think about this we can help to a certain degree: first, by not sending him off as though he were a nuisance and in our way; second, by offering our time and attention. Just having someone who knows (sitting down somewhere, over a cup of tea, not standing in a busy corridor) explaining to him exactly what is happening to his partner, and to the pregnancy, is a help. (Figure 23.1.) And third, by assuring him that his problems during this difficult time are important to us.

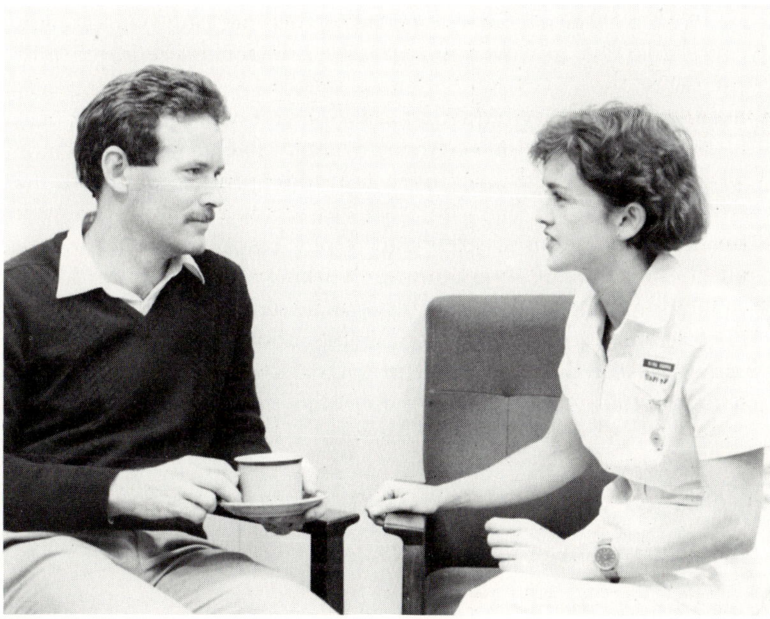

Figure 23.1
The man should always be given a full explanation of what is happening to his partner, and to their pregnancy

Abortion

Abortion is the termination of a pregnancy before the foetus is viable. It is believed that between 10 and 20 per cent of pregnancies end in spontaneous abortion, most of them during the first twelve weeks.

Spontaneous abortion

Causes

- abnormality of the embroyo or foetus is the most common cause of early abortion and is often due to chromosomal defects
- abnormalities of the uterus, resulting in a distorted uterine cavity or restriction of growth and expansion of the uterus, eg fibroids, congenital malformations, uterine prolapse or retroversion
- damage to the cervix, from deep tearing during childbirth or surgical procedures (dilation, amputation)
- maternal diseases and ingestion of drugs: diseases include acute viral infections, high fevers, and inoculations, eg against smallpox. Chronic nephritis and heart failure may result in foetal anoxia. Errors in the metabolism of folic acid, which is necessary for foetal development, will result in foetal death. Certain drugs, especially cytotoxic agents, will interfere with the normal process of rapid cell division. Prostaglandins will cause abortion by stimulating uterine contractions
- trauma, but usually only when applied directly to the uterine cavity. Sexual intercourse, especially when orgasm occurs, might cause abortion in a woman who has a history of repeated miscarriages
- hormonal factors, eg reduction in the output of progesterone, may be blamed for abortion occurring at ten to twelve weeks, the time when the placenta takes over hormone production from the corpus luteum
- psychosomatic causes: stress and strong emotions are known to affect the uterine functioning, working through the hypothalamic-pituitary system. Most gynaecologists can quote case-histories of stress-related spontaneous abortions, and they can usually also tell of successful pregnancies occurring (in women with previously bad histories) after anxieties have been removed

Types of spontaneous abortion

Four types are shown in Figure 23.2.

Threatened abortion

Bleeding from the uterus is noticed. In 50 per cent of cases the bleeding is slight, gradually ceasing after a few days, and the pregnancy proceeds normally. Even so, the woman may continue to worry about the effect of the bleeding on the baby. She can usually be assured that were the foetus damaged, the pregnancy would generally not continue; it is wise to ask the doctor to add his reassurance. The treatment is bed rest and sedation for at least forty-eight hours, with careful observation of the colour and type of all

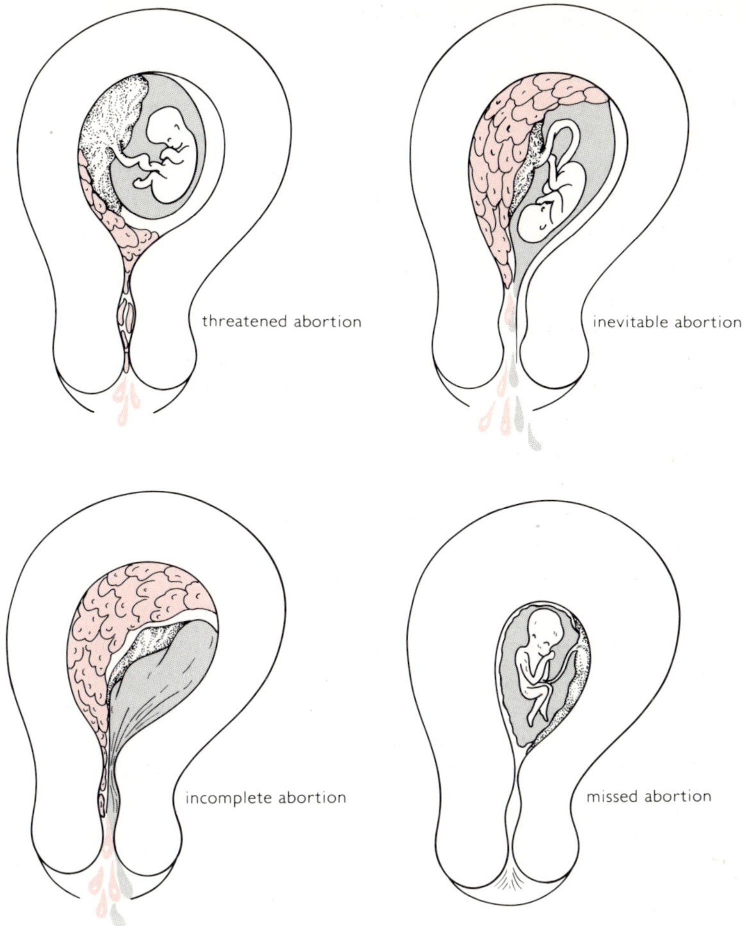

Figure 23.2
Types of abortion

vaginal loss. Enemas and laxatives should not be given. An ultrasound scan is performed at this stage, and may be repeated two weeks later. The couple are advised against having intercourse for this period.

The woman in hospital should use pans rather than go to the toilet, and all pads should be kept for inspection before disposal. If the bleeding persists and is accompanied by pain and cervical dilatation, the abortion is then typed as 'inevitable'.

Inevitable abortion

Ineviable abortion is characterised by moderate to severe blood loss, uterine contractions causing cramping pains, and cervical dilatation. Its management consists of:

- complete bed rest
- careful measurement and observation of all matter passed vaginally. Forceps should be used to separate any clots to see whether

or not they contain foetal tissue. All matter passed is saved and sent off for laboratory examination.

- frequent and accurate recording of vital signs (temperature, pulse, respirations, blood pressure)
- relief of pain, which may suddenly become severe
- withholding of food, possibly fluids as well, because a general anaesthetic may be necessary
- administration of ergometrine, if ordered, to contract the uterus
- taking a specimen of blood for Hb, typing and cross-matching.

If abortion does not occur within twenty-four hours, the uterus is evacuated, using ovum forceps, a curette or a suction cannula; all material obtained is sent away for histological examination. Antibiotics are frequently prescribed at this stage.

While attending to all of these important physical aspects of care, the nurse must consider the emotional needs of both the woman and (usually) her partner. Privacy and some flexibility in the hosptial routine should be arranged to allow them to be together during this difficult time.

Complete abortion

Complete abortion has occurred when all the products of conception—the foetus, membranes, and placenta—have been expelled. Bleeding and pain will then cease, the cervix closes, and the uterus involutes. Figure 23.3 shows an embryo of eight weeks expelled as a complete sac.

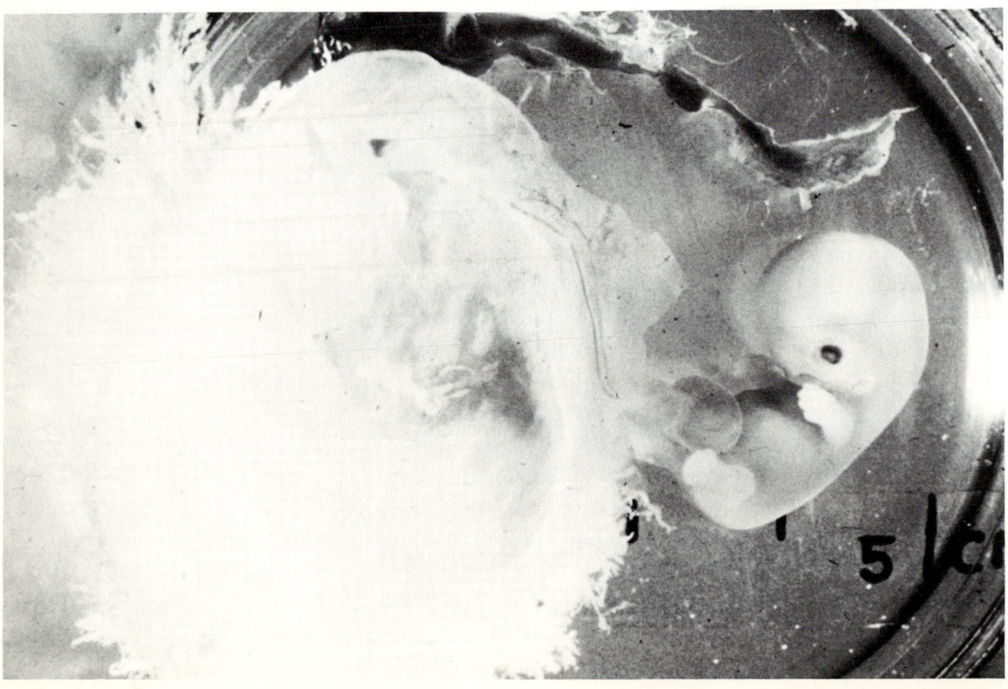

Figure 23.3
An embryo of eight weeks gestation (spontaneous complete abortion)

Incomplete abortion

Incomplete abortion refers to the retention of part of the products of conception, almost always the placenta, which does not separate as readily in early pregnancy as it does at term. The bleeding does not progressively decrease and the cervix remains open.

Treatment, nursing care and observation are as described for inevitable abortion. The evacuation of the uterus, however, is performed immediately after diagnosis to prevent further blood loss. The woman is usually kept in hospital for a further two days to be observed for bleeding. Special attention is given to vulval hygiene. In some cases, suppression of lactation may be necessary. Anti-D gamma globulin would be given to an Rh-negative woman.

Missed abortion

Missed abortion occurs when, after a threatened abortion, the bleeding stops but the products of conception die and are retained. After several weeks a brown discharge may be seen and the external signs of pregnancy disappear. Hypofibrinogenaemia may occur. Clotted blood from placental haemorrhages sometimes fills the uterus to form a carneous mole. Spontaneous evacuation eventually occurs at about eighteen weeks and many doctors feel that it is safer to wait for this. But the woman is often, understandably, anxious for it to be removed sooner, when she realises that the foetus is dead. It is a very difficult situation.

Treatment

If the uterus is less than fourteen weeks in size, it can be emptied by suction curettage with intravenous egometrine given at the same time. When the uterus is larger than 'fourteen weeks' in size, prostaglandins or oxytocin are given by intravenous infusion to induce labour.

Abortion due to cervical incompetence

Abortion due to cervical incompetence usually occurs around the twentieth week of pregnancy. The cervix dilates painlessly and the foetal sac protrudes. In a subsequent pregnancy, abortion is prevented by the insertion (under anaesthesia) of a purse-string suture around the cervix at the junction of the vaginal rugae and the smooth cervix (Shirodkar's suture). This suture is left until the thirty-eighth week of pregnancy, when it is divided. Labour then follows quickly and is usually short and relatively painless. The success rate is up to 80 per cent in cases of genuine cervical incompetence.

Where this treatment is not successful or is unsuitable, a more complicated ligature, using a polyvinyl suture, may be inserted at the level of the internal os, at a time when the woman is not pregnant. The suture is non-recoverable, and so the woman will need a caesarian section for delivery of any subsequent foetus.

Habitual abortion

This term is used when a woman has had three or more consecutive spontaneous abortions. The causes are multiple and often there is more than one factor involved. General ill-health, chronic disease or infection, anxiety, cervical incompetence, and states of hormonal imbalance are all possible causes. When careful investigation results in the elimination of even one of these factors, the next pregnancy will often continue successfully to term. Deliberate rest has some of the best results.

Induced abortion

Thereapeutic abortion is now a legal procedure in some parts of the world. In Australia, it is allowed in those cases where the mental or physical health of the mother would be threatened more by the continuation of the pregnancy than if the pregnancy were to be terminated. Included under this heading are the following circumstances:

- severe cardiovascular disease
- pulmonary disease, active tuberculosis
- chronic renal disease
- malignancy, especially of the breast or cervix
- psychiatric conditions, the severity of which may be difficult to assess
- following infections in early pregnancy with conditions known to cause foetal malformations, eg rubella, cytomegalovirus, toxoplasmosis
- Rh isoimmunisation, which has previously resulted in a severely affected baby
- where there is a strong likelihood that the child will be affected by an hereditary condition or where previous children born to the couple have been deformed.

Methods to induce abortion

Before the fourteenth week

Suction evacuation involves aspiration of the uterine contents through a hollow curette connected to controlled suction apparatus. Before eight weeks, this can be done with minimal cervical dilatation and under local (paracervical) anaesthesia. After eight weeks, cervical dilatation and a larger curette are necessary to ensure complete emptying of the uterus, and it needs to be done under general anaesthesia. Suction evacuation has superseded traditional uterine curettage for this purpose because it involves less risk of perforation. It is often performed as an outpatient procedure.

After the fourteenth week

The following may be used:
Hypertonic saline, injected via the abdominal route. Twenty per cent salt solution usually kills the foetus and causes strong contractions. Its dangers are possible damage to abdominal tissues and the peritoneum and blood electrolyte imbalance. It can be fatal to the mother if it enters a vein.
Prostaglandins, which stimulate contractions. They may be given by slow intravenous infusion or injected into the amniotic sac. Their use may need to be supplemented by an oxytocin infusion. The whole process requires extreme care in observation, monitoring and control of dosage, to prevent such calamities as rupture of the uterus. It sequires hospital admission.
Abdominal hysterotomy, which is in fact a miniature caesarian section. It allows the uterus to be completely evacuated when other methods would not achieve this, or would be dangerous. It does, however, carry the risks of laparotomy. It is most often used when the pregnancy is well into the second trimester and where the woman is to be sterilised as well.

Risks of induced abortion

Therapeutic abortion is not without its risks. As well as the specific risks noted above, haemorrhage, perforation of the uterus, damage to the cervix, Rh isoimmunisation and infection leading to infertility may occur. Antibiotics are given routinely in many centres, but because of the trend towards outpatient abortion, treatment largely depends upon the woman's continued usage of the drugs.

It is difficult to generalise about the psychological effects following therapeutic abortion. Statistics show very little because post-operative follow-up is inadequate. Some women appear to have quite severe reactions of depression and withdrawal from society; certainly the stability of many a marriage has suffered. Careful counselling is an absolute necesssity for anyone contemplating this step.

What does a nurse say when directly asked for advice by someone considering therapeutic abortion? Unless she has expert knowledge and insight into the particular situation, she does *not* deliver a verdict; the responsibility is too great. She does, however, urge and assist that person to consult someone with expertise and experience. She knows of the existence of pregnacy support services for those who might need them; and, most importantly, she reads and listens to information about this controversial, moral, religious and ethical problem, and decides for herself whether or not she is willing to be involved professionally in therapeutic abortion. Those who hold conscientious objections to the procedure cannot be made to participate in abortion procedures and their refusal to participate will not be held against them.

Septic abortion

Infection may complicate any type of abortion, as the normal resistance of the genital tract is virtually absent at this time. Criminal abortions (illegally induced backyard abortions) still cause the most serious infections due to lack of aseptic precautions. The other factor involved is the presence of products of conception, dead placental tissue, within the uterus. The infection may invade the endometrium and spread directly or indirectly to cause peritonitis, salpingitis, and septicaemia.

Symptoms

Malaise, high fever, tachycardia and headache are usually present. An offensive vaginal discharge may be present, but not always. Pelvic examination is painful.

Management

A high vaginal swab is taken for culture, and antibiotic therapy is commenced. Retained products are evacuated by curettage (or, if after twelve weeks, by oxytocin infusion) but, unless there is severe bleeding as well, curettage is delayed for twelve to twenty-four hours to allow the antibiotics to act. This lessens the risk of organisms entering the bloodstream and possibly causing bacteraemic (endotoxic) shock or disseminated intravascular coagulation (DIC). Both are serious and often fatal complications of septic abortion.

Ectopic pregnancy

Ectopic pregnancy occurs when a fertilised ovum embeds in a site other than the uterine cavity. The pregnancy is rarely able to survive for longer than six to ten weeks, either because the site is unsuitable for satisfactory development of the placenta, or because there is insufficient room to accommodate the growing pregnancy (Figure 23.4).

Figure 23.4
Ectopic pregnancy

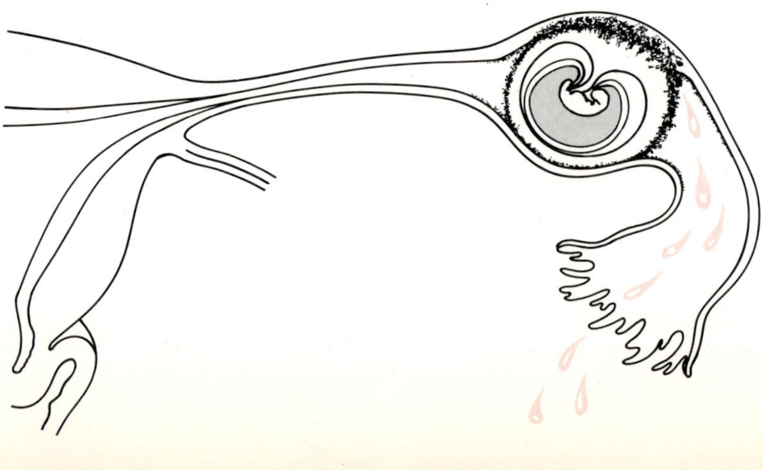

Sites of ectopic implantation

The site may be:

- a fallopian tube
- the cervix
- the abdominal cavity
- an ovary
- a broad ligament.

Tubal pregnancy is by far the commonest of these, and so is the only one discussed here in detail; the others are rare. Abdominal pregnancies occasionally go to term to be delivered by laparotomy; the placenta has attached itself to whichever organs would supply its needs, and so its removal poses great problems, especially the danger of haemorrhage.

Tubal pregnancy

Tubal pregnancy will result in one of three outcomes:

Death of the ovum in the early stages; it then is either completely absorbed or remains as a tubal mole.

Tubal abortion, the most common outcome, with the ovum (and possibly blood) being expelled from the tube into the uterus or out into the peritoneal cavity. This usually results in its death; very occasionally it implants again and develops as a secondary abdominal pregnancy.

Tubal rupture: erosion and finally rupture of the tube occurs when the ovum continues to grow past the stretching ability of the muscular tube. The rupture of the tube is usually accompanied by rupture of one or more large arterioles, so there can be considerable blood loss which drains to the pouch of Douglas to form a pelvic haematocele.

Causes

- partial obstruction of the tube. There is enough room for the passage of spermatozoa, but not enough for the fertilised ovum. Obstruction is most often the result of old inflammation, tuberculous or other salpingitis, but is also caused by diverticuli, previous tubal surgery, kinking and pressure or adhesions from outside
- tubal endometriosis
- delay in the passage of the ovum to the uterus, eg unilateral development of the Mullerian system combined with ovulation from the opposite ovary

Signs and Symptoms

Pregnancy: amenorrhoea, early breast changes, uterine enlargement (due to hormonal influence) and the other signs of early pregnancy are usually present; the pregnancy may have been confirmed as positive. Sometimes the woman is unaware that she is pregnant.

Pain, in the lower abdomen, which is caused by distension of the tube or by blood irritating the peritoneum. Peritoneal irritation can give rise to shoulder-tip pain when the woman is lying down. Severe abdominal pain is commonly accompanied by fainting in cases of ruptured tubal pregnancy.

Vaginal loss, brown or red in colour and usually slight but persisting. It has two possible sources: from the tube via the uterus, or from the breakdown of the decidua as a result of oestrogen withdrawal after the death of the embryo.

Evidence of internal blood loss: the slow bleeding that follows tubal abortion or the leakage prior to rupture may cause anaemia but it is the severe bleeding that can follow tubal rupture that gives rise to collapse and shock. The abdomen is extremely tender and is distended.

Management

The woman is admitted to hospital. Shock, if present, is treated, and intravenous fluids commenced while waiting for blood cross-matching. In those cases where there is real doubt about the diagnosis, a laparoscopy may be performed. Otherwise the treatment is immediate laparotomy, excision of the affected tube, and removal of clots from the pelvic cavity. Sometimes an effort is made to conserve the tube, especially where the other tube is absent or known to be damaged.

The post-operative period is usually without complications. Once the bleeding has ceased and blood volume restored, the danger has passed. It has, however, been a sudden, urgent and frightening experience and it has resulted in the ending of what might have been a very much wanted pregnancy.

Hydatidiform mole

Very occasionally and for no known reason, an early pregnancy develops abnormally and the uterus fills with a mass of grape-like vesicles (see Figure 23.5) which produce enormous quantities of the hormone *chorionic gonadotrophin*. The vesicles grow from the chorionic villi, which project from the outer cell mass of the blastocyst and which are normally destined to become the placenta. The embryo dies and disappears.

The uterus is larger than normal for the period of gestation, and is soft and rounded. The foetal heart is not heard, nor are foetal parts felt. Hyperemesis may occur and pre-eclamptic toxaemia appears early. There may be episodes of slight, dark vaginal bleeding and, rarely, grape-like vesicles are passed vaginally. The urine pregnancy test is strongly positive.

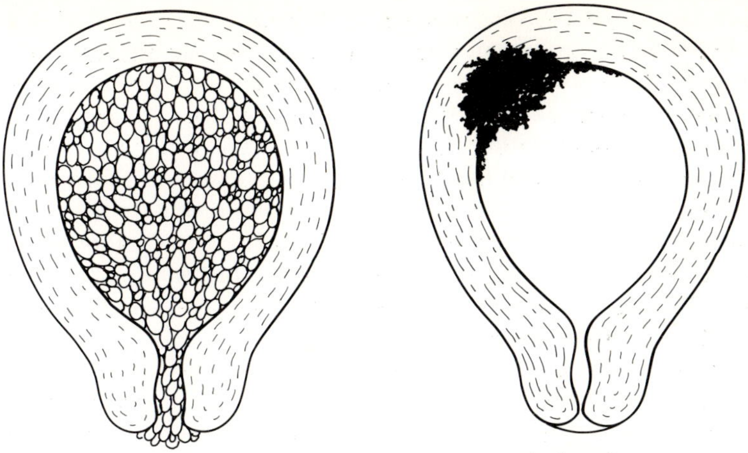

Figure 23.5
Hydatidiform mole and choriocarcinoma

Diagnosis is aided by ultrasonography (which can be used as early as eight weeks), the use of diluted urine for pregnancy tests, and X-ray of the abdomen to confirm the absence of a foetal skeleton.

Hydatidiform mole occurs on an average in about one in 750 pregnancies in Australia. Its incidence in South-East Asia and in the Far East, however, is far greater. It occurs more frequently in the older age group (over 35 years) and in women who have had more than one baby, although it can happen in any pregnancy.

Treatment

Once hydatidiform mole is diagnosed, it must be removed immediately because some (5 per cent) of these moles develop into malignant trophoblastic disease—choriocarcinoma. Spontaneous delivery does occur in some cases, but may not be complete. The uterus has to be *emptied* and this can be achieved by the methods described for therapeutic abortion. Hysterectomy is usually performed when the woman is over the age of forty.

Follow-up

After discharge from hospital, frequent (at first, weekly) follow-up examinations are essential. These will continue for two years, their frequency depending on the findings at each visit. The woman is warned against starting another pregnancy during this time, and family planning advice or referral is usually necessary. The doctor will observe for persistent bleeding which may indicate retained products, and for the return of normal menstruation which would be suppressed by elevated levels of HCG (human chorionic gonadotrophin). Chest X-rays are performed regularly until the urinary HCG levels are normal, to exclude pulmonary metastases of choriocarcinoma.

The routine pregnancy test cannot be used for follow up as it is not sufficiently accurate. Precise measurements of the urinary excretion of HCG over twenty-four hours are performed weekly until the levels are within the normal range for the non-pregnant woman. After this the levels are measured monthly for twelve months or longer. HCG levels drop very rapidly after a normal pregnancy, usually within two to three days. Following a hydatidiform mole the return of these levels to normal can take from two to six months. If a progressive decline does not occur (or if the decline is followed by a rise), courses of methotrexate are given. Methotrexate is a folic acid antagonist, and trophoblastic (placental) tissue has high folic acid requirements. The treatment is given in hospital and daily white cell counts are performed.

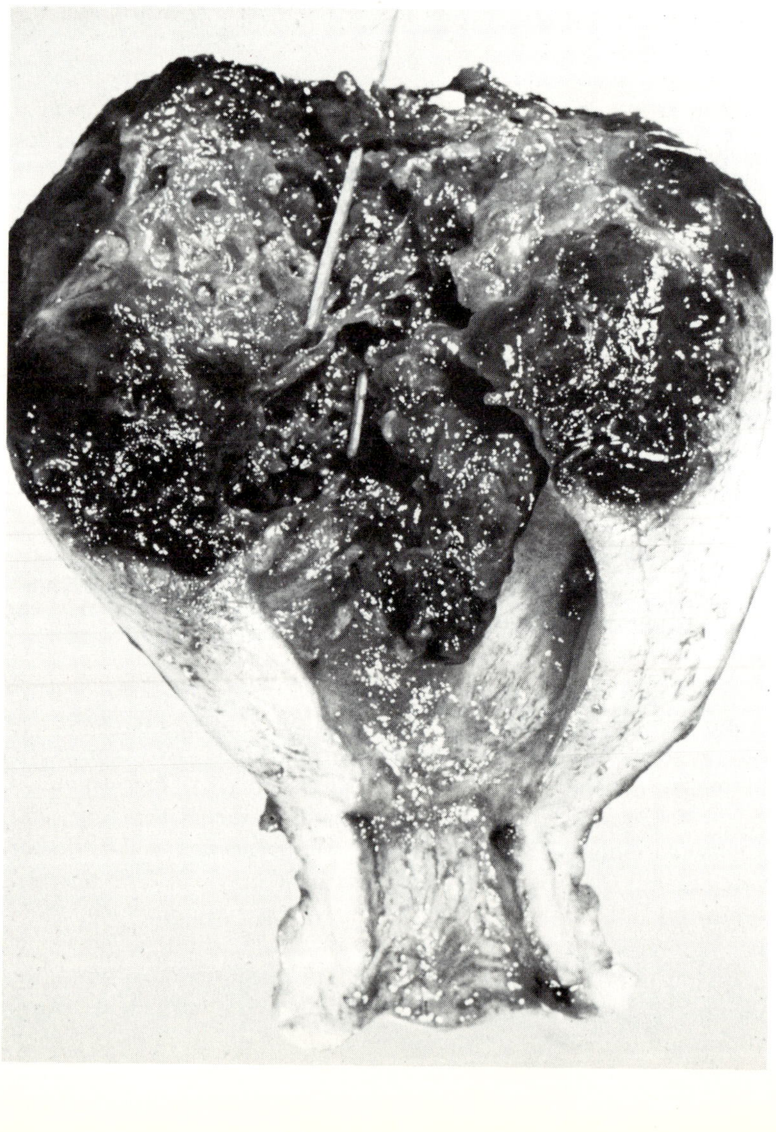

Figure 23.6
Uterine perforation by invasive mole

Choriocarcinoma

Choriocarcinoma arises when there is invasion of the uterine wall by malignant trophoblastic tissue. It is rare, but is the feared consequence of hydatidiform mole. It can also arise after an apparently normal pregnancy or uncomplicated abortion, but in more than 50 per cent of cases it is preceded by a mole pregnancy. Because an early spontaneous delivery of a hydatidiform mole can resemble an uncomplicated abortion, the importance of saving any products of conception that have been passed, for histological examination, is emphasised.

Choriocarcinoma spreads rapidly once it starts, directly (Figure 23.6) and via the bloodstream. Metastases occur in the brain, the liver and the lungs. It was nearly always fatal, but methotrexate and other cytotoxic agents have had good results, with the metastases and the primary growth in the uterus disappearing.

Hydatidiform mole can, indeed, be a pregnancy that has gone wrong.

24 The infertile couple

Infertility is the inability to achieve or establish a pregnancy. It is believed to occur in about 10 per cent of marriages, and can be due to factors arising in the male partner, the female partner, both partners or in the particular combination of one female with one male. But it is the woman who does not become pregnant, so it is almost always the woman who seeks advice first.

Infertility investigations are not usually undertaken until the couple have been trying (to achieve pregnancy) for a period of eighteen months. Where the couple are concerned about their age, however, investigations would be started earlier than this.

Once the investigations are started they may go on for several months. Many of the investigations involve processes that are embarrassing or worrying to the couple, and they can get very distressed about the whole business. But infertility investigation and treatment does have very positive aspects; in at least one third of cases, causes are discovered and can be treated successfully.

Factors necessary for establishment of pregnancy

Pregnancy is established when an ovum, fertilised by a spermatozoon, finds a suitable place in which to embed and from which it can obtain its needs to continue living.

This may not be as simple as it sounds. Although only one ovum is necessary, it must be released into the peritoneal cavity and it must find its way into the fallopian tube. Although only one spermatozoon will actually fertilise that ovum, millions are necessary to break down the outer shell (zona pellucida) of the ovum so that that one can get through. Then, the ovum and sperm must have access to each other, ie the genital tract must be patent. They must meet when they are still alive—both will die or degenerate (under normal conditions) unless fertilisation takes place within a limited time after their release. If fertilisation is successful, the zygote can live for up to seven days on its own reserves; in fact, it needs this time to develop sufficiently to form the chorionic villi through which its basic needs can be supplied. But after this time it must embed in a place that has been prepared to supply its needs. So the factors necessary for the successful establishment of pregnancy are:

- ovulation must take place
- spermatozoa must be present (in sufficient quantity and quality)
- intercourse must take place at, or close to, the time of ovulation
- the genital tract must be patent
- there must be a suitable place for the fertilised ovum to embed. (Figure 24.1 illustrates these factors.)

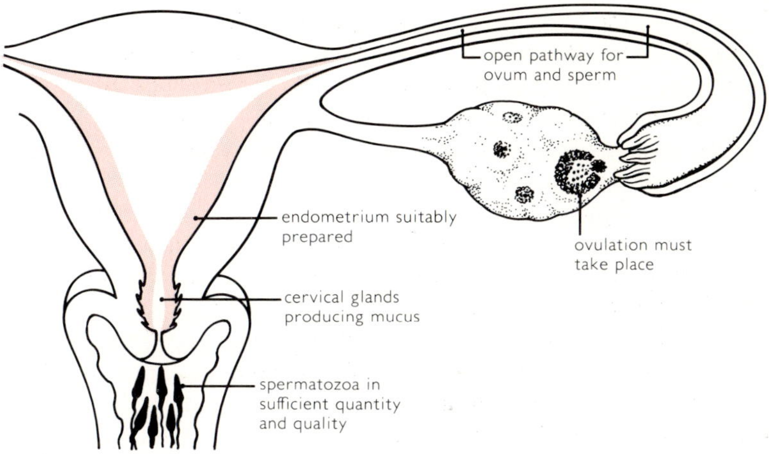

Figure 24.1
Factors necessary for establishment of pregnancy

Causes of infertility

Ovulation must take place

Anovulation may be due to the absence or underdevelopment of the ovaries, to ovarian surgery or irradiation, or to the lack of responsive ova occurring as a natural event (responsive ova decrease in number from the age of twenty-five onwards), or as a result of cytotoxic drugs. Pituitary and hypothalamic conditions and other endocrine factors inhibit ovulation by their failure to release the gonadotrophins or their releasing factors. Post-pill infertility is an example of the continued suppression of these hormones. The causes of failure to ovulate are discussed fully under the heading 'Amenorrhoea' in Chapter 12.

Spermatozoa must be present in sufficient quantity and quality

After they have been deposited in the vagina, the sperm must survive their journey to the upper genital tract. Vaginal acidity can kill large numbers of sperm, as can lubricant agents used during intercourse. The cervical mucus may be impenetrable to sperm; it has to be of a certain consistency to allow them to travel through it.

The sperm themselves must be alive, motile and present in their hundreds of millions (200 to 600 million spermatozoa are usually found in a single 2–4 mL ejaculation specimen of seminal fluid).

Absence of sperm can result from chromosomal, hypothalamic, pituitary and testicular disorders. Specific causes include: testicular atrophy (as may occur after mumps orchitis), undescended testicles, irradiation and cytotoxic drugs. Obstruction of the male genital tract can be due to adhesions following infections (especially gonorrhoea and tuberculosis) or to surgery. Deficiency in the quantity and quality of sperm may be due to some of the causes above, especially when the condition has affected only one side. Chronic infection of the accessory organs, the epididymus and the prostate, may affect the sperm count and quality, as may varicoceles, which are varicosities of the spermatic cord. Excessive warmth near the testes interferes with spermatogenesis; certain occupations or the wearing of tight underpants may have this effect. Other factors that may contribute to male infertility are excesses in work, alcohol consumption and smoking.

Intercourse must take place at, or close to, the time of ovulation

First of all, intercourse must take place. Apareunia (where intercourse does not occur at all) can be due to congenital disorders such as imperforate hymen or absence of the vagina, to vaginismus, or to lack of knowledge on the part of either partner about the act of intercourse. Dyspareunia can decrease the frequency of intercourse or it can result in premature withdrawal and ejaculation outside the vagina.

Ovulation mucus: when intercourse has taken place properly and sperm have been deposited in the vaginal vault, they require the presence of a particular quality and consistency of cervical mucus to assist their passage. This mucus, which is clear, slippery, stretchy and rather like egg-white, is present only when the oestrogen levels in the blood are at a certain peak, just prior to ovulation.

Survival of the ovum: the ovum will live for only twelve to twenty-four hours after its release unless it is fertilised. Although they have been known to survive for longer periods, even up to one week, sperm, under normal conditions, usually lose their fertilising power within seventy-two hours. This means that unless intercourse takes place within the space of the four to five days around the time of ovulation, it will probably not result in pregnancy.

The genital tract must be patent

Complete vaginal and cervical strictures do occur, but are uncommon. Obstruction of the fallopian tubes is the main problem. The lumen of the tube is incredibly narrow. Obstruction may be the result of salpingitis caused by gonorrhoea, tuberculosis or widespread pelvic infection. Adhesions from surgery, endometriosis and old inflammation can cause kinking of the tubes or closure of their fimbrial ends. Trauma to the tubes, whether accidental or deliberate, will usually result in their obstruction.

There must be a suitable place for the fertilised ovum to embed

The endometrium must be prepared to receive the fertilised ovum. Following ovulation the corpus luteum produces significant quantities of progesterone, which acts on the endometrium, which had been previously built up under the influence of oestrogen. Progesterone produces a state of increased vascularity and causes the endometrial glands to secrete glycogen and mucus for the immediate nourishment of the embedding ovum. Unless ovulation occurs, this will not happen.

Embedding and establishment of pregnancy may not be successful in cases of deficiency of endometrial thickness, abnormal hormone ratio, adenomyosis, infection (even of a low grade), and disturbances of blood supply. Other intrauterine factors include congenital malformations, fibroids and polyps, and intrauterine foreign bodies.

Other causes of infertility

General ill-health, malnutrition, anaemia, overwork.
Immunological factors: it is known that spermatozoa are antigenic and that there must normally be some mechanism active in women to prevent immune reactions. If that mechanism does not operate the woman may form antibodies that will cause rejection of the sperm. A lot of research is currently being carried out on this problem.
Psychological factors: obvious or hidden emotional factors can influence a couple's ability to achieve pregnancy. These can operate without necessarily inhibiting , but still having some effect. Minor psychological problems are undoubtedly made worse when the couple are anxious about their inability to conceive (or when the results of conception, pregnancy, labour and childbearing are feared).

When their calendar is marked with the dates upon which they must 'perform' and when they restrict intercourse to these days only, or when their intention during intercourse is more to become pregnant than to express their love for each other, there is indeed a greater strain and tension produced. This tension might inhibit orgasm, cause occasional episodes of impotence or generally affect the overall health of the couple, with the ultimate result of lowering their potential to achieve pregnancy.

Investigations and treatment

History

At the first visit, a detailed history is taken. In addition to the questions that are usually asked at a routine gynaecological examination, the doctor will try to assess the woman's attitude to pregnancy and her feelings about infertility. As well, he will ask about specific gynaecological symptoms she has had in the past, about contraceptive methods that have been used, and about her attitude to, and enjoyment of, intercourse. He will test the woman's knowledge and understanding of the menstrual cycle and ovulation.

Examination

A general medical and pelvic examination is performed and any obvious local condition treated; occasionally the doctor will find that the woman is still a virgin.

Before the woman goes home, she may be given a temperature chart to complete, with instructions on how to take and record her daily temperature. Alternatively, or as well, she may be referred to a family planning clinic specialising in the ovulation method, to begin instruction in the interpretation of cervical mucus changes.

Factors relating to her general health, nutrition and lifestyle are discussed; blood tests, eg for haemoglobin, may be ordered.

An appointment is made for her return, (accompanied by her partner if possible) in one or two months, after which specific investigations will probably be started.

Tests for ovulation

Temperature charting

The completion of a series of basal body temperature charts over a number of cycles will indicate ovulation by showing a rise in temperature of 0·5°C. This elevation continues until just before menstruation, and is due to the thermogenic effect of progesterone; thus it indicates the formation of the corpus luteum.

Plasma progesterone

Blood is taken during the second half of the cycle to estimate the plasma level of progesterone, as an indication of ovulation.

Examination of cervical mucus

Mucus examined in the preovulatory phase will show a fern-like pattern when dried and examined under a microscope. After ovulation, progesterone causes this ferning pattern to disappear.

Vaginal wall smear

This may be taken to demonstrate cell maturation or inhibition as a basis of hormonal activity.

Endometrial biopsy

A sample of endometrium can be obtained, without dilating the cervix, through a fine suction cannula or small Novak's curette, and can be done as an outpatient procedure. Secretory changes in the endometrium will confirm ovulation.

Urine collection

Urine collection over twenty-four hours will reveal pregnanediol in the urine if ovulation has occurred; it will be absent before ovulation.

Treatment of anovulation

If ovulation is proved to be absent, attention is given to causative factors (see Chapter 12). Ovulation can be induced in certain cases by the administration of ovulation-stimulating drugs, such as gonadotrophins extracted from cadaveric human pituitary glands (HPG) or the urine of postmenopausal women (HMG), or clomiphene citrate. Clomiphene is an anti-oestrogenic compound and is thought to act by lowering the oestrogen levels in the body to the point where the hypothalamus responds by an increased output of FSH and LH releasing factors. These in turn cause ovarian activity to occur, with the stimulation of ovarian follicles to maturity and ovulation, sometimes with more than one ovum being released. Small doses of oestrogen may be given in conjunction with clomiphene to maintain the suitability of the cervical mucus. Clomiphene is a potent drug and is always given in controlled doses; its effects are monitored very carefully. This treatment is usually only given in large centres or by doctors who specialise in fertility treatment.

Tests for sperm quantity and quality

Once it is proved that ovulation is occurring in the woman, the next step is to find out if the spermatozoa from the male are satisfactory. Some men may find this a difficult question to face, and occasionally the woman will try to talk her doctors into continuing investigations on *her*, so that her partner does not have to find out if, in fact, he is the one responsible.

Seminal examination is carried out on either a specimen of ejaculated semen obtained by coitus interruptus (or by masturbation) or on a post-coital specimen of the woman's cervical mucus (Hühner's test).

Examination of ejaculate

The whole ejaculate is collected in a clean, dry, glass container with a tight lid; it needs to be examined within two hours. As it must be kept cool during this time, the man is warned to carry it in a bag or in an outside, rather than an inside, pocket. The semen is measured for volume and is then examined under a high-power microscope. A total sperm count is made and percentages of motile and abnormal spermatozoa are estimated.

A second semen analysis is always done at a later date, in case errors in collection have occurred.

Post-coital (Hühner's) test

This gives broader information and to many couples, because of aesthetic or religious reasons, is a more acceptable investigation. It is done only during the ovulating phase and is carried out as soon as possible (within two hours) after intercourse. The couple are instructed to have intercourse as naturally as possible, without using any douches, creams or lubricants. The woman should remain lying on her back for some time before getting up. She then goes to the doctor or laboratory where a specimen of mucus from the cervical canal is removed.

The mucus is examined microscopically and the number of active and motile sperm counted; the ability of the sperm to penetrate the cervical mucus is noted. If death of the sperm occurs as soon as they enter the mucus it could be due to a state of cervical immunity to those spermatozoa.

Treatment of male infertility

Infertility caused by seminal factors is managed by a specialist in this field.

Azoospermia (complete absence of sperm) is difficult to treat. Gonadotrophin therapy and clomiphene are used in some cases. Microsurgery to repair damaged or obstructed tubes may be successful.

Death of sperm from cervical immunity can sometimes be overcome if the man uses a condom during intercourse for at least six months. As well, the woman might be prescribed prednisone for the same period.

Oligospermia (where the sperm are deficient in quantity or quality) is sometimes treated by giving androgens over a long period, at least six months. Surgical correction of any varicocele or division of known adhesions is made.

Factors relating to improvement of lifestyle and habits that might contribute to the condition are discussed. Especially important is the prevention of prolonged exposure of the scrotum to heat.

Artificial insemination, using the semen from the husband (AIH) or from an outside donor (AID), may be the answer to a diagnosis of male infertility, if this procedure is acceptable to the couple.

Tests for tubal patency

These tests are performed during the first half of the menstrual cycle, usually on about day 10 of a 28-day cycle. If there is any possibility that pregnancy might have occurred between the time the test was ordered and time it is due to be done, the test is postponed, or, at the least, a pregnancy test is done.

Laparoscopy

Laparoscopy has reduced the necessity for many of the other investigations for infertility. It allows direct visualisation of the ovaries, tubes and uterus, showing evidence of recent ovulation, patency and freedom of the tubal fimbriae, and abnormalities such as endometriosis, swelling or adhesions.

Tubal patency can be demonstrated by the introduction of dyed saline through the cervix and uterus, and observation of its spill through the distal ends of the tubes.

The commoner tubal patency tests, tubal insufflation and hysterosalpingogram, are performed as outpatient procedures but, because of their nature, require full aseptic precautions. A careful explanation given before the procedure will help the woman who might be bewildered. Such things as the sterile set-up, her legs being up in stirrups, and the scrubbing and gowning by the doctor can be rather frightening, especially when her only preparation might have been (in the case of hysterosalpingogram) 'We'll get an X-ray done'!

Tubal insufflation (Rubin's test)

In this procedure, carbon dioxide is passed through the genital tract under pressure (but never of more than 200 mm mercury). The gas is introduced through a cannula with a leakproof seal, into the cervix. The cannula is connected by tubing to a manometer that registers pressure in mm of mercury, and may be read rather like a blood-pressure machine. Some manometers trace a graph as well. The pressure gauge is watched as it rises and then drops when the gas escapes into the peritoneal cavity. If there is an obstruction, the pressure will remain high. The doctor will, as well, listen to the abdomen for the sound of gas coming through the tubes. Following the procedure, when the woman sits or stands upright, she may experience shoulder pain owing to the collection of gas under the diaphragm and this is another sign that the gas has managed to get through at least one tube. It is also another factor that should be remembered when explaining the procedure beforehand.

Tubal insufflation, as well as being diagnostic, is occasionally therapeutic. The gas and the pressure may 'blow out' tiny adhesions or obstructions that might have caused the problem.

Hysterosalpingogram

This is an X-ray using a radio-opaque substance which is injected through a tight-fitting cervical cannula (Figure 24.2). The substance will outline the uterine cavity and the tubes, and will spill out into the peritoneal cavity if there is no obstruction. X-rays are taken during and after the procedure and again, in some places, twenty-four hours later. The hysterosalpingogram shows the side and site of blockage, if there is one, and it also shows up any abnormalities in the size and shape of the uterine cavity (Figure 24.3).

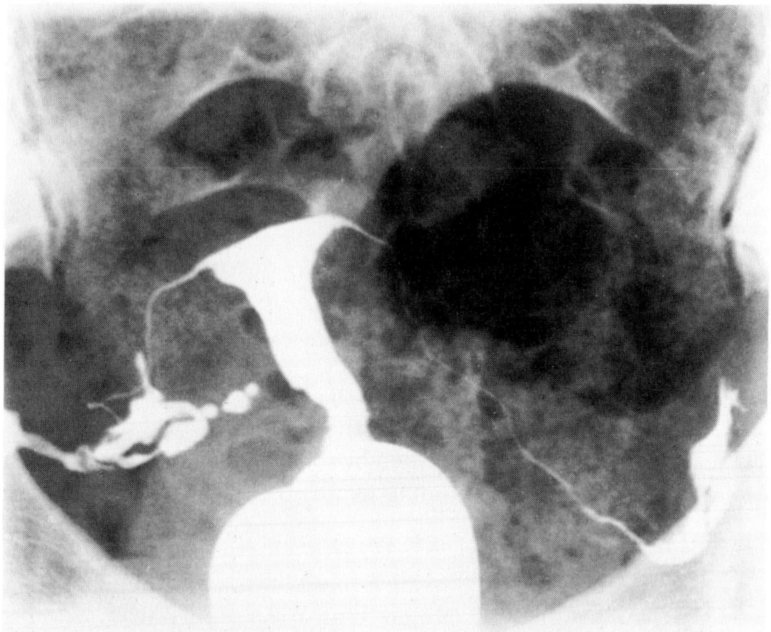

Figure 24.2
X-ray (hysterosalpingogram) showing bilateral tubal patency

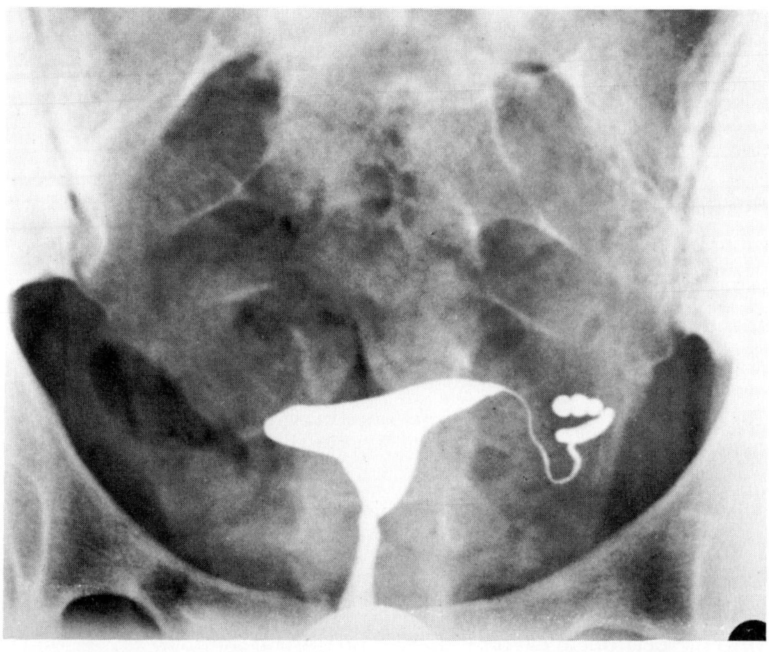

Figure 24.3
X-ray (hysterosalpingogram) showing right cornual obstruction and left fimbrial occlusion (hydrosalpinx)

Test for uterine factors causing infertility

Many of the causes of these uterine factors will be eliminated by pelvic examination, endometrial biopsy and hormonal assessments. A hysterosalpingogram will show distortion of the uterine cavity by fibroids, bands (synechia), polyps, foreign bodies or developmental disorders. A dilatation and curettage may be performed to remove a non-receptive or hyperplastic endometrium and to see if the new endometrium which grows up from the basal layer will be more suitable for the establishment of a pregnancy.

Treatment

Treatment is relevant to the cause. Antibiotics may be ordered to combat low-grade but persistent endometritis. Hormonal treatment may correct endometrial hyperplasia and adenomyosis. The act of dilating the cervix may allow better drainage of the uterus. Fibroids, if discovered, may be removed by myomectomy.

Investigations and treatment of pyschological causes of infertility

These investigations are, in effect, begun at the very first visit of the woman who presents complaining of infertility, by the questioning that is part of the history taking. When the doctor is able to interview the man as well, he is likely to get a clearer picture of any pressures and problems that may exist. If he is able to interview each one separately as well as together he may discover facts about the one of which the other is quite unaware. If these are simple, he may be able to help the couple to communicate these things to each other. If the situation is difficult, he will certainly, and soon, refer the couple to a doctor who specialises in psychosexual medicine.

For many couples, the mere fact of being investigated for infertility has its own effect. To some, it may greatly increase the slightest emotional problem. However, there are many accounts of couples who have been 'trying too hard' and who eventually decide to adopt a baby; they discontinue their efforts and investigations, and conceive their own child in a remarkably short time. And to just as many others, investigations mean that something is being done at last and these people, by relaxing and worrying less about their infertility, may achieve the same result.

In-vitro fertilisation (IVF)

Techniques for this procedure are improving continually, with increasing success. IVF involves:

- removal from the ovary of mature ova just before ovulation
- fertilisation, outside the body (in vitro means in glass), by a sufficient number of spermatozoa

- preparation of the uterus to a suitable state to receive a fertilised ovum
- transferring the fertilised ovum at exactly the right stage of development (when it is at the four to sixteen cell stage), to the prepared endometrium.

In-vitro fertilisation is aided by:

- chemical stimulation of ovulation, usually using clomiphene
- laparoscopy or ultrasound for ovum location and removal
- suitable methods of storing spermatozoa
- hormonal stimulation of the endometrium, so that it resembles the secretory phase, to receive the fertilised ovum.

There are considerable legal and ethical problems surrounding IVF. The issues of surrogate motherhood and the storage of deep frozen embryos as standbys in case first transplants fail are just two that are presently being considered, together with the financial cost.

Infertility management in the future

Research is bringing about a multitude of changes in medicine in general. Infertility problems that were once considered untreatable are now being conquered daily. Microsurgery has brought about great hope for women (and men) with tubal obstruction problems. In-vitro fertilisation has been successful for many women with severe tubal blockage and it may also be one answer to immunological causes of sperm rejection.

Although more and more pregnancies are being terminated by one method or another, more and more couples are demanding answers and solutions to the problems of infertility. What used to be accepted as final—infertility of unknown cause—is no longer readily accepted by couples or by their doctors. Everything should be done to allow every chance for the woman to conceive, maintain and deliver children; this is the function for which every organ and structure in the reproductive system was designed.

Further reading

E L Billings, J J Billings and M Catarinch, *Atlas of the Ovulation Method*, Advocate Press, Melbourne, 4th edn, 1980

K Dunn, J Leeton, *Birth Control*, Pitman, Melbourne, 1982

M M Garrey et al, *Gynaecology Illustrated*, Churchill Livingstone, Edinburgh, 2nd edn, 1979

J Hailes, *The Middle Years*, Pitman, Melbourne, 2nd edn, 1984

L Madaras and J Patterson, *Womancare*, Avon Books, New York, 1981

A Kilmartin, *Understanding Cystitis*, Pan Books, London, 1973

L Lanson, *From Woman to Woman*, Penguin Books, Harmondsworth, 1975

M Storch and C Carmichael, *How to relieve Cramps and other Menstrual Problems*, Workman, New York, 1981

I Mackay, N Beischer, L Cox and C Wood, *Illustrated Textbook of Gynaecology*, W B Saunders, Sydney, 1983

Index

abdominal
examination, 66
hysterectomy, 192–3
hysterotomy, 233
operations, 192–5
pregnancy, 235
skin preparation, 202
wound care, 207
abortion, 227–34
fibroids and, 161
tubal, 235
acquired immune deficiency syndrome (AIDS), 133
adenocarcinoma
endometrial, 162
vaginal, 148
adenomysis, 4, 170, 243
adnexae, 4
adolescence, 41–5
adreno-genital syndrome, 89–90
aging, changing caused by, 38–9, 46–8
AIDS (acquired immune deficiency syndrome), 133
amenorrhoea, 97–100
possible responses to, 13
Turner's syndrome and, 88
developmental disorders and, 94–5
amenorrhoea-galactorrhoea syndrome, 99
anatomy, 20–31
androgens, 87
anorexia nervosa, 44, 99
anteflexion of uterus, 174
anti-prostaglandins, 106
apareunia, 4, 242
arrhenoblastoma, 167
arteries, pelvic, 30
artificial insemination, 154
artificial vagina, 63
Asherman's syndrome, 100
atrophic changes, 47
azoospermia, 4, 242, 246

backache
chronic cervicitis and, 121
dysmenorrhoea and, 105
fibroids and, 161
prolapse and, 179
Bartholin's glands, 20
abscess of, 114
cyst of, 114, 146
inflammation of, 114, 116
marsupialisation of, 114, 198–9
basal temperature charting, 215, 244
Billings ovulation method, 216–18
bimanual examination of uterus, 70
biopsy
cervical, 152
endometrial, 163
vulval, 148
bladder
fistula, 182
hypertonic, 184
loss of tone, 183
management after surgery, 126–7
bladder neck weakness, 184–6
physiotherapy for, 185
surgery for, 186, 198
bowel
management after surgery, 206
preparation, pre-operative, 203
breasts
examination of, 67, 74
premenstrual, discomfort of, 108
broad ligament

anatomy of, 27–8
new growths of, 164

caesium insertion, 155
Candida albicans, 119
candidiasis, 119
cap, cervical, 220
carcinoma, *see* individual organs
cardinal ligaments, 28
carneous mole, 231
caruncle, urethral, 4, 146, 187
cauterisation, diathermic, 77–8
cervical
cap, 220
immunity to sperm, 246
incompetence, 231
mucus, 25, 37, 216, 242
smear, 81, 152
cervicitis, 120
cervix
amputation of, 181, 198–9
anatomy of, 25
benign growths of, 149
biopsy of, 152
carcinoma of, 150
ectropion of, 121
'erosion' of, 120
examination of, 67
incompetent, 231
infection of, 120
polyps of, 104, 149
chancre, 4, 128
chancroid, 134
chemical contraceptive agents, 221
chemical pessaries, 77
childbearing, changes caused by, 39
childhood, reproductive system in, 38
chlamydia, 127
'chocolate cysts', 127
choriocarcinoma, 239
chromosomes, 4, 86–7
chronic epithelial dystrophies, 116, 136, 139
circumcision, male, cervical carcinoma and, 150
climacteric, 4, 38–9, 46–52
bone changes after, 47
dyspareunia and, 49
gynaecological problems during, 49
hormone replacement in, 50–1
management of symptoms in, 50–2
menopause and, 47
ovulation and, 47
postmenopausal bleeding and, 52
virilising changes, 48
clitoris, 21
clonidine, 51
clomiphene, 100, 245
coitus, 5
abortion and, 229
cervical carcinoma and, 150
after climacteric, 49
interruptus, 219, 245
pain or difficulty with, 142–5
after surgery, 192–9, 210
colpoperineorraphy, 180
colporrhaphy, 180–1
effects of, 196–7
colposcopy, 82, 152
conception, 5
factors necessary for, 240
condom, 126,134, 219, 246
condylomata acuminata, 115
condylomata lata, 128
cone biopsy, 153
cone excision, 5, 153
congenital malformations, *see* developmental disorders
consent forms for surgery, 202
contact bleeding, 103, 121, 152
contraception, 211–25
corpus albicans, 33
corpus luteum, 33, 36–7
cysts of, 165
cryosurgery, 78
for chronic cervicitis, 121
for stage 0 cervical carcinoma, 153
for venereal warts, 115
cryptomenorrhoea, 93
culdoscopy, 82
culdotomy, 124
curettage, dilatation and, 196
Cushing's syndrome, 91
cystitis, 187

'honeymoon', 188
cystocele, 5, 175–81
cysts, *see* individual organs
cytology, 5
  cervical, 152
  endometrial, 163

danocrin, 172
deodorants (vaginal, vulval), 73, 136
dermoid cysts
  ovarian, 165
  vaginal, 148
developmental disorders, 94–5
  see also individual organs
diabetes
  endometrial carcinoma and, 162
  monilial vaginitis and, 119
  oestrogen replacement therapy and, 50
  pruritus vulvae and, 137
  vulvitis and, 113
diaphragm, contraceptive, 220
diathermic cauterisation, 77
dilatation and curettage (D & C), 196
discharge from hospital after surgery, 210
discharge, vaginal, *see* vaginal discharge
Doderlein's bacillus, 23
dorsal position, 65
douching, vaginal, 5, 78–9
  for contraception, 218
  dyspareunia and, 142
  intracavity irradiation and, 157
  natural defence against infections and, 79
  pelvic peritonitis and, 124
  pre-operative, 203
  procedure for, 78–9
dysmenorrhoea, 5, 104–7
  chronic cervicitis and, 121
  chronic salpingitis and, 123
  endometriosis and, 171
  possible responses to, 9
  uterine malformations and, 64
dyspareunia, 5, 142–5
  chronic cervicitis and, 121
  chronic salpingitis and, 123
  endometriosis and, 171
  infertility and, 242
  possible responses to, 16
  retroverted uterus and, 175
  after sterilisation operations, 224
  after vaginal repair, 181
dysuria
  frequency and, 187
  gonorrhoea and, 126
  Herpes simplex genitalis and, 132

ectopic pregnancy, 5, 234–6
  migration of ovum and, 96
  pelvic peritonitis and, 124
  tubal rupture and, 235
ectropion, cervical, 121
embryo, development of reproductive organs in, 92
endocervicitis, 121
endocervix, 5
endometrial
  cysts (of ovary), 166
  lavage, 163
endometriosis, 5, 170–3
  deep dyspareunia and, 142, 171
  dysmenorrhoea and, 107, 171
  infertility and, 171, 243
  sites of, 171
endometritis, 121
endometrium
  carcinoma of, 162
  climacteric changes in, 47
  cyclic changes in, 34–6
  hyperplasia of, 101
  non-responsive, 98, 100
  polyps of, 158
  structure of, 25
endotoxic shock, 234
enterocele, 5, 179
episiotomy, 5
  prevention of prolapse and, 178
  scarring and dyspareunia, 142
epithelial dystrophies, 116, 136, 139
'erosion', cervical, 5, 120
examination, pelvic, *see* gynaecological examination
examination under anaesthesia, 70, 196

exenteration, pelvic, 154

fallopian tubes
absence of, 96
anatomy of, 25–6
infections of, 121–4
ligation of, 222
occlusion of, 242
pregnancy in, 234
reconstruction operations for, 223
tumours of, 164
family planning, 211–25
feminising tumours, 167
feminism, 91
fern test of cervical mucus, 244
fertilisation, 5, 240–2
fibromyomata, 5, 158–62
intrauterine devices and, 225
menorrhagia and, 102
fistulae, 182–3
foetus, 5
follicle stimulating hormone (FSH), 32–5, 46, 98, 245
follicular cysts, 165
folliculitis (vulval), 113
fornices of vagina, 23, 69, 174
fourchette, 20
fractional curettage of endometrium, 163
frequency of micturition, 127, 187, 188
gonorrhoea and, 126
frigidity, 142
fundus of uterus, 5
furunculosis (vulval), 113

galactorrhoea, 101
gamete, 6
Gardnerella vaginalis, 120
genital herpes, 130–3
gentian violet solution, 76, 119
germinal epithelium, 27, 32
gestation, 6
gonad, 6, 87
gonadal sex, 87
gonadotrophins
chorionic gonadotrophin, 33, 237
follicle stimulating hormone, 32–5, 46, 98, 245
luteinising hormone, 33
gonorrhoea, 126–7
bartholinitis and, 114
salpingitis and, 122
tubal obstruction and, 127, 243
graafian follicle, 33, 37
gravid, 6
gynaecological (pelvic) examination, 61–74
under anaesthesia, 70, 196
indications for, 64
gynaecomastia, 89, 91

habitual abortion, 232
haematocele, pelvic, 235
haematocolpos, 93
haematoma, pelvic, 209
haematometra, 93
Haemophilus vaginalis, *see Gardnerella*
haemorrhage, *see also* specific sites
after abortion, 233
menstrual, 103
postmenopausal, 52
post-operative, 208–9
haemorrhoids, dyspareunia and, 142
hermaphroditism, 87
Herpes simplex virus, 130–3
cervical carcinoma and, 130
high vaginal swab, 234
hirsuitism, 6, 91, 100, 168
Hodge pessary, 175
'honeymoon' cystitis, 188
hormonal sex, 87
hormone feedback system, 34
hormone-producing tumours, 91, 167
hormone therapy
climacteric symptoms and, 50
senile vaginitis and, 118
senile vulvitis and, 116
Turner's syndrome and, 89
hot flushes, 47
Hühner's test, 246
hydatidiform mole, 6, 236–8
hydrosalpinx, 123

hymen, 22
  imperforate, 92
  rigid, 142
hypertension, endometrial carcinoma and, 162
hypertonic saline, induction of abortion with, 233
hypomenorrhoea, 100
hypothalamus
  hormone releasing factors and, 35
hysterectomy
  abdominal, 192–3
  bilateral salpingo-oophorectomy and, 192–3
  vaginal, 198–9
  Wertheim's, 194–5
hysterosalpingogram, 247
hysterotomy, abdominal, 233

imperforate hymen, 92
  incision of, 93
impotence (male), local anaesthetics and, 143
inclusion cysts, 6, 146, 148
incompetence of cervix, 231
incomplete abortion, 231
incontinence of urine, 182–7
  possible responses to, 16
induced abortion, 232–3
infancy, reproductive system in, 38
'Infant Hercules' syndrome, 90
infertility, 6, 240–50
  endometriosis and, 171
  fibroids and, 161
  possible responses to, 18
  salpingitis and, 123
injuries to urinary structures, 209–10
insufflation of uterine tubes, 247
intercourse, sexual, *see* coitus
internal os, 24
intersex conditions, 86–91
intracavity irradiation, 153–8
intractable pruritus, 139
intrauterine contraceptive devices, 224–5
introitus, inelasticity of, 142
inversion of uterus, 176
in-vitro fertilisation (IVF), 249–50
isthmus of uterus, 24

jaundice, pruritus vulvae and, 137

karyotype, 6, 88
Klinefelter's syndrome, 89
kraurosis vulvae, 137

labia majora, 21
labia minora, 21
lactation, 6
  amenorrhoea and, 99
laparoscopy, 198–9
  infertility and, 247
leucorrhoea, 6
  see also vaginal discharge
leukoplakia, 6
  see also chronic epithelial dystrophies
levator ani muscles, 30
ligaments, pelvic, 27–9
lithotomy position, 66, 191
Lugol's iodine, 152
luteinising hormone, 33–7
lymphadenoma, pruritus vulvae and, 137

Manchester repair, 181, 198–9
Marshall-Marchetti operation, 186, 198–9
Meigs' syndrome, 167
menarche, 6, 41
  delayed, 92, 98
menopause, 6, 47–9
menorrhagia, 6, 101–3
  fibroids and, 102
  intrauterine devices and, 225
  possible responses to, 10
  uterine malformations and, 95
menstrual
  cycle, 33–4
  disorders, 97–107
  loss, 34
menstruation, 6, 34
methotrexate, 238
metronidazole, 118
metrorrhagia, 6, 103–4

possible responses to, 12
micturating urethrocystogram, 84
mid-stream urine collection, 84
'mini-pill', 212
miscarriage, *see* abortion
missed abortion, 231
mitosis, 86
mole
carneous, 231
hydatidiform, 6, 236–8
tubal, 235
monilial vaginitis, 119
mons pubis, 20
motility of spermatozoa, 6, 242, 246
mucinous cystadenoma, 166
mucus, ovulation, *see* ovulation
Mullerian ducts, 92
myomata, *see* fibromyomata
myomectomy, 194–5
myometrium
adenosis of, 170
anatomy of, 25
changes due to age and childbearing, 38–9

Nabothian follicles, 69, 120, 150
natamycin, 118
natural family planning, 215–18
Neisarria gonorrhoeae, 126
nerves, pelvic, 31
nystatin pessaries, 119

obesity
endometrial carcinoma and, 162
pelvic examination and, 70
oestrogen
actions of, 37
sources of, 36
oligospermia, 246
oophorectomy, 194–5
oophoritis, *see* salpingo-oophoritis
operations, 190–9
oral contraceptives, 212–14
monilial vaginitis and, 119
pelvic surgery and, 201
post-pill amenorrhoea, 99
premenstrual tension and, 110
pruritus and, 136
sexually-transmitted diseases and, 126
osteoporosis, 47
ovarian cystectomy, 194–5
ovarian hormones
actions of, 36–8
ovaries
absence of, 96
anatomy of, 26–7
changes due to age, 38–9
polycystic, 99, 116
prolapse of, 143, 175
'streak', 88
tumours of, 164–8
overflow incontinence, 183
oviducts, *see* fallopian tubes
ovulation, 6, 32–3
mucus, 216–18, 242
temperature changes at, 214, 244
tests for, 244–5
ovulation method (Billings), 216–18
ovum
embedding of, 243
release of, 32
survival of, 242
oxytocic, 6
infusion for abortion, 233

packing (vaginal)
pre-operative, 204
post-operative, 209
procedure, 79–80
secondary vaginal haemorrhage and, 209
pan-hysterectomy, 192–3
Papanicoloau smear, 81, 152
papillomata
cervical, 150
vulval, 146
paraurethral (Skene's) glands, 20, 127
pediculosis pubis, 115
pelvic
abscess, 124
examination, *see* gynaecological examination

floor, 29
haematocele, 235
haematoma, 209
infections, 111–35
nerves, 31
peritonitis, 124
veins, 31
perineal body, 30
perineal care after surgery, 207
perineorrhaphy, 7, 181, 196–7
perineum, 22
peritonitis
pelvic, 124
post-abortal, 234
pessaries, 7
chemical, 77
Hodge, 175–6
insertion of, 80–1
retroversion and, 175–6
ring, 81, 180
supporting, 81, 180
uterovaginal prolapse and, 179
'pessary test', 175–6
physiology, 32–9
physiotherapy (pelvic floor)
dyspareunia and, 144
stress incontinence and, 185–6
'pill', the, *see* oral contraceptives
pituitary gland
amenorrhoea and, 98–8
hormones of, 32–3
hypothalamus and, 32
menorrhagia and, 101
prolactin from, 99
placenta, 7
hydatidiform mole and, 236
retained, 121, 231, 234
podophyllin, 77, 116, 147
polycystic ovaries, 99, 166
polymenorrhagia, 101
polymenorrhoea, 101
polyps
cervical, 104, 149
endometrial, 158
pooling of blood in the vagina, 208
positions used in gynaecology
dorsal, 65
genupectoral (knee-chest), 83
lithotomy, 66, 191
Sims', 65
Trendelenburg, 192
post-coital bleeding, 103, 152
postmenopausal bleeding, 52
post-pill amenorrhoea, 99
post-operative care, 203–10
post-operative complications, 208–10
pregnancy
abdominal, 235
ectopic, 234–6
termination of, 232
tubal, 234–6
premenstrual tension, 108–10
pre-operative care, 200–3
presacral neurectomy, 172
procidentia, 178–9
progesterone, actions of, 36–8
progestogen therapy
endometrial carcinoma and, 164
endometriosis and, 172
premenstrual tension and, 110
prolapse, uterovaginal, 175–81
operations for, 180
pessary treatment for, 81, 180
prostaglandins, 106, 233
pruritus vulvae, 7, 137–41
chronic vulvitis and, 116
intractible, 139
possible responses to, 15
psychological factors in, 137
pseudocyesis, 7
pseudohermaphroditism, 87
psoriasis, vulval, 137
psychogenic bladder, 188
psychological sex, 87
puberty, 7, 41–2
pubocervical ligament, 29
punch biopsy, 153
pyosalpinx, 123

radical vulvectomy, 152, 148–9, 196–7
radiotherapy
endometriosis, for, 173
vulval carcinoma, for, 148
radioactive insertions, 155–8

rectocele, 7, 179, 181
red degeneration of fibromyomata, 161
retained products of conception, 121, 231, 234
retention cysts
cervical, 69
ovarian, 165
retroflexion of uterus, 7, 174
retrograde menstruation, 172
retroversion of uterus, 7, 174–6
dyspareunia and, 175
reversible sterilisation, 223
rhythm method of family planning, 135
ring pessary, 81, 179
round ligaments, 28
Rubin's test, 247

salpingectomy, 194–5
salpingitis, 121–4
salpingo-oophoritis, 121–4
scabies, 137
scanty menstruation, 100
Schiller's test, 152
semen, 7, 241–2
analysis of, 245
senile vaginitis, 117
septate uterus, 94
septate vagina, 94
septic abortion, 234
sex determination, 86–7
sexual intercourse, *see* coitus
sexually transmitted diseases, 125–35
AIDS, 133
chancroid, 134
chlamydia, 127–8
education about, 134
gonorrhoea, 126–7
Herpes simplex genitalis, 130–3
misconceptions about, 125–6
non-specific urethritis, 134
prevention of, 134
screening for, 134
syphilis, 128–30
Sheehan's syndrome, 99
Shirodkar's suture, 231
shock
endotoxic, 234
toxic shock syndrome (TSS), 124–5
Sims' position, 65–6
Sims' speculum, 64
Skene's ducts, 20, 127
Skene's glands, 20, 127
skin preparation, pre-operative, 202–3
smegma, 150
soft sore (chancroid), 134
speculum, 7
bivalve, 64
Sims' 64
spermatozoon, 7, 241–2, 245
spermicidal agents, 221
spirochaete, 128
spontaneous abortion, 228–32
'spotting'
endometrial carcinoma and, 163
ovulation and, 103
squamocolumnar junction of cervix, 25
staging of cervical carcinoma, 151
Stein-Leventhal syndrome, 91, 99, 166
sterilisation operations, 221–4
stilboestrol, vaginal adenocarcinoma and, 148
'streak' ovaries, 88
stress incontinence, urinary, 184–7
demonstration of, 68–9, 185
stroma, 7
suction evacuation of uterus, 232
superficial perineal muscles, 30
supporting pessaries, 80–1, 179–80
prolapse and, 180
retroversion and, 175–6
syphilis, 128–30

tampons, 7, 125
sensible use of, 125
toxic shock syndrome (TSS) and, 124–5
temperature charting, 215, 244
teratomata, 165
termination of pregnancy, *see* induced abortion
threatened abortion, 228
threshold for bleeding, 34
thrombosis after surgery, 208
thrush, vaginal, *see* monilial vaginitis

toxic shock syndrome (TSS), 124–5
transformation zone of cervical canal, 150, 152
Trendelenburg position, 117
Treponema pallidum, 128
trichomonal vaginitis, 118
Trichomonas vaginalis, 118
true hermaphroditism, 87
true incontinence, 182
tubal
  diathermy, 221
  insufflation, 247
  ligation, 194–5, 221
  obstruction, 243
  pregnancy, *see* ectopic pregnancy
  reconstruction operations, 223
tuberculosis
  chronic endometritis and, 121
  tubal obstruction and, 243
tumours, *see* individual organs
Turner's syndrome, 88

ultrasound, 85
unicornuate uterus, 95
ureters, damage to, 209
urethral caruncle, 146, 187
  dyspareunia and, 142
urethral
  prolapse, 142, 187
  sling operations, 181, 198–9
  syndrome, 188
urethritis
  dyspareunia and, 142
  gonorrhoea and, 126
  non-specific, 134
urethrocele, 7, 179, 181
urethroplasty, 198
urge incontinence, 184
urinary incontinence, 182–7
  possible responses to, 16
urinary retention, 183
urogenital sinus, 92
uterosacral ligament, 28
uterovaginal prolapse, 176–81
uterus
  absence of, 95
  adenomyosis, 170
  anatomy of, 24–5
  benign tumours of, 158–62
  bicornuate, 95
  carcinoma of, 162–4
  changes due to age and childbearing, 38–9
  development of, 92
  didelphys, 95
  displacements of, 174–80
  duplicated, 95
  examination of, 70
  fibromyomata, 158–62
  hypoplasia of, 95
  infantile, 95
  infection of, 121
  inversion of, 176
  ligaments of, 27–9
  malformations of, 94–5
  prolapse of, 176–81
  retroversion of, 174–6
  septate, 95
  unicornuate, 95

vagina
  absence of, 94–5
  adenocarcinoma of, 148
  anatomy of, 22–4
  artificial, 95
  atresia of, 94
  benign tumours of, 148
  changes due to age and childbearing, 38–9
  deodorants for, 113, 136, 142
  development of, 92
  dilators for, 95, 143–4
  douching of, 78
  duplicated, 94
  endometriosis of, 171
  examination of, *see* gynaecological examination
  foreign bodies in, 117
  fornices of, 17, 23
  infections of, 116–20
  lubricants for, 67, 143
  malformations of, 94–5
  packing of, 79–80, 203, 204
  prolapse of, 179

repair of, *see* colporraphy
secretions of, 23
septate, 94
treatments (creams, paints, pessaries), 77
vault of, 23
vaginal hysterectomy and repair, 198
vaginismus, 143–5
vaginitis, 116–20
varicocele of spermatic cord, 246
vasectomy, 222–3
vault, vaginal, 23
veins, pelvic, 31
venereal diseases, *see* sexually transmitted diseases
venereal warts, 115
ventrosuspension operations, 194–5
endometriosis and, 172
retroversion and, 176
vesicles, in hydatidiform mole, 236
vestibule, 20
viable, 7
villi, chorionic, 236
virilising tumours, 91, 167
virilism, 91
virus infections
abortion and, 228
cervical carcinoma and, 150
Herpes simplex genitalis and, 130
voiding, post-operative, 204–6
vulva
anatomy of, 20–2
benign tumours of, 146
biopsy of, 147
carcinoma of, 147
care of after surgery, 206
changes due to age and childbearing, 38–9
dystrophies of, 116
examination of, 67
hygiene of, 93, 114, 124
infections of, 112–16
leukoplakia of, 116, 137
pruritus of, 137–141
tumours of, 146–7
warts of, 115, 146
vulvectomy, radical, 116, 152
vulvo-vaginitis, 112

warts
venereal, 115
vulval, 115, 146
Wertheim's hysterectomy, 154, 194–5
Wolffian ducts, 92
womb, *see* uterus
'womb stones', 161
wound care after surgery, 207–8

yoghurt, for monilial vaginitis, 119

zona pellucida, 240
zygote, 7, 86, 240